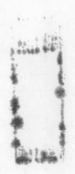

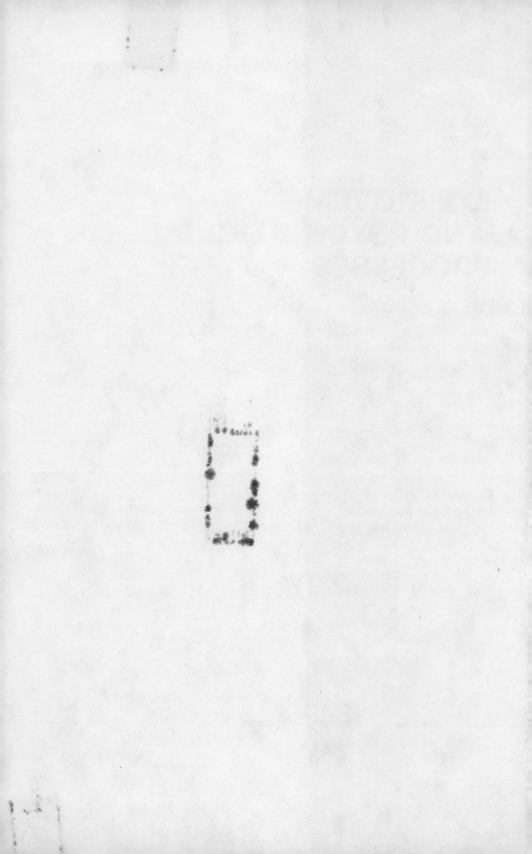

EYE MOVEMENTS AND PSYCHOLOGICAL PROCESSES

COMMITTEE ON VISION
ASSEMBLY OF BEHAVIORAL AND SOCIAL SCIENCES
NATIONAL RESEARCH COUNCIL

SPONSORED BY THE
U.S. ARMY HUMAN ENGINEERING LABORATORY

edited by

RICHARD A. MONTY

U.S. ARMY HUMAN ENGINEERING LABORATORY

JOHN W. SENDERS

UNIVERSITY OF TORONTO

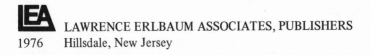 LAWRENCE ERLBAUM ASSOCIATES, PUBLISHERS
1976   Hillsdale, New Jersey

DISTRIBUTED BY THE HALSTED PRESS DIVISION OF

JOHN WILEY & SONS

New York   Toronto   London   Sydney

This symposium was supported under the auspices of the Office of Naval Research Contract # N00014-75-C-0406 to the National Academy of Sciences/National Research Council with funds provided by the U. S. Army Human Engineering Laboratory.

Lawrence Erlbaum Associates, Inc., Publishers
62 Maria Drive
Hillsdale, New Jersey 07642

Distributed solely by Halsted Press Division
John Wiley & Sons, Inc., New York

Library of Congress Cataloging in Publication Data

Main entry under title:
Eye movements and psychological processes.

    Papers from a symposium sponsored by the U. S.
Army Human Engineering Laboratory, held in Princeton,
N. J., Apr. 15–17, 1974.
    Includes bibliographies and indexes.
    1. Visual perception–Congresses.   2.   Eye–
Movements–Congresses.   I.   Monty, Richard A.
II.   Senders, John W., 1920–   III.   United States.
Army Human Engineering Laboratory.
BF241.E9   617'.846   76–13442   April 9, 1976
ISBN 0-470-15029-7

Printed in the United States of America

Contents

Foreword

This volume had its origins in a request, by Dr. Richard A. Monty and Professor John W. Senders representing the U.S. Army Human Engineering Laboratory, Aberdeen Proving Ground, that the Committee on Vision of the National Research Council assist them in planning a conference on eye movements.

The Executive Council of the Committee on Vision acted on this request at its meeting in November, 1973, by appointing Dr. William Collins as Chairman of a Planning Committee. The purpose of the Planning Committee was to define some of the scientific problems, both basic and applied, and to select a realizable objective for a symposium. The Planning Committee included members of the Committee on Vision: William Collins, Richard Monty, John Senders, Leonard Matin, Frances Volkmann, Julian Hochberg, and David Robinson. The report and recommendations of the Committee were approved by the Executive Council.

The collaborative efforts of Dr. William A. Benson, Executive Secretary of the NRC Committee on Vision, Dr. Richard A. Monty, and Professor John W. Senders resulted in the symposium presented herein. The organization of the present volume follows that of the conference. The editing of manuscripts was the responsibility of Dr. Monty and Professor Senders.

CONRAD G. MUELLER
Chairman, Executive Council
NAS–NRC Committee on Vision

This volume is dedicated to Guy T. Buswell and Miles A. Tinker, early investigators of eye movements, whose efforts covered so much of the ground that sometimes it seems that there remains for us only the investigation of fine detail.

The gaze of man is free to move around
From place to place where'ere the eye does will.
It flicks about to give the mind its fill
and make the image whole within the head.
It seeks with lightning speed the source of sound
And follows smoothly anywhere it's led.

From deep within the brain the signals come
To stabilize the world of visual space
Against all violent motion of the face;
And does it all with simple rule of thumb.

JOHN W. SENDERS

Preface

During the last ten years, the quantity of research on eye movements as they pertain to psychological processes has been increasing at a rapid rate. It was this trend that led us to propose to Dr. John Weisz, the Director of the U.S. Army Human Engineering Laboratory, that we conduct a symposium on this topic. Dr. Weisz was enthusiastic about this concept, so we approached the Committee on Vision of the National Research Council and asked for their assistance and expertise. The resulting symposium was conducted at the Nassau Inn in Princeton, New Jersey on April 15–17, 1974.

Our purpose was to bring together investigators representing different theoretical positions and methodological approaches to present their recent findings, to debate the theoretical points of view, and to identify and discuss the major research problems. An attempt was made to invite participants ranging all the way from promising graduate students through the established authorities in the field. The result was an intensive three-day session with meetings from early morning until late into the evening with much opportunity for formal and informal group discussion. The edited papers and transcripts of our discussions are the contents of this book.

We wish to thank the U.S. Army Human Engineering Laboratory for sponsoring the symposium, and the Committee on Vision of the National Research Council for assistance rendered. In particular, we wish to thank John D. Weisz, Director of the Human Engineering Laboratory, who made this symposium possible, William Benson, Executive Secretary of the National Research Council Committee on Vision, for handling the myriad administrative details surrounding the conference, and Jacob A. Barber, Office of the Deputy Chief of Staff for Personnel, Department of the Army, who contributed significantly to expediting the conference schedule. We also are indebted to the other members of the program planning committee, namely, William Collins (Chairman), Leonard

Matin, David A. Robinson, and Frances C. Volkmann, for their substantial contributions toward defining a workable, meaningful symposium format. With awe we pay thanks to Ira P. Maisel of the Leavitt Recording Service for the fantastic endurance demonstrated in recording and transcribing the first draft of the symposium proceedings, and to Joseph Mazurczak, who patiently tape recorded the entire symposium. A special word of thanks goes to Dennis F. Fisher, a well-endowed young psychologist, who worked with us continuously from the beginning to the end of the entire process. Whenever we could not be reached to handle some bothersome detail surrounding this meeting, Dennis F. Fisher was there to fill the gap. Special thanks go also to B. Diane Eberly, the charming young secretary who was responsible for all the typing and record keeping surrounding the meeting itself as well as for typing most of the final draft of this manuscript.

RICHARD A. MONTY
JOHN W. SENDERS

Part I

THE PHYSIOLOGY
OF EYE MOVEMENT CONTROL:
THE VESTIBULAR, PURSUIT, SACCADIC
AND VERGENCE SYSTEMS

As indicated in the introduction to this volume, the function of the conference was to bring together people from diverse disciplines to report upon and to discuss the present state of knowledge and of ignorance with respect to the relationship between eye movement and psychological processes. Because of the diverse backgrounds ranging from pure mathematics to pure psychology, it was felt that some common base of knowledge and understanding of the underlying physiology of eye-movement control should be presented in order to avoid extended discussions stemming from ignorance, illusion, myth, and fantasy about how the eye moves and what the exact nature of the machinery is that causes it to move from one place to another. This session, therefore, dealt with the four semiindependent forms of eye movement. These are: the *vestibular*, dealing with the relationship between vestibular inputs and reflexive eye movements stemming from these; the *pursuit,* almost invariably manifested in the presence of externally moving targets with some defined range of angular velocity; the *saccadic,* which occur predominantly in the refixation of the eyes from point to point in the visual field (and which have a totally different time course from the pursuit movements); and the *vergence,* which occur with changes in distance of the point of regard of the two eyes with respect to the observer. Each of these topics was treated in detail.

The chairman of this first session was Dr. David A. Robinson of the Johns Hopkins University.

I.1

The Vestibular System
for Eye Movement Control[1]

Geoffrey Melvill Jones

McGill University

Quite recently the system for the vestibular control of eye movements has begun to emerge as a large and a controversial topic. However, for myself, the most remarkable feature of this system still remains its versatility and effectiveness in our everyday life. Imagine, for example, the "engineering" accomplishment of a system which allows one to "keep one's eye on the ball" when running and weaving at top speed in a football game, or to hold the eye on successive "stepping stones" during an exhilarating run down a mountain path. Normal vision alone could certainly not accomplish such feats since not only does normal head movement contain sinusoidal frequencies considerably higher than the upper limit of our visual tracking system, but also much higher head angular velocities are encountered than could be compensated by means of vision alone.

These phenomena are readily demonstrated by first shaking this page through small angles at about 3–4 Hz in front of the stationary head. Visual tracking is obviously not sufficient to fixate the retinal image and the writing appears blurred. Then, holding the page still, but shaking the head at the same frequency and amplitude (rotationally about a vertical axis) relative to the page, one sees the writing sufficiently clearly to read; the vestibuloocular reflex introduced by head movement produces automatic stabilization of the eyes with, in these circumstances, a gain very close indeed to one (Benson, 1970). Interestingly such autostabilization occurs in all three orthogonal degrees of freedom; that is, during head rotation in both sagittal and frontal planes of the skull as well as the

[1] This work was supported by Canadian Defence Research Board Grants Nos. 9910-37 and 9310-92.

horizontal one (e.g., Melvill Jones, 1964; 1965; and 1966), a fact also readily demonstrated by the same simple means of personal verification.

The Mechanical End Organ

By far the most important origin of these vestibuloocular responses is the system of six semicircular canals. Figure 1 is a diagram of what is generally considered to be the essential functional components of a semicircular canal. In order for the canal to function at all there must be continuity of fluid flow around the full circle of the endolymphatic tubular structure. Then, since the whole labyrinth is fixed to the skull, when the head is angularly accelerated, say to the right, the fluid will tend to be left behind due to inertia of the fluid mass. Three important features of the resulting pattern of flow should be noted here, all of which stem directly from the very small size of the system, especially the very thin diameter of the endolymphatic canal ($\frac{1}{3}$ mm in man).

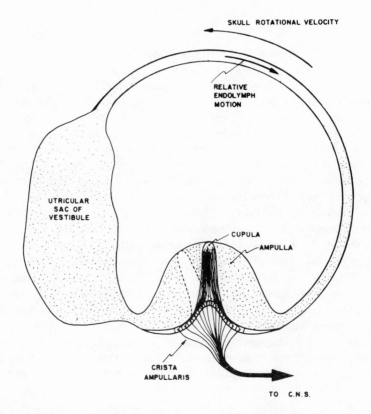

FIG. 1. Diagram of essential mechanical components of a semicircular canal. (After Jones & Milsum, 1965.)

First, due to this very small size, viscous forces become large compared to the inertial ones which drive the flow (i.e., the Reynold's number of the system is very small, numerically <1). Such flow as occurs is therefore strictly stream-lined, or laminar, in character. As a result the relative *velocity* of fluid flow (V) is strictly proportional to the inertial driving force and hence also to the head angular acceleration (α):

$$V \propto \alpha$$

Consequently, bearing in mind the linearity of this relation, the time integrals of these functions, namely $\int V \, dt$ and $\int \alpha \, dt$, must also be proportional to one another.

But

$$\int V \, dt = D \quad \text{and} \quad \int \alpha \, dt = \omega$$

where D = relative angular *displacement* of fluid and ω = head angular *velocity* relative to space. Thus, since

$$\int V \, dt \propto \int \alpha \, dt,$$

so also

$$D \propto \omega.$$

In turn, since the cupula appears to be watertight (Dohlman, 1938) and hence cupular angle (θ) is proportional to fluid displacement (D) around the endolymphatic tube, we may draw the further conclusion that

$$\theta \propto \omega.$$

Stated in words this important conclusion shows that the mechanical response of the canal, manifest as cupula angle, serves as an integrating angular accelerometer; that is, as an angular speedometer, registering at every instant the angular *velocity* of the head relative to *inertial space*. One interesting and topical outcome of this conclusion is that mechanical components of the canals should operate as angular speedometers just as effectively in the zero gravity environment of outer space as on Earth.[2]

Second, the relatively very high viscous damping associated with the low Reynold's number ensures rapid response of the speedometer action, the time constant of which has been estimated as between 3 and 5 msec (Jones & Milsum, 1965).

Third, because of the heavy viscous damping to be expected in such a small system of tubes, the actual fluid displacements incurred must be very small

---

[2] At this point in his talk Dr. Melvill Jones produced a one foot diameter closed circular tube containing a relatively viscous silicon fluid and some suspended visible particles from which it was possible to show that the above mathematical relations really do hold.

indeed (Oman & Young, 1972). For example, it has been calculated that in the cat horizontal canal a neurophysiologically measured threshold stimulus of $2°/sec$ head rotation would be expected to cause a corresponding angular deflection of the cupula around 1.2×10^{-3} degrees of arc (Melvill Jones & Milsum, 1971). Obviously in this case the cupula would never move outside the available range of movement in the ampulla (Fig. 1) and hence avoidance of mechanical saturation would also seem to be a direct outcome of the very small size of the system.

Errors of Canal Response

Although during most naturally occurring head movements the mechanical response of the canals faithfully registers the vector of head angular velocity in a wide range of animal species (Jones & Spells, 1963; Jones & Milsum, 1965), it is nevertheless well known that abnormally prolonged patterns of rotation lead to "erroneous," or misleading, patterns of canal response. A mechanical source of such errors lies in the elasticity of the cupula. Thus, whereas rapid angular acceleration of the head to a steady speed of rotation would cause deflection of the cupula to a given point of deviation (per-rotational stimulation), continued rotation at that speed would allow time for its elastic restoration to the zero, or datum, position (Fig. 2). Then, on suddenly decelerating the rotation back to a stationary condition, the cupula would be forced out again through an equal but *opposite* angle, generating in turn a false sensation of reversed rotation known clinically as the postrotational response. Finally this erroneous response would

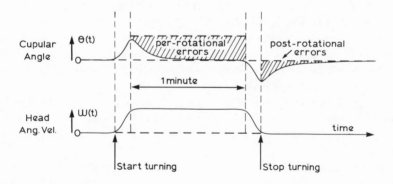

FIG. 2. Diagramatic representation of per- and postrotational errors to be expected in the mechanical response of the canal.

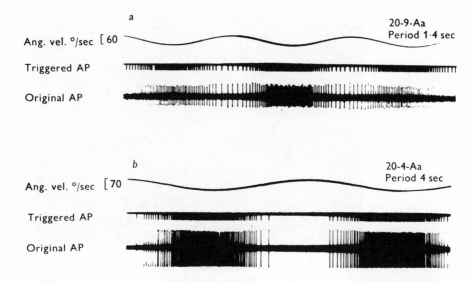

FIG. 3. Unit neural responses in vestibular nuclei of decerebrate cats during sinusoidal horizontal rotation. The upper trace in each set of records gives turntable angular velocity, upward deflection indicating right-going velocity. (After Melvill Jones & Milsum, 1970.)

itself decay (exponentially) to zero as cupular elasticity slowly forced the fluid back to whence it came.

Neural Response

Of considerable interest is the fact that at least some components of neural response received in the brain correspond very closely to the mechanical end-organ responses described above. For example, Fig. 3 shows unit neural responses recorded from two separate nerve cells located in the cat vestibular nucleus, obtained during sinusoidal head rotation within the range of natural movement. In the upper set of records, firing frequency (i.e., frequency of action potentials (AP)) was modulated all around the cycle of sinusoidal rotation, the response always being approximately in phase with head *angular velocity*. The lower set of records shows similar response in a neural unit suppressed below its threshold of firing during the "inhibitory" phase of the cycle of stimulation.

Figure 4 shows the computer-averaged response of another similar unit during sinusoidal rotation at a much lower frequency (1/16 Hz). Two features are noteworthy: first, the response is very smoothly modulated in the same (i.e., sinusoidal) fashion as the stimulus; second, this neural response is seen to be

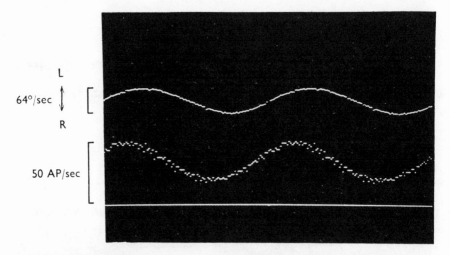

FIG. 4. Computer-averaged stimulus (top trace = angular velocity) and response (middle trace = unit firing frequency) of a canal-dependent cell in the cat vestibular nucleus obtained during horizontal sinusoidal rotation. The bottom (straight) line gives zero firing frequency. (After Melvill Jones & Milsum, 1971.)

phase-advanced relative to the stimulus angular velocity, as would be expected in the mechanical response of the end organ, due to the continuous influence of the effects of cupular elasticity at this abnormally low frequency of head movement.

Figure 5 shows the similarly computed response of another unit during the latter half of a stimulus such as that depicted in Fig. 2. The exponential pattern

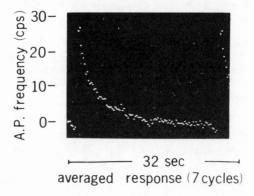

FIG. 5. Postrotational response of a unit similar to those in Figs. 3 and 4. At the moment of arresting a prolonged steady turn, the cell burst into vigorous activity and thereafter the firing frequency decayed exponentially to its original resting level. (After Melvill Jones, 1970.) Compare with the final portion of the diagram in Fig. 2.

of decay in neural firing frequency is seen to replicate that to be expected from the mechanical response of the end organ in these circumstances. This particular unit was suppressed below its threshold of firing during and after the subsequent stopping stimulus (not shown in the figure).

A word of caution is needed here, to point out that not all neural signals exactly follow the expected end-organ response. Thus there certainly are dynamic terms in the transduction from mechanical to some neural components, for example both a fast adaptive term (Shimazu & Precht, 1965; Fernandez & Goldberg, 1971)—probably responsible for the introduction of a "lead" characteristic that appears at higher frequencies of oscillation (Fernandez & Goldberg, 1971; Benson, 1970)—and a slow adaptive term (Malcolm & Melvill Jones, 1970).

The Elementary Vestibuloocular Reflex Arc

How are these brainstem signals fed forward to drive the oculomotor system? Figure 6 illustrates one component of the elementary connections now known to exist, passing in this instance from the two horizontal canals to drive the lateral and medial rectus muscles of one eye.

On turning to the left, the spontaneous neural activity in primary afferent neurones (on average 80–100 AP/sec) is increased on the left side and decreased on the right side. Inhibitory commissural connections ensure that this reciprocal influence is properly carried from one side to the other (Shimazu & Precht,

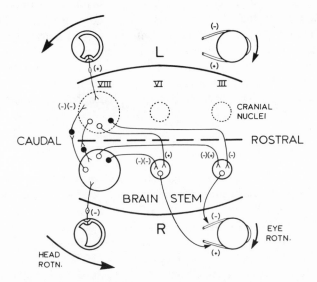

FIG. 6. Essential neuronal components constituting the elementary vestibuloocular reflex arc. (After Melvill Jones & Gonshor, 1975.)

1966). Among other things, such commissural connections would maintain reciprocally organized bilateral ascending influences in the event of unilateral dysfunction in peripheral components. In addition, they probably improve signal-to-noise ratio and linearity of over-all response, as in any differentially organized information processing system (Melvill Jones, 1967). From the left (medial) vestibular nucleus, excitatory interneurones ascend to the right VI nucleus to synapse monosynaptically on abducens motoneurones, innervating the right lateral rectus muscle. Inhibitory interneurones also arise from this site and ascend to synapse directly on contralateral medial rectus motoneurones, thus establishing appropriate reciprocal motor drive to antagonistic muscles, rotating the eye in a compensatory direction in the same plane as the horizontal canals. A reversed ipsilateral innervation, also conveyed monosynaptically, drives a corresponding compensatory rotation of the ipsilateral eye (not shown in Fig. 6). Similar patterns of reciprocal innervation arise from the right canal and nucleus. Thus the elementary reflex arc is essentially disynaptic and brings excitatory, inhibitory, disfacilitatory, and disinhibitory influences to bear on the oculomotor system.

In reality, similar connections have been demonstrated for each orthogonal (i.e., right angular) pair of canals and parallel muscles, although detailed connections are perhaps somewhat more difficult to visualise. The relations may be followed through, however, when it is appreciated that, for example, the right anterior and left posterior canals approximately parallel the actions of the superior and inferior recti of the right eye and the inferior and superior obliques of the left eye. It then remains only to remember that head rotation downward and to the right in the plane of those canals excites the right anterior and suppresses the left posterior primary afferents, for all logistically correct connections to be derived. An extensive series of recent neurophysiological experimental studies has indeed demonstrated that all such functionally appropriate disynaptic connections do indeed exist (for review articles see Precht, 1972; Ito, 1972; and more recently Precht & Baker, 1972; Ito, Nisimaru, & Yamamoto, 1973a and 1973b).

Additional Neural Pathways

Despite these tight relations between logistic requirements and the actual layout of reciprocally acting disynaptic pathways, it turns out that other neural systems are heavily involved in the organization of oculomotor response to vestibular stimulation. Lorente de Nó (1931, 1933) showed that more terminals project onto oculomotor neurones from the reticular formation (RF) than from the medial longitudinal faciculus (MLF). Presumably not all these RF projections are influenced by vestibular inputs, although Robinson (1968) has made the interesting suggestion that some RF mechanisms might be utilized by more than one afferent input. For example, the paramedian pontine RF (PPRF) has been shown to exhibit burst-type activity in advance of saccadic bursting of oculomotor neurones (Cohen & Henn, 1972) and, therefore, may well participate in the generation of saccadic eye movements. An important question is, does the PPRF participate in the formulation of saccadic bursts resulting from different sources of neural command—e.g., voluntary, optokinetic, and vestibular? As pointed out by Robinson, it would seem uneconomic to employ different saccade-generating systems in each case.

Furthermore, bearing in mind the fact that a saccade-generating network presumably needs to integrate either the incoming drive, or a copy of the output of the oculomotor system, or both, it would seem reasonable to postulate that the same network might also serve to integrate a component of vestibuloocular drive concerned with smooth pursuit. Certainly it seems evident that such an integrative function is called for to account for proven dynamic relations between oculomotor neurone firing frequency and vestibularly induced smooth pursuit eye movement (Skavenski & Robinson, 1973).

One may guess that in all probability the role of the RF in vestibularly driven eye movements will prove to be more extensive than can yet be claimed from experimentally proven facts. For example Pompeiano & Morrison (1965), have shown that during certain phases of sleep, vestibularly driven nystagmus may disappear without change in the input-output characteristics of the monosynaptic junction between primary vestibular afferents and second-order neurones projecting rostrally from the vestibular nuclei presumably to innervate motor neurones in the oculomotor nuclei. Perhaps functional inactivation of parallel polysynaptic RF pathways may be responsible. However that may be, it is well known that certain relatively long-latency vestibuloocular responses, of a much less specific kind than the disynaptic ones, can be induced in the absence of the MLF, but not in the absence of the RF (Szentágothai, 1950).

More recently it has been shown that other long-latency responses may also be accounted for by vestibulocerebellovestibular pathways (Precht, 1972; Baker, Precht, & Llinás, 1973). Thus both primary afferent and second-order vestibular neurones project to the vestibulocerebellar cortex (e.g., Brodal & Torvik, 1957; Precht & Llinás, 1969; Ito, 1972). In turn the activated Purkinje cells project their direct inhibitory (or indirect disfacilitatory) influence back to secondary vestibular neurones identified as running rostrally to innervate oculomotor neurones (Angaut & Brodal, 1967; Precht, 1972; Ito, 1972).

What function could these "feed forward" cerebellar influences play in vestibuloocular control? From current research findings it seems highly probable that one function may be to bring about adaptive changes induced by alteration of the visual environment. For example, it has recently been shown (Melvill Jones & Gonshor, 1972; Gonshor & Melvill Jones, 1973 and 1976; Melvill Jones & Gonshor, 1975) that prolonged exposure of human subjects to a reversed visual field brings about effective reversal of the vestibuloocular reflex tested in the dark.

Figure 7 illustrates three responses, all obtained as a result of sinusoidal rotation in the dark. Records (a) were obtained on a control day. Records (b) and (c) were obtained 3 days and 18 days, respectively, after commencing prolonged, continuous exposure to vision reversal produced by horizontally oriented dove prisms. The prisms were suitably mounted in a pair of goggles that

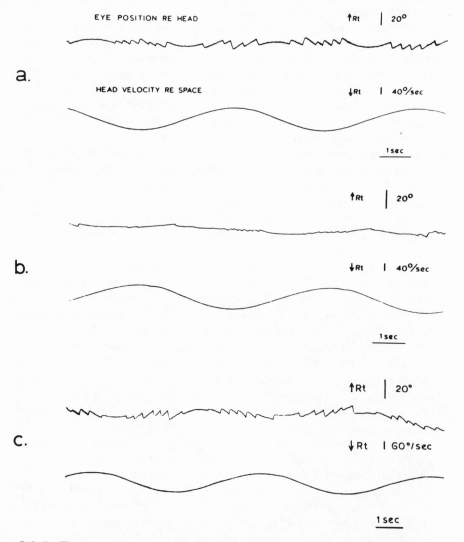

FIG. 7.   Three sets of records obtained from the same human subject (a) during a control run, (b) after wearing reversing prisms continuously for 3 days (c) after 18 days reversed vision. Note the change of phase relation between eye and head traces in (a) and (c). (After Melvill Jones & Gonshor, 1975.)

prevent vision except through the prisms themselves. In each set of records, the lower trace gives the angular *velocity* of the turntable obtained from a tachometer and the upper trace shows the induced (nystagmoid) reflex response, measured as eye angular *displacement* relative to the head by means of horizontal, DC-coupled electrooculography. The control response (a) shows a typical record of normal compensatory nystagmus. The response at 3 days (b) was substantially suppressed and very variable. However, by the 18th day (c) the response had largely recovered both its magnitude and its typically nystagmoid form, but was reorganized in an effectively *reversed* direction.

It is tempting to infer that a relatively simple explanation of this rather striking exhibition of central plasticity may be available in the feed forward inhibitory cerebellar pathway outlined above. It is only necessary to assume a sufficient increase in effectiveness of that inhibitory pathway relative to the direct monosynaptic excitatory one, for reversal of the ongoing signal to have been brought about at the stage of second-order interneurones in the MLF.

Figure 8 illustrates diagramatically the essential components of such a mechanism. During normal head rotation the influence of the direct (+) pathway would outweigh that of the indirect transcerebellar one (−), and the resulting oculomotor drive would generate properly compensatory eye movements. However this oculomotor response would be directly opposite to that required for retinal image stabilization when looking at the outside world through the reversing prisms. Retinal afferents resulting from consequent image slip would then in some way be required to increase effectiveness of the transcerebellar pathway until the negative influence of that pathway outweighs the positive influence of the direct one. In this way the same primary afferent signal could be made to cause an appropriately reversed oculomotor response (Gonshor & Melvill Jones, 1976).

No doubt the matter is not so simple as this. Nevertheless the potential plausiblity of Fig. 8 is enhanced by the recent demonstration of modulation of Purkinje cell activity in the vestibular cerebellum by image movement stimuli on

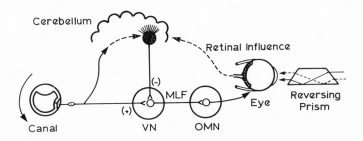

FIG. 8. Schematic diagram of a possible adaptive mechanism. (After Gonshor & Melvill Jones, 1976.)

the retina (Maekawa & Simpson, 1972, 1973). Additional evidence further supports the basis of this simple mechanism. Thus such adaptive change as has been demonstrated in the cat appears to be substantially reduced, or abolished, by cerebellectomy (Robinson, 1975). Similarly, visually induced adaptive change in the vestibuloocular reflex of the rabbit has recently been shown to be abolished specifically by removal of the floccular lobe of the vestibular cerebellum (Ito, Shiida, Yagi, & Yamamoto, 1974). Furthermore, a changed relationship between optokinetic stimuli and head rotation has been shown to bring about changes in vestibular second-order neuronal activity, generally appropriate for causing reduced relative movement of the retinal image and the retina itself (Dichgans & Brandt, 1972; Henn, Young, & Finley, 1974).

Oculomotor Responses to Linear Accelerative Stimuli

It seems clear that although the most important effect of vestibular stimulation upon the oculomotor system is mediated through rotational stimulation of the canals, linear accelerative stimuli can also generate significant, though less marked, oculomotor response. First, static reorganization of the gravitational vertical relative to the head can produce very small, but systematic, counter-rotation of the eyes about the visual axis (Miller, 1962; Miller & Graybiel, 1971). More marked eye movements result from dynamic reorientation of the gravitational vector relative to the head. Thus, prolonged "barbecue-spit" rotation about a horizontal axis continues to generate involuntary nystagmus in the absence of vision long after elastic restoration of the cupulae would be expected to have eliminated the normal mechanical response of the canals (Guedry, 1965; Benson & Bodin, 1966). That such response is specifically due to rotation of a linear acceleration vector relative to the head rather than angular movement of the canal was confirmed both by Benson Guedry, and Melvill Jones (1970), and by Correia and Money (1970).

For example, Fig. 9 shows the averaged profile of nystagmus slow-phase velocity (i.e., slopes of slow-phase sweeps) induced in an intact conscious cat during a pattern of movement described as parallel swing rotation (PSR). In this motion the animal's center of gravity is made to describe a circular path in a horizontal plane, but without inducing angular movement of the animal. In these circumstances a rotating centripetal acceleration vector is made to sweep around the animal without generating the normal rotational stimulation of the canals.

Again, purely linear accelerative body movements conducted in a horizontal plane have been shown to generate involuntary nystagmoid eye movements (Jongkees, 1967; Niven, Hixson, & Correia, 1966). However, it is important to note that in all the above quoted experiments the stimulus included change of direction of the linear acceleration vector either by rotating such a vector around the animal, or as a consequence of vectorial summation of the imposed accelera-

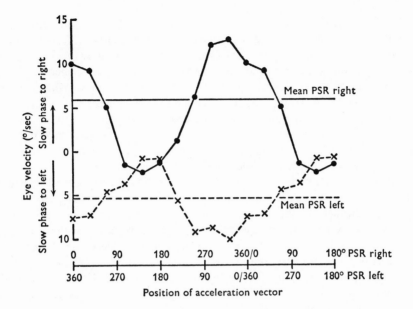

FIG. 9. Mean slow-phase eye angular velocity in a conscious intact cat subjected to PSR motion (see text), averaged from six consecutive cycles. (After Benson, Guedry, & Melvill Jones, 1970.)

tion with that of gravity. As shown by Benson, Guedry, and Melvill Jones (1970), in these circumstances the oculomotor response could be accounted for at least in part by some form of activation of specifically canal-dependent second-order neurones in the vestibular nuclei. The question, therefore, still remained, can linear accelerative stimuli generate reflex oculomotor response without change in direction of the acceleration vector?

Recent experiments of Melvill Jones, Downing, and Rolf (1973) have examined this question by exposing human subjects to patterns of purely vertical acceleration, using the NASA vertical movement simulator at NASA Ames Research Centre Laboratories. Systematic, although weak, eye movements were found in the absence of vision. A special feature of this response was that its phase dependence upon change of stimulus frequency proved similar to that of otolith-dependent vestibular neural units in cats subjected to somewhat similar sinusoidal linear accelerative stimuli (Melvill Jones & Milsum, 1969). The probability, therefore, seems high that these eye movements were induced by purely unidirectional linear accelerative stimulation of the vestibular otolith system. That appropriate neural pathways exist for such a response has been demonstrated by several investigators (e.g., Schwindt, Richter, & Precht, 1973; Hwang, Poon, & Cheung, 1974).

The conclusion must therefore be drawn that both rotational and linear accelerative stimuli can provide functionally effective inputs to the oculomotor system. It is nevertheless important to appreciate that, whereas there is always a unique relation between angular head movement and the required compensatory eye rotation in the skull, this is patently not so for linear movements. Angular eye movements can never properly compensate for linear head movements, since in these circumstances the required compensatory angular velocity of the eye depends upon the radial distance separating the visual object from the eye. Presumably this would account for the relatively large part played by canal, as compared to otolith, inputs to the oculomotor driving system.

Taking a broad overview, the vestibuloocular reflex system is seen as a medium through which automatic stabilization of the eye relative to inertial space is achieved throughout the normal range of naturally occurring angular head movements. Apparently the system is capable of extensive adaptive change, always acting in such a way as to reduced retinal image slip during head movement. Good autostabilization then provides the essential "base" on which to superimpose other purposeful eye movements, despite the presence of on-going movement perturbations due, for example, to locomotor activity or even transportation in jolting man-made vehicles.

DISCUSSION

STEINMAN: How accurate is the compensation of this system for movement when you allow vestibular as well as retinal information to come in?

MELVILL JONES: In the normal situation the vestibuloocular response in the absence of vision is highly frequency dependent. If I am turning at about 0.5 Hz the ratio of compensatory angular velocity of the eye to angular velocity of the head is about .6. However, at about 1 Hz the ratio is about 1. Interestingly, at higher frequencies the gain of the system may become greater than 1.

ROBINSON: Wasn't your question about open eyes?

STEINMAN: Both open and closed. From what you say the velocity is not going to be too well compensated because of the errors in amplitude ratio.

MELVILL JONES: That's a very good point. What I have been describing is the response of the vestibuloocular system. It is surely the case that visual fixation is capable of handling frequencies below $\frac{1}{2}$ Hz. At these lower frequencies you don't need a gain of 1 in the vestibuloocular system and the over-all gain is boosted to 1 by the direct retinal input. At higher frequencies, where visual tracking is incapable of handling the situation, the gain of the vestibulo-ocular reflex rises so that approximate image stabilization is obtained without the need for supplementary stabilization from the visual tracking system.

STEINMAN: Is the gain really 1 at those low velocities or is it .9? Is it known what the degree of compensation is from measurements of high-accuracy electro-oculograms?

MELVILL JONES: Presumably you are talking about minutes of arc. So far as I know it is not yet possible to answer this question, partly because the outcome is highly dependent on the kind of image that the subject is looking at and partly because, as already discussed, it is also dependent upon the frequency of oscillation.

GOULD: How long do the subjects wear prisms every day?

MELVILL JONES: All day. The prisms are put on and remain on until the end of the experiment. The only time they are taken off is at night when the lights have been switched off and the subject is in bed. However, they had to be particularly careful to put them on before opening their eyes in the morning because of the very rapid reversion which can occur.

FRY: To what extent does inhibition figure in this compensation. I have heard that if one gives an acceleration in one direction immediately followed by acceleration in the opposite direction, the input from the second inhibits the first so that there is no vestibular response. That would mean that high-speed oscillation of the vestibular mechanism would be nonfunctional. Is that true?

MELVILL JONES: No, I do not think so. I believe what you describe may be related to the fact that if one closes the eyes and suddenly turns the head to the right, there is a fair probability that the first eye movement will be a saccade in the noncompensatory direction. This may very well be related to the useful function of having the eyes move first in the direction of a stimulus which is to be fixated in order that it can be seen before the head comes into line with it. This can lead to a rather confusing feature that might be called an anticompensa-tory response associated with violent vestibular stimuli that throw the eyes in the "wrong" direction. Thus, rapid alternations of head position with the eyes closed, and without an afterimage to be observed, leads to movement of the eye which is the opposite of compensatory movement.

I.2

The Physiology
of Pursuit Eye Movements

David A. Robinson[1]

The Johns Hopkins University

A great variety of animals, from man to the crab, respond to movements of the visual surround with following eye movements. In spite of the fact that this type of eye movement is found in quite primitive animals and must have developed early in evolution, the anatomical pathways that serve this reflex remain obscure. There are very few places in the primate brain, for example, where stimulation produces smooth movements (not counting the vestibuloocular pathways), there are no restricted locations where a lesion can abolish smooth movements, and no cells whose activity is principally related to optokinetic eye movements have been observed in the brain stems of alert animals. Consequently, very little is actually known about the neurophysiology and neuroanatomy of pursuit or following eye movements. We're not much better off when it comes to the descriptive physiology of these movements. In spite of many studies in man there are many areas left unexplored and there exist no theoretical models which can satisfactorily unite and explain what information we do have.

Fortunately, good progress has been made in describing the optokinetic behavior of the simpler system of the rabbit. Clearly, animals with foveate vision have more complicated requirements than those without (the fovea is, in fact, the main complicating feature of primate eye-movement control) and Collewijn (1972) has utilized this fact to produce a remarkably accurate control-systems model of the rabbit's optokinetic system. It's more likely that the evolution of the fovea caused the optokinetic system of afoveate forebears to be modified

[1] The author's research is supported by grant EY00598 from the Eye Institute, National Institutes of Health, U. S. Public Health Service.

rather than scrapped and replaced, so one might suppose that some aspects of the system seen in the rabbit might also be found in the human oculomotor system, however overlaid they might be with newer circuits.

Collewijn's model is shown in Fig. 1. On the sensory side it is characterized by neurons in the rabbit's retina that detect the direction and speed with which images slip across the retina. They are called directionally selective units. The discharge rate of these units is proportional to retinal slip velocity $\dot{e}$, which is the derivative of the difference between the position of some arbitrarily chosen point (the target) θ_T that moves with the visual surround and the position of the eye, θ.

One of the major physiological contributions to this model was the discovery by Oyster, Takahashi, & Collewijn (1972) that there were two main classes of directionally selective units, one group that responded to slip velocities from below .01°/sec to about 1.0°/sec (DSU–LV, Fig. 1), and another that responded up to above 10°/sec (DSU–HV, Fig. 1). The velocity of .01°/sec, or 36°/hr, is about twice the velocity at which the stars move across the sky. This was the first demonstration of neural apparatus capable of detecting such slow drifts. Both types of cells cut off at sufficiently high velocities, that is, they fail to respond at all to the motion, which corresponds to the fact that the rabbit makes no optokinetic response to sudden displacements of the visual field. The low-velocity cell group gives the system a high forward path gain which results in fast, accurate tracking of stripes so long as they move at velocities less than 1.0°/sec. Beyond this. the high-velocity cell group provides only a low gain so

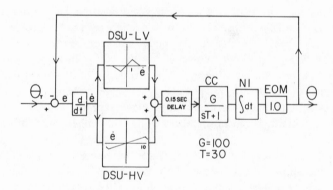

FIG. 1. A slightly modified diagram of Collewijn's model of the rabbit's optokinetic system. Symbols are: θ_T, position of an arbitrary point that moves with the visual surround; θ, eye position; e, retinal error; $\dot{e}$, retinal slip velocity; DSU–LV and –HV, low-velocity and high-velocity (respectively) directionally selective neurons in the rabbit's retina; CC, a central controller characterized by a gain G and a time constant T (in Laplace transform notation); NI, neural integrator; EOM, the extraocular muscles, globe, and suspensory tissues.

that tracking is inadequate and sluggish when the visual surround moves more rapidly than 1.0°/sec.

On the motor side of the reflex, it's been fairly well established that, over the bandwidth in which we're interested, the discharge rate of eye muscle motoneurons is proportional to eye position (see Robinson & Keller, 1972 for a review). Consequently, the conversion of motor nucleus activity to eye position (EOM, Fig. 1) can be simply represented as having a gain of 1.0. All control systems analysts agree that the eye movement command is generated by an integrator which converts a central command (a step) for a desired eye velocity into the movement (a ramp) which has that velocity. Such an integrator is known to exist in the central pathway of the vestibuloocular reflex (Skavenski & Robinson, 1973; Carpenter, 1972) and there is some circumstantial evidence that this neural intergrator is shared by all conjugate eye movement systems: saccadic, pursuit, and vestibular. The point here is that not only are neural integrators a necessary hypothesis in models of the oculomotor subsystems, but there is growing support in neurophysiology that they can be demonstrated as real neuronal circuits. So the neural integrator NI in Fig. 1 is not merely an ad hoc trick devised for the purposes of simulation but probably will soon be isolated and demonstrated in the pons as research rapidly makes progress in this area.

What really remained for Collewijn to explore was the properties of the elements that lay between the visual system and the integrator. The system in Fig. 1 is, of course, a negative feedback control system and its principal virtue, which is the main purpose of all feedback systems, is to maintain the appropriate relationship between input and output in spite of large variations of the parameters of the internal elements. Consequently, the only way to get a good look at the properties of the forward path is to open the feedback loop. This was done by sewing a metal ring onto one eye of the rabbit and holding it so it could not move. This eye saw the moving stripes. The opposite eye was covered and its movement measured. Thus, the visual system was stimulated in the absence of eye motion and the covered eye gave the system's open-loop response.

When the stripes moved at less than 1.0°/sec, nystagmus developed in the covered eye. The slow-phase velocity reached a steady-state level with a time constant of about 30 sec. This level was almost 100 times the velocity of the stripes. Consequently, the central part of the reflex (CC, Fig. 1) had a time constant of 30 sec and the open loop gain was 100. The model in Fig. 1 produces a remarkably faithful reproduction of just about every experimental test one can think of for the rabbit's optokinetic system.

It now remains to find the central controller in the nervous system and discover how it works. Optokinetic nystagmus (OKN) persists in the rabbit after removal of the visual cortex and the cerebellum. For a long time the superior colliculi were suspected to mediate the reflex but careful removal, which does not encroach on the pretectum, still spares OKN. However, lesions of the pretectum seriously interfere with OKN and stimulation of it produces OKN with very low threshold currents. This is a relatively unexplored area of the brain but, no doubt, future research will reveal just what role it plays in the circuit of Fig. 1.

The most important aspect of Collewijn's work is that it clearly reveals the function of the rabbit's optokinetic system. Having no fovea, rabbits do not pursue small objects moving against a stationary backdrop. To evoke following eye movements, all or most of the visual surround must be in motion. But rabbits never find themselves surrounded by a rotating visual scene in nature (if they rotate their heads in a stationary surround, of course, the vestibuloocular reflex provides the needed eye movements). Early on, physiologists tended to study this system quite out of context. Its very name, optokinetic reflex, suggests that its purpose was thought to be to track a moving visual environment. However, since this situation never arises naturally, it would seem a waste of time to develop a system for which there is no function. In fact, it's pretty clear that the purpose of the reflex is to hold the rabbit's eyes still.

Now this might seem odd because if one needs a system to actively hold an eye still, it implies that there must be disturbances that would otherwise make it move. The source of such disturbances might not seem obvious if one has not had experience in communication and control systems where noise and component drift and their suppression are a constant problem. Obviously, eye position control, even in the rabbit, is the end product of a lot of data processing by neural circuits and it would be unrealistic to suppose that these circuits are free from noise and drift. They are not.

The noise in the rabbit's optokinetic system was studied by Collewijn and van der Mark (1972) by again opening the feedback loop in Fig. 1. This can be done, in this case, simply by turning out the lights. In the dark, the rabbit's eyes began to drift about over quite large amplitudes (e.g., $20°$) at velocities of up to $1.0°/sec$. The predominant components in this noise were of low frequency although a spectral analysis of the noise has not been done. Instead, these authors sampled eye velocity periodically and constructed histograms of velocity in open-loop and closed-loop conditions. In the former case, the range of the histogram was about $\pm 1.0°/sec$. When vision was permitted, feedback greatly reduced the velocity spread, illustrating quantitatively what was qualitatively obvious by inspection of the eye position records: without feedback, the rabbit's eyes drifted all about; with feedback, the rabbit's eyes were locked onto the visual scene and drifted almost not at all.

From this we can conclude that the function of this reflex is not to make the eye move but to hold it still. An interesting corollary is that the velocity range of the noise is $1.0°/sec$ and the velocity range of the sensitive groups of directionally selective units is also $1.0°/sec$. Obviously, the latter have been tailored by evolution to deal with the former. One lesson from this work is that nature did not invent the optokinetic system to track moving stripes, and while OKN can be a valuable research tool, it is only profitable as such if one keeps firmly in mind that it is the response of a system attempting to do something for which it was never designed.

Now one might still ask, what is the point of holding the eye still? It's not immediately obvious that a little eye drift can interfere with the rabbit's behavior sufficiently to justify the evolution of an optokinetic system. There are three possibilities. Retinal slip can interfere with visual acuity. Hold a pencil tip just over this printed page, fixate on it and then slowly move the page relative to the pencil and try to read. One tends to cheat in this experiment because it is so natural to track the printed words (that is, hold them stationary on the retina) in order to see them clearly. If one can resist this temptation, it's clear that it is very difficult to make out letters and words when they move across the retina at rather low velocities. So it's tempting to suppose that the rabbit's ability to recognize pattern and form is much better when retinal slip is kept very small, that is, well below $1.0°/sec$.

However, this should not be considered obvious; a lateral-eyed bird in flight has no possibility of maintaining the images of the visual world through which it is flying stable on its retina and it makes no attempt to do so. Yet it avoids small twigs and captures small insects on the wing so it can "see" these things quite well despite the fact that their images are slipping over the retina at fairly high speeds. No doubt different kinds of visual analyzers must be developed to suit the life styles of different animals.

A second reason for stability is this: rabbits do need the ability to spatially localize seen objects. If they do this by adding retinal location to eye-in-head position to locate an object with respect to their body, they must know the position of the eye in the head. It's thought presently (e.g., Skavenski, Haddad, & Steinman, 1972) that this is done by outflow; that is, from an efference copy of the eye position neural command. If neural noise caused an "involuntary" eye movement, it could dissociate actual eye position from efference copy and spatial localization would be incorrect.

The third possibility was suggested to me by J. Pola at this meeting. If a fox 300 ft away is trotting across a field at 2 miles/hr, it crosses the rabbit's visual field at $.6°/sec$. If the rabbit's eye were stationary, only motion-detection cells related to the fox would be stimulated and it would be easily detected. If the rabbit's eye were drifting at $1.0°/sec$, all motion detectors would be stimulated and the rabbit's brain would have to detect a relative slip of $.6°/sec$ between one cell group and its surrounding cells. That's not impossible but it's obviously simpler (and less noisy) in the first case than in the second.

The point of this discussion is that it cannot be automatically assumed that eye stabilization is an obviously desirable thing in itself. The rationale for the evolution of the rabbit's optokinetic system will not be clear until we know more about the perceptual and behavioral benefits derived from it.

Can Collewijn's model help us to understand optokinetic and pursuit eye movements in man? So far, it hasn't. There are two major changes found in man; he is frontal-eyed and he has a fovea. Consider the first of these. The main novel feature that arises when an animal's eyes start to turn forward in evoluation is the area of binocular overlap that emerges in front of the animal. There must have been some benefit from this, probably depth perception, that acted as an evolutionary pressure to turn the eyes even further forward. Even without a fovea, this raised a new problem; when a frontal-eyed animal translates through its environment at a constant velocity and looks to one side, the images seen by its eyes do constitute a real optokinetic stimulus. This is just the situation in looking out a train window, hence the old-fashioned term, train nystagmus. Note that this situation does not constitute an optokinetic stimulus for the rabbit.

Consequently, the system that formerly was only asked to hold the eyes still is now asked to track the moving scene. That's only a problem because of the velocities involved. If a man walks at 3 miles/hr and looks sideways at objects 10 ft away, they represent an optokinetic stimulus of 25°/sec. Such situations are not unnatural; carnivores and ungulates in hot pursuit or flight (respectively) must find themselves in even worse situations. As a result, it became necessary to push the linear range of the optokinetic system upward. This represents no particular design problem in Fig. 1, merely the evolution of directionally selective units that continue working to higher slip velocities. However, the domestic cat, for example, has only extended its velocity range to about 5°/sec (unpublished observations by myself). It's never been clear to me that cats really possess a pursuit system. They track small objects of interest primarily with saccades.

The question of the velocity range in primates is, of course, thoroughly obscured by the development of the fovea (by which I mean any localized area of the retina where visual acuity is better than elsewhere) which confounds optokinetic movements (by which I shall mean movements evoked by motion of the entire visual field) with pursuit movements (by which I shall mean foveal tracking of a small target moving against a stationary scene).

This points out a dichotomy that is echoed throughout the subject of smooth-pursuit movements: there seem to be, in man, at least two systems. Neurologists often distinguish them as cortical vs. subcortical. A variety of animals produce OKN without a visual cortex. This is not surprising in most subprimates (e.g., cat), especially those without a fovea (e.g., rabbit), because of the now well-recognized visual abilities of the superior colliculi in the brain stem. It's more surprising in the monkey where most visual behavior is obviously mediated through the visual cortex. There are even a few reports that cortically blind men can also respond to optokinetic stimuli (ter Braak, Schenk, & van Vliet, 1971) although this is rare and moot. The implication is, in the monkey at any rate, that the visual cortex is necessary for pursuit but not for optokinetic movements.

A second feature of the dichotomy is automaticity. One can elect to pursue or not to pursue a moving target. One has little or no such control over optokinetic following. When the entire visual world moves, it is difficult or impossible to suppress following movements. Conversely, it is equally difficult or impossible (for most people) to make smooth movements across a stationary visual scene. There are well-known exceptions to this. One makes smooth movements during REM sleep (Fuchs & Ron, 1968). Many people can smoothly track their hand in the dark (Steinbach, 1969). The simplest demonstration is to use an afterimage (Kommerell & Klein, 1971). If one has, say, a 5° circular afterimage centered on the fovea, and one "pays attention" to the left edge (2.5° off the fovea), one's eye will start to slide smoothly off to the left. With a little practice, by "paying attention" or turning the "mind's eye," as opposed to the eyeball itself, in various directions by various eccentricities, one can generate smooth eye movements in any direction over a wide range of velocities. All this is done, obviously, without any retinal image slip at all. These exceptions have interesting and important theoretical implications but they are still exceptions and do not change the fact that optokinetic movements have a surprisingly automatic quality. The implication is that anything that automatic must be subcortical.

The problem with this simple idea is that, if we use, by analogy, the example of the rabbit, we must assume that such a subcortical system must be used for fixation, that is, to keep the eye from wandering once it is put somewhere. Yet, somehow, the idea that we use a subcortical system to maintain fixation seems absurd. It probably is.

The third feature of the dichotomy is fovea versus periphery. In fact, my definition of the terms optokinetic and pursuit are based on this distinction. The reason it seems silly to suppose that fixation is subcortical is that fixation is foveally dominated and that implies a cortical function. When we watch a long pass thrown on the football field, we reduce to zero the retinal slip of the football's image on the fovea (that is, we track it) despite the fact that the rest of the visual scene, stadium and spectators, is slipping across our retinas at high velocities. Certainly then, when image slip in the periphery is pitted against slip on the fovea, the latter wins hands down.

This can be easily demonstrated in the laboratory. If even a tiny stationary fixation point is provided together with a background of moving stripes, a subject instructed to fixate the point can almost completely suppress any eye drift that might otherwise have been induced by the stripe motion. Conversely, one can hold the stripes still and move the point. A subject can track the point as well as he could if the stripes were not present. This is hardly a new observation but it is now being examined more carefully and quantitatively by Murphy and Kowler (1974) in R. Steinman's laboratory.

Let's examine the idea that fixation is foveally dominated and cortically mediated in primates from a neurophysiological standpoint. In Fig. 1, an important element is the set of directionally selective units which sense retinal slip, the sine qua non of slip detection. They seem to shift more and more from brain stem to cortex as one goes up the phylogenetic scale. As we've seen, they are found in the rabbit retina. In cat, it was thought for a long time that while they were seen in the superior colliculus (e.g., Sterling & Wickelgren, 1969) they were not to be found in the retina. That now appears to be incorrect (Stone &

Fukuda, 1974) although these so-called W cells, which are directionally selective, are smaller and scarcer than the more common X and Y cells. In the monkey, no one has yet found directionally selective units in the retina and there are very few of them even in the superior colliculus (Schiller & Koerner, 1971). There are, of course, many such units in the visual cortex (as is also the case in rabbit and cat), so there appears to be a migration of these cells from brain stem to cortex in primates with the suggestion that, if they are used for fixation, then fixation is cortical in primates.

But a quantitative problem arises. In order to limit retinal slip to the order of .1°/sec, as seen in the slow drifts of human fixation, the visual system must be capable of detecting such velocities. Now the great majority of cells in visual cortex are motion-sensitive and many are directionally selective to motion as well. But the physiologists who record from them are usually not interested in this problem and seldom explore the velocity range over which such cells respond. The velocities usually reported are around 5–50°/sec. Units that respond well in this range may not respond at all to .1°/sec. Recently, however, B. Dow, at the National Eye Institute, National Institutes of Health, found, almost by accident, cells in the foveal region of monkey visual cortex that did respond to low velocities in this range (unpublished observations). While this demonstration is neither necessary nor sufficient to indicate that fixation is cortical, it certainly helps to build up the case.

Alternatively, one can turn to the brain stem and try to show that fixation cannot be mediated by visual units there. In several interesting new lines of investigation, experimenters have discovered regions in the brain stem where cells respond more or less directly to visual stimuli. Maekawa and Simpson (1973), for example, in the rabbit, have traced a retinal projection from the accessory optic tract to the inferior olive and relayed to the vestibulocerebellum (e.g., flocculus and nodulus) on climbing fibers. Westheimer and Blair (1974) have found cells, in the monkey, in the nucleus of the transpeduncular tract, thought to be the termination of the accessory optic tract, that respond to moving visual stimuli. This could conceivably suggest that, as in the cat, there are directionally selective units in the monkey retina after all, whose small cell and fiber size has allowed them, so far, to escape detection. Although our knowledge of the receptive field properties of these units is rudimentary, it does seem clear that they have very large receptive fields (e.g., 60°) and seem to be concerned with the movement of the general visual environment and not with the movement of small objects on local regions of the retina. In the monkey or the cat, no cells have been found in the brain stem, with the exception of the superior colliculus, that appear to be possible candidates for mediating foveal pursuit. So again, the notion is reinforced that fixation in primates is cortical and foveal.

Of course the directionally selective units seen in the brain stem and cerebellum raise the question of why they are there at all. I believe that some of their function has to do with certain forms of adaptation and homeostasis. Let me give an example. If, say, some internal disturbance unbalances the drives from the two horizontal semicircular canals (e.g., a minute vascular lesion in the VIIIth nerve or vestibular nucleus) an unwanted nystagmus would occur. When this in fact happens in patients, the nystagmus, which is seen unchecked in the dark, is suppressed by mechanisms with at least three different time courses. Both the optokinetic and pursuit systems act to suppress it immediately when visual feedback becomes available in the light. Over the next few hours and days, a repair mechanism is obviously at work rebalancing the vestibular unbalance, and nystagmus in the light is entirely suppressed and becomes diminished even in the dark. Finally, over a period of months, the job is complete and the patient has recovered. There is good reason to believe that the vestibulocerebellum and vestibular nuclei are important circuits for this repair process. In order to effect this repair the oculomotor system must be able to detect that something has gone wrong. Continuous unidirectional image slip on the retina is not only an important undesirable consequence of such a problem, but is also the most sensitive way to detect it. Therefore, the repair mechanism in the brain stem or cerebellum clearly needs the input from directionally selective visual neurons. The cells described above may very likely be involved, then, in some such parametric-adaptive process and not at all intended for the purpose of following stripes on an optokinetic drum.

Ironically, the repair mechanism may be unable to distinguish between an internal lesion that would create nystagmus and an optokinetic drum stimulus. After all, such a stimulus is thoroughly unnatural and evolution would scarcely have provided for it. In this case, the repair mechanism, in its effort to null out persistent retinal slip, would be fooled into making nystagmus instead of suppressing it. It could be just such a process that accounts for the OKN in a monkey without its visual cortex and which has led to the erroneous assumption that there is a subcortical optokinetic system in primates. Obviously it would be a bad conceptual mistake to lump such an adaptive repair mechanism and the rabbit's "fixation" system together. Their purposes, function, bandwidth, linear range, and circuitry are quite different.

My feeling at the moment, then, is that in man, fixation, foveal pursuit, and optokinetic following are all cortical, but the interpretation of optokinetic experiments can easily be confounded by the accidental stimulation of brain-stem adaptive mechanisms. These responses are slow and may respond only to full- or large-field stimulation. Consequently, their contamination can best be avoided by observing the response of the eyes to a given stimulus motion within the first few seconds of its onset. The response to any stimulation that persists for minutes (a completely unnatural situation) will undoubtedly contain the results of stimulating adaptation processes.

Before leaving this subject, one must point to the remarkable finding by Westheimer and Blair (1973b) that removal of the cerebellum in the monkey appears to abolish both pursuit and OKN! It certainly does not abolish the latter in cat or rabbit. This raises a series of interesting questions: Are we much too facile in extrapolating results across species? (There's a clear warning here.) And just what is the role of the cerebellum in eye movement control? This is a new and rapidly developing field of investigation.

We still have before us the task of describing and modeling the system or systems responsible for fixation, pursuit, and optokinetic movements in man. Until we do this, we'll not get very far in interpreting neurophysiological results. Here is a problem that illustrates how badly off we are in just not having good quantitative descriptions to work from. When we track a target, do we match eye and target velocity exactly or do we keep slipping behind the target? In the context of Fig. 1, let G be the forward-path gain. Then the closed-loop gain is $G/(1 + G)$. In the rabbit, the steady-state value of G for retinal slips less than $1.0°/\text{sec}$ is 100. The closed-loop gain is then .99; that is, the eye velocity is 99% that of target velocity. If G were only 10, then eye velocity would be 91% of target velocity. If G were 7, 6, or 5, the ratio would be 87.5%, 86%, and 83%, respectively. It's hard to believe that this ratio is actually not well known for human tracking. Steinman, Skavenski, and Sansbury (1969) are the only group to try to measure it accurately. They report about 80–90%, indicating that G is somewhere between 5 and 9—not very high. These results are quite important and it would be nice to see them confirmed or modified by further, more thorough investigation.

Koerner and Schiller (1972) have attempted to measure G in the monkey in much the same way that Collewijn did for the rabbit, by stimulating an immobilized eye. Since the system is nonlinear, G depends on stripe velocity, decreasing as the latter increases. They found G to be as high as 10–30 for retinal slip velocities down to about $2°/\text{sec}$. Lower velocities were not investigated. Unfortunately, it's not clear with this full-field stimulus whether one is stimulating a pursuit or an optokinetic system and, since stripe motion of long duration was used (as was also true in Collewijn's study), one is not sure to what extent fast tracking systems or slow adaptation systems were stimulated. These experiments need to be repeated within the context of functional control systems models.

Almost nothing has been done in exploring the dynamics of the responses to foveal versus peripheral motion. Examples of the latter situation are experiments in which the foveal area is devoid of stimuli and stripes move only in the periphery. The cleverest way to do this these days is by visual feedback; that is, one has a computer-generated display of stripes, measures eye position, and blanks out the display in the vicinity of the fovea. This creates an artificial central scotoma. However one does this, it is possible to produce OKN by peripheral stimulation (Cheng & Outerbridge, 1973), but the dynamics (latency, time constants, open-loop gain, etc.) have not been investigated. Again, the differentiation for adaptive processes has not been considered.

Assuming that these responses are not purely adaptive, one might ask, given a foveal fixation (or tracking) system, why one needs a peripheral fixation (or tracking system). There are at least two possibilities. One is that it is vestigial; that is, there is a little rabbit left in all of us. Obviously the fovea dominates the periphery and can easily suppress any optokinetic drive that comes only from the periphery, but when the fovea is out of the way, the old (brain stem?) system is released and can function. Experiments designed to test this have not been done. A second hypothesis concerns night vision when illumination levels are scotopic. The impoverished visual system might need all the help it can get through stabilization of the eye on the surround, yet it is now deprived of foveal (photopic) vision. Consequently, it must rely on a scotopic fixation system.

What I hope emerges from all this discussion is that this system is wide open for further investigation. There are many questions begging to be answered and hypotheses begging to be tested and, as I said before, the interpretation of neurophysiological data must, by and large, await these descriptive experiments and theories before they will fall into place and give us explanations instead of just more and more (and more) data.

Finally, I'd like to briefly indicate some of the interesting complications we will encounter in making these models. A major simplistic assumption in Fig. 1 is that, in the absence of vision, the brain has no notion of where the eye is in the orbit. This is probably quite wrong, and many have hypothesized an internal signal called efference copy, a replica of the signal sent to the eye muscles which tells the brain at least where the eye ought to be. Young, whose discussion follows immediately, proposed that this information be used in the interesting way shown in Fig. 2. If one takes retinal error velocity $\dot{e}$ and adds to it a signal $\hat{\dot{\theta}}$ proportional to the efference copy of eye velocity, one recreates, centrally, a signal proportional to target velocity with respect to the (stationary) head, $\hat{\dot{\theta}}_T$. This is the desired eye velocity in the head, so it is passed to the eye muscles

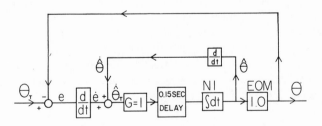

FIG. 2. A modification of Fig. 1 that uses an internal signal $\hat{\theta}$ which is an efference copy of eye position or eye velocity, $\hat{\dot{\theta}}$, to recreate the internal representation of target velocity in space, $\hat{\dot{\theta}}_T$. This is equivalent to an open-loop system, since positive and negative feedback cancel, so forward path gain G must be 1.0. Other symbols are as in Fig. 1.

after integration, with a gain of 1.0. An enormous control systems advantage of this arrangement is that the delay of .15 sec in Fig. 1, which can lead to stability problems, is now unimportant because the internal positive feedback just cancels the external negative feedback and the system in Fig. 2 behaves just as if neither feedback path were present at all. The system behaves as if it were open loop and so, of course, it could never become unstable. Thus, the two main attractions in considering Fig. 2 are that stability is not a problem and that the psychophysical percept of target velocity in space, $\dot{\theta}_T$, is explicitly shown as an important control variable.

L. Young, who will continue to pursue the pursuit system, will discuss this model, developed by S. Yasui and himself. Although I'm not sure I agree with their interpretation of how visual and vestibular information are combined and how afterimages affect the behavior of the vestibuloocular reflex (these differences lie beyond the scope of this discussion), I do find the model in Fig. 2 attractive and worth exploring. One aspect of it, however, should be commented on. Negative feedback has as its major function the purpose of making system performance relatively independent of internal and external disturbances. Fortunately, the oculomotor system is free from external disturbances (external forces applied to the eyeball) but it is not free from internal disturbances. Effectively removing the negative feedback as in Fig. 2 also removes all the advantages of negative feedback. If the forward gain in Fig. 1 dropped by 50%, very little would happen to closed-loop performance. If the same thing happened (to $G = 1$) in Fig. 2, the closed loop gain would also drop by 50%. All protection against parameter drift is lost in Fig. 2. This need not imply that Fig. 2 is an untenable scheme but it does mean that one must make the additional hypothesis that some form of parametric-adaptive control must exist before this "open-loop" characteristic can be tolerated by any real biological system.

Note that Figs. 1 and 2 are not mutually exclusive; the former could still apply to an afoveate system that is overlaid by a foveal system similar to that of Fig. 2. In fact, the main problem in this whole area is that we have so little good data available that it is really impossible to evaluate models properly. The smooth-pursuit system in man is not simple and grows more complex the longer one examines it. My guess is that for at least the next five years, progress will not be made in the neurophysiology of this system but in the design and analysis of experiments that will allow us to construct better theoretical models: a process for which nothing stands in the way except some hard work.

DISCUSSION

WURTZ: Is it a viable hypothesis at this time that the primate has retained the rabbit's stabilization system over the whole retina and has added on the tracking system in the fovea: specifically, in your "TV scotoma" paradigm, do you get drift from the loss of the stabilization due to the fovea, which has now been taken out? Possibly without any visual target on the fovea, there would be a drift.

ROBINSON: Yes, Murphy and Kowler in Steinman's laboratory have done experiments like this. What you are saying is: suppose one looks at the center of a perfectly blank circle, can one let the periphery do the stabilization? I think the answer is that stabilization is still very good under those conditions. Isn't that right?

STEINMAN: Yes, it is.

ROBINSON: So we can use peripheral information to get fairly good fixation control. The problem that remains is whether that peripheral control is cortical, subcortical, or both. Still, the monkey might be sort of halfway between the rabbit and man; it would be interesting to try and train a money to pay attention to something on his fovea and then to neglect it and pay attention to something on his periphery to see whether monkeys are more like man or more like rabbits.

STEINMAN: I would like to make two comments. First of all, the stabilization level with slow control is optimal with an annulus or disk that's on the order of half a degree. There is stability with a peripheral annulus, but it is not as good.

The second comment is with respect to the velocity-matching question. There has been some recent activity in my laboratory in measuring tracking gain. Murphy and Kowler have some data, which leads me to say, with considerable confidence, that you can get 88% velocity matching and as high as 95%. (I am talking now about tracking a point against a dark or a homogeneous field.) However, velocity matching is certainly not 100%. The original measurements we had, in which subjects were matching by only about 85%, were done before we knew that we had the option of adjusting the tracking velocity to fractions of target velocity. So we were probably doing that unconsciously to some extent in the early experiments. We are now working hard trying to velocity-match, with just a point target, but 95% is the best we can do.

We have not done what you have suggested, namely, have an acuity target where the subject's task is to resolve it while tracking. This might guarantee that he would use the fast foveal system and perhaps match.

I.3

Eye Movements during Afterimage Tracking under Sinusoidal and Random Vestibular Stimulation [1]

Syozo Yasui

California Institute of Technology

Laurence R. Young[2]

Massachusetts Institute of Technology

Smooth-pursuit eye movements can be elicited in the absence of a moving image on the retina, and bring into serious question the entire notion that the purpose of the smooth movement system is stabilization of the retinal image (Steinbach & Held, 1968; Young, 1971). We suggest that smooth eye movements serve the role of driving the eyes conjugately at a speed related to the *perceived target velocity*. As indicated in Fig. 1, the assumption of a corollary discharge path, together with a connection from perceived velocity to eye velocity, is an alternative to the retinal feedback path for oculomotor control (Yasui & Young, 1975; Yasui, 1974). One way of demonstrating the existence of this path is by use of a standard stimulus to initiate smooth eye movements. In this case, we used standard vestibular stimuli. By generating a visual target which is stationary on the retina, using a foveally centered afterimage, we were able to observe the change in slow-phase eye movements when a perceived target (the afterimage) was actively tracked by the subject (Kommerell & Taumer, 1972; Heywood & Churcher, 1971, 1972; Grüsser & Grüsser-Cornehls, 1972). Observation of an

[1] This work was supported by NASA Grant NGR 22-009-025 and was also presented at the Symposium on Basic Mechanisms of Ocular Motility and Their Clinical Implications, Stockholm, 1974, and is in press in a book by that name, G. Lennerstrand and P. Bach-y-Rita, eds., Pergamon Press, 1975.

[2] Presented by Laurence R. Young.

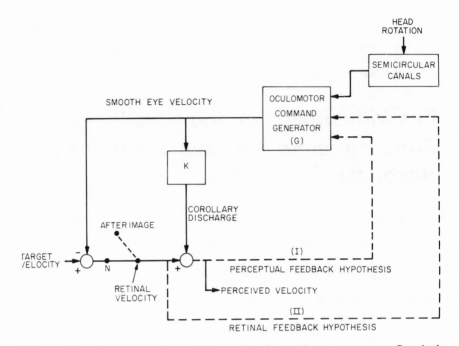

FIG. 1. Schematic representation of the control of smooth eye movements. Perceived velocity of the target is assumed to generate a smooth eye movement via loop (I). The effect of the eye movement in changing retinal velocity is partially cancelled by the corollary discharge of gain K.

increase in the speed of slow-phase eye movements when the subject perceived the target motion (during afterimage tracking) supports the notion of the activation of a positive (regenerative) feedback loop from eye movement, to perceived target velocity, to change in eye velocity.

The smooth portion of the horizontal vestibuloocular reflex was analyzed in terms of the frequency response, relating slow-phase eye velocity to angular velocity of a rotating chair under four different cases: (1) sinusoidal rotation about a vertical axis in total darkness; (2) sinusoidal rotation during afterimage tracking; (3) pseudorandom head rotation in total darkness; (4) pseudorandom head rotation during afterimage tracking. The frequency of oscillation for the sinusoidal test was varied randomly in the range from .025 to .7 Hz. Peak angular velocity was also varied, but never exceeded 40°/sec. Alertness was maintained through a mental arithmetic task. After several oscillation periods in the dark, a monocular foveal afterimage was produced by a fixated flash bulb. Subjects attempted to fixate the target and indicate its direction of motion using a three-position switch. Eye movements were recorded using a photoelectric limbus tracking method. The frequency of response of slow-phase eye velocity relative to the chair velocity (vestibuloocular reflex transfer function) was calculated from the sinusoidal eye movement trace by hand for the sinusoidal cases, and from the MITNYS eye velocity program (Tole & Young, 1971; Allum, Tole, & Weiss, 1975) for the pseudorandom chair motion.

The vestibuloocular reflex recorded prior to the initiation of the afterimage agreed with published results for sinusoidal stimulation (Benson, 1970). After the flash was made and the afterimage appeared, the fast-phase movement almost disappeared and eye movements tended to become smooth. The apparent motion of the visual afterimage relative to the subject was in phase with the smooth eye movements, as expected. The cumulative eye position (sum of slow phases) and slow-phase velocity under afterimage tracking conditions were always greater than those of tracking in the dark prior to the flash.

The frequency response comparing the vestibuloocular reflex gain and phase under conventional vestibular stimulation (eyes open in the dark, indicated by "no vision") and the afterimage tracking for the same vestibular stimulation are shown in Fig. 2. The frequency response clearly shows the significant effect of the afterimage tracking in increasing the gain and advancing the phase of the vestibuloocular reflex ($p < .05$), as predicted by the hypothesis of a regenerative feedback loop involving perceived velocity. For example, at .7 Hz, the slow-phase velocity under afterimage tracking was approximately twice as large as that for motion in the dark under the same vestibular stimulus. The phase

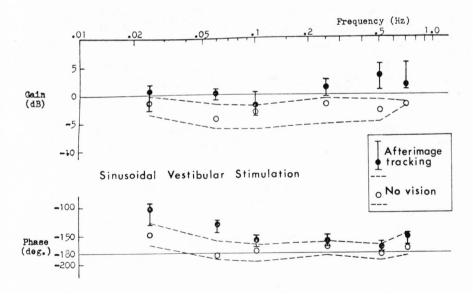

FIG. 2. Frequency response comparison (based on sinusoidal head rotation) between afterimage tracking eye movement and vestibular nystagmus slow phase in complete darkness without afterimage. Median data points and ± one standard deviation are shown (four subjects).

advance of up to about 40° with afterimage tracking held for all frequencies, and was most prominent at the lowest frequencies tested.

Figure 3 is a frequency response for the pseudorandom input vestibuloocular reflex under the conditions of rotation in the dark with and without the presence of an afterimage. There appears to be no substantial difference between the frequency response of the vestibuloocular reflex in the dark for sinusoidal and for pseudorandom inputs. Unlike normal visual–oculomotor tracking (Stark, Voissius, & Young, 1962), prediction due to target periodicity is apparently not involved in the nonvisual oculomotor response, at least in the relatively low frequency range tested. Eye-movement amplitude ratios become somewhat greater during afterimage tracking over the frequency range investigated, although the difference is not as conspicuous as in the previous sinusoidal comparison, nor is it quite as consistent throughout the frequency range. Nevertheless, the fact that the presence of an afterimage and the generation of a perceived angular velocity of this afterimage increased the angular velocity of eye movement for random as well as sinusoidal tracking indicates that the important factor is perceived visual motion and not its predictability.

The observation that the presence of an afterimage during vestibular stimulation increases the velocity of slow-phase eye movements is in support of the theory that such slow-phase movements are generated, at least in part, by the perceived velocity of the target. Since the target is immobilized on the retina, this perceived velocity is clearly not generated by retinal slip, but rather by a mechanism related to the eye movement, such as corollary discharge. As an example, movement of the head to the left generates a slow-phase eye movement

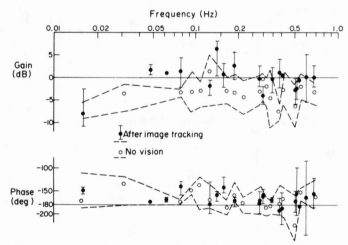

FIG. 3. Frequency response data for two types of smooth eye movement under pseudorandom vestibular stimulation: smooth eye movement during visual tracking of vestibularly induced afterimage apparent motion versus normal vestibular nystagmus slow phase in the dark.

to the right, based on the vestibular stimulation. This right eye movement produces an apparent motion of the foveal afterimage to the right relative to the subject. This perceived target motion presumably then generates an increased eye velocity to the right through the positive feedback loop (I) in Fig. 1. The fact that the system is not unstable indicates that the loop gain of this positive feedback loop must be less than unity, which is consistent with the theory that the cancellation associated with the outflow mechanism is less than complete and is, in fact, probably only of the order of 60 or 70%. Note that the gain of the vestibuloocular reflex during afterimage tracking exceeds unity (0 dB) in the midfrequency range for both sinusoidal and pseudorandom tracking, although the gain of the human vestibuloocular reflex in the dark is only approximately .6 in the midfrequency range.

DISCUSSION

HALLETT: There is another method whereby one can elicit smooth pursuit movement in the absence of a moving visual stimulus. Lightstone (1973) reported that if one uses a voluntary saccade to trigger a step displacement of the target, and if the displacement is in a predicted direction and extent, then the second saccade must be delayed by a full reaction time (assuming that the subject is instructed to fixate the target) and one observes a smooth pursuit movement of no appreciable latency at about 5° per sec.

I.4

The Neurophysiology of Saccades[1]

Albert F. Fuchs

University of Washington

Most of our normal viewing life is spent examining a stationary visual environment and the eye movement that we use for such exploration is the saccade. Saccades are apparently the only voluntary eye movement present at birth and provide the human infant with its sole means of exploring his new visual world. Some examples of the saccadic scan paths of reading and searching are shown in the accompanying paper by Dennis Fisher. A saccade serves to rapidly shift the direction of gaze from one object in the visual field to another, with "seeing" actually impaired during the saccadic trajectory. The saccade is probably the most rapid somatic movement that any muscular system in the body can produce. For example, a 40° human saccade takes about 100 msec to execute whereas a 40° flexion of the forearm would require more than 300 msec. Unlike an arm movement, however, the saccade is said to be ballistic in nature so that, once begun, its velocity or goal cannot be modified.

In the usual laboratory situation, a saccade is elicited by having the subject fixate a target spot which rapidly jumps to one side. A monkey's response to a 10° horizontal target step (Fig. 1) serves to demonstrate most of the properties of the saccade and its control system. After an average reaction time or latency of about 200 to 250 msec, the eye accelerates rapidly, to reach its maximum velocity of about 550°/sec about midway in the trajectory; thereafter, the eye decelerates with a similar trajectory to land on the target with almost no overshoot or ringing. If the target step is greater than about 20°, the saccade falls

[1] This study was supported by grants RR00166 and EY00745 from the National Institutes of Health, U. S. Public Health Service.

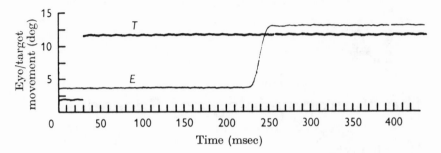

FIG. 1. A typical saccadic response (E) of a trained monkey to a step change in target position (T).

about 10% short of the required distance and a second saccade follows after another reaction time to put the eye on target (Fuchs, 1967).

There are at least four noteworthy features of this response.

1. A position error seems necessary to elicit a saccadic eye movement. Earlier investigators (Rashbass, 1961; Young, 1966) demonstrated that target steps of less than .3° (i.e., within the functional confines of the fovea) did not elicit saccades, and postulated the existence of a saccadic "dead zone." Recently, however, Steinman, Haddad, Skavenski, and Wyman (1973) have shown that steps as small as 3.5 min of arc are sufficient to cause a saccade.

2. A relatively long delay (200–250 msec) elapses between the visual stimulus and the resulting saccade. About 150 msec can be accounted for by the time it takes visual information to reach the cortex (about 80 msec) and the latency to elicit a saccade by cortical stimulation (about 70 msec). Further processing during the reaction time has been studied by causing the stepped target to step once again before the saccade occurs. Suffice it to say that the saccade to the original step can be canceled as little as 80 msec prior to its scheduled occurrence (Wheeless, Boynton, & Cohen, 1966; Komoda, Festinger, Phillips, Duckman, & Young, 1973).

3. We are unaware of the occurrence of saccades although we often emit as many as 2 or 3 per second (e.g., during reading). The rapid dislocation of the visual world during a saccade must be dealt with either by a purely visual phenomenon such as masking (Brooks & Fuchs, 1975) or by a corollary discharge from the oculomotor system which suppresses vision during saccades (Volkmann, Schick, & Riggs, 1968).

4. Since each of the preceding three features is scheduled for separate sessions later in the conference, I am left to discuss the final feature: the saccadic trajectory itself and specifically the neurophysiology that underlies it. First of all, however, it is important to characterize the saccade completely so that we

can pinpoint the changes in neural firing and muscle force that ultimately reflect themselves in the saccadic trajectory.

A saccade is usually defined by its duration and maximum velocity, both of which increase with saccadic amplitude (Fig. 2). For normal saccades executed at random around a structured visual field (S.F., Fig. 2), monkeys require an additional millisecond in duration for every degree of increase in amplitude (humans require 2 msec/deg). A similar relationship applies for the fast phases of vestibular nystagmus (Ron, Robinson, & Skavenski, 1972) elicited in a structured visual field (data points and Ny. S.F., Fig. 2). If structure is removed from the visual field either by placing the monkey in the dark or in a Ganzfeld, the duration of both voluntary saccades (Gnz., Drk.) and the "involuntary" fast phases of nystagmus (Ny. Drk., Ny. Gnz.) increases; however, both increase by essentially similar amounts. These data suggest that the fast phases of vestibular nystagmus (and also optokinetic nystagmus) are saccades. The maximum velocity achieved during a human saccade increases with amplitude up to 20°; for larger saccades, a velocity saturation occurs at between 500 and 700°/sec (Fig. 2, right); monkey saccades saturate at 1000°/sec. The characteristic relating maximum velocity and saccadic amplitude can be extrapolated backward to include the small microsaccades of fixation (Zuber, Stark, & Cook, 1965). Similarly, if

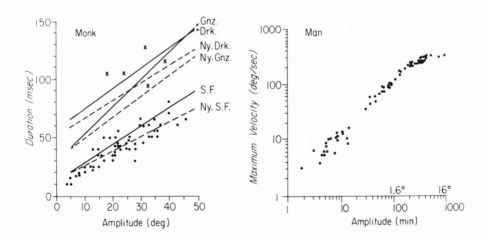

FIG. 2. Saccadic duration (from monkeys; Ron et al., 1972) and maximum saccadic velocity (from man; Zuber et al., 1965) plotted against saccade amplitude. Solid lines in the left graph refer to voluntary saccades elicited on a structured field (S.F.), on a Ganzfeld (Gnz.), or in the dark (Drk.). Dashed lines refer to the fast phases of vestibular nystagmus under similar conditions. The data points in the left graph demonstrate the spread for the Ny. S.F. condition.

the S.F. duration–amplitude relationship is extrapolated back to zero, the intercept of 15 msec also correctly corresponds to the duration of a 10-min microsaccade suggesting that the microsaccades of fixation may be generated by the same neural mechanism or at least are limited by the same mechanics as the larger saccades.

The neurophysiology of the saccade has been approached by starting at the saccadic trajectory itself and working back into the brain sequentially from the forces that move the eye, to the motoneurons that cause the muscles to contract, to the possible neural structures that provide inputs to the moto-neurons. The forces that move the eye have been very elegantly described by Robinson (1964) who used a tightly fitting suction contact lens both to apply horizontal external forces to the eye and to measure forces exerted by the eye during a variety of eye movements. If a step of force is applied (Fig. 3A, dashed

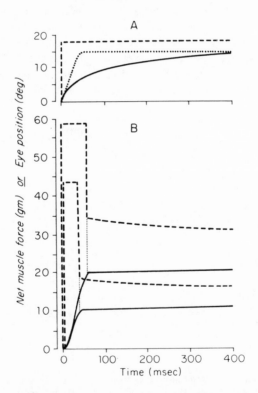

FIG. 3. The net muscle force associated with saccadic eye movements under different conditions (modified from Robinson, 1964). The upper set of curves compares a normal saccade (dotted curve) with the eye movement (solid curve) resulting when a step of force (dashed curve) is applied to the globe through a suction contact lens. The lower set of curves shows the predicted net forces (dashed curves) associated with a 10° (lower solid trace) and 20° (upper solid trace) saccade.

curve), the eye, to a first approximation, responds along an exponential trajectory with a time constant of 150 msec (Fig. 3A, solid curve). Clearly, a step in net force is not adequate to provide an actual saccade (Fig. 3A, dotted curve). By further applying a variety of isometric and isotonic constraints to the tracking eye, Robinson (1964) was able to construct a model that predicted the net force on the eye during saccades (Fig. 3B). Just prior to a $10°$ movement (lowest two traces), there is a rapid increase in force to a level (43 g) much greater than that required to keep the eye in its deviated position (15 g). The duration of the force is approximately equal to the duration of the saccade. During a $20°$ saccade (Fig. 3B, upper traces), the net force is greater and is applied for a longer time appropriate to the longer duration of the larger saccade. Once again the net force during the saccade exceeds that required to keep the eye deviated. However, the excess force is approximately equal (23–25 g) for both saccades, suggesting that a separate group of muscle motor units fire during saccades to provide a pulse of constant force whose duration reflects the duration of the saccade (Robinson, 1964). Histological evidence indicates that the rectus muscles are composed of a variety of muscle fiber types ranging from very fast singly innervated fibers to very slow multiply innervated types. While it is tempting to ascribe the excess pulse of force to contraction of the fast twitch fibers, very little physiological evidence is available to support such a hypothesis.

The net force applied to the globe during a horizontal saccade is generated by the synergistic operation of the two horizontal rectus muscles. Some evidence concerning muscle activity during the saccade has come from measurement of the human electromyogram (EMG) which reports the summed electrical activity of muscle fibers. During a lateral saccade, the lateral rectus muscle exhibits a burst of activity of saccadic duration, but the medial rectus (the antagonist) exhibits a complete cessation of activity for the duration of the saccade (Björk & Kugelberg, 1953). Therefore, the pulse of force during a saccade (Fig. 3) is the result of a carefully coordinated activation of the agonist muscle and the simultaneous relaxation of the antagonist muscle, each for the precise duration of the saccade.

The EMG activity reflects the firing patterns of motoneurons which innervate the rectus muscles. Over the last several years, several different laboratories have recorded motoneuron activity in the unanesthetized monkey trained to make saccadic eye movements. Each group agrees that there is only one type of motoneuron in the three oculomotor nuclei; each motoneuron participates in every type of eye movement with a discharge pattern that can be predicted for saccadic, smooth pursuit, vergence, and vestibular eye movements. The stereotyped firing pattern associated with saccades is demonstrated in Fig. 4 from extracellular recordings in the abducens nucleus whose neurons innervate the lateral rectus muscle (Fuchs & Luschei, 1970). When the eye fixates, motoneurons discharge at a very steady rate which increases as the eye shifts fixation to a more lateral position. About 7 msec prior to and during a lateral saccade

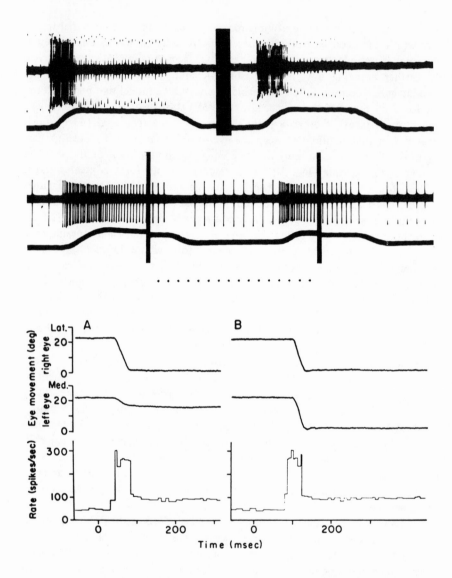

FIG. 4. Discharge patterns of abducens neurons associated with horizontal saccades in the unanesthetized monkey. The upper two panels represent discharge patterns from one motoneuron, the middle three panels represent discharge patterns from a second motoneuron. The lowest trace in each panel shows the eye movement with upward deflections representing lateral eye movements. Time marks occur at 10-msec intervals (Fuchs & Luschei, 1970). The lowest panel represents the discharge rate of a left abducens neuron (in analog form) during a normal conjugate saccade (B) and a conjugate saccade in which the excursion of the left eye was limited (A) (Keller & Robinson, 1971).

between fixation points, the motoneuron emits an intense burst of spikes whose frequency greatly exceeds the final fixation frequency. If the saccade exceeds 5°, the burst firing frequency reaches rates of up to 800 spikes/sec, the maximum rate at which these units can fire. The duration of the burst of spike activity is approximately equal to the duration of the saccade as can be clearly seen in the second motoneuron (middle panels). Therefore, during a lateral saccade, an agonist motoneuron emits a pulse of spikes which is superimposed upon a step change in firing frequency associated with the fixation change. When the eye looks medially so that the same motoneuron now innervates an antagonist muscle, the discharge ceases completely during the saccade. Since the antagonist muscle is essentially passive during the saccade and does not resume activity until the eye has landed, the net pulse step of force is created only by the pulse-step activity in the agonist motoneuron (compare Fig. 4 with Fig. 3). Therefore, the characteristics of the neural pulse step, when played through the dynamics of the muscle and viscoelastic load of the eye, are alone sufficient to bring the eye to its final position in a deadbeat fashion.

The carefully choreographed pulse step of neural activity is not generated by local feedback circuits. By applying a tightly fitting contact lens, Keller and Robinson (1971) were able to prevent the eye from moving, hence preventing the muscle and its afferent endings from stretching during an intended saccade. In part B of the lower half of Fig. 4, the usual pulse step of activity was recorded from the left abducens nucleus during a leftward saccade. In part A, the left eye was allowed to move only one-third its usual distance, a condition which severely alters the afferent feedback from the muscles, yet the pulse step of neural activity associated with the saccade remained unchanged.

Continuing to follow the saccadic information into the central nervous system, we now need to know the source of the pulse-step signal to the motoneurons. In this conference, both Melvill Jones and Robinson have already implicated the pontine reticular formation as an important staging area for vestibular and smooth pursuit movements. For the following reasons, it must also be vital for the generation of the horizontal saccade: (1) lesions of the pons cause complete ipsilateral gaze paralysis (Goebel, Komatsuzuki, Bender, & Cohen, 1971); (2) electrical stimulation of the pons yields short-latency saccades; (3) both anatomical and electrophysiological studies have described direct pathways from the pontine reticular formation to the oculomotor nuclei; (4) on the other hand, higher structures thought to be important in saccade generation (e.g., the superior colliculus, the frontal eye fields) send efferents to the pons rather than directly to the various oculomotor nuclei.

Two different hypotheses have emerged to describe the pattern of the pontine input signal to motoneurons. The first suggests that the burst associated with saccades and the stepwise change in activity associated with different fixations are generated by separate groups of pontine neurons (Luschei & Fuchs, 1972);

the motoneuron simply adds the two firing patterns together. The upper two traces of Fig. 5 show a pontine unit which exhibits a burst of activity for each lateral saccade. A burst precedes the saccade by 5–8 msec (a 5-msec example shown) and the burst duration increases with saccade duration (see last two saccades in upper panel). Oblique saccade directions are also represented in the pons; the third and fourth panels illustrate another unit whose most intense burst begins before (8-msec example shown), and lasts the duration of, saccades having right and downward components. Because these neurons lie in the appropriate brainstem area and since the burst, on the average, begins before the burst in motoneurons and lasts the duration of the saccade, it is likely that they provide the pulse input to the motoneuron for the saccade. The lowest panel illustrates another pontine unit whose step changes in firing rate with lateral eye fixations could be added to the burst changes in the upper panel to produce the pulse-step pattern in abducens motoneurons.

The second hypothesis suggests that the pontine input provides only step changes in activity and that the motoneuron membrane itself differentiates the step to provide the burst seen in motoneurons. By impaling a motoneuron with a microelectrode, Barmack (1974) was able to pass current across the membrane in an attempt to simulate the effects of synaptic inputs having different patterns. When a small step of current was applied, cat abducens motoneurons emitted a burst of spikes (Fig. 6A). Larger steps of current caused bursts of longer duration and, in addition, some sustained activity which seemed to increase with current strength. The discharge patterns produced by intracellular current injection (Fig. 6, A, B, C) resemble motoneuron firing patterns except for two significant differences. First, contrary to the steady burst associated with saccades in normal motoneurons (Fig. 4), the synthetic burst obtained by current injection falls exponentially with a time constant $\leqslant$20 msec (Fig. 6, right-hand graph). Second, a step injection of current fails to produce the remarkably regular firing associated with fixation in normal motoneurons (Fig. 6). Therefore, although the properties of oculomotor neuron membranes may contribute to motoneuron discharge characteristics, the differentiator action alone is not sufficient to account for the saccadic pulse-step activity.

As was mentioned earlier, several parts of the oculomotor system believed to be concerned with saccades send efferents to the pons, possibly to drive the neurons illustrated in Fig. 5. Recently, one of these structures, the superior colliculus, has been studied rather extensively (Schiller & Koerner, 1971; Schiller & Stryker, 1972; Schiller, Stryker, Cyander, & Berman, 1974; Goldberg & Wurtz, 1972a, b; Wurtz & Goldberg, 1972a, 1972b) and suggestions have been made regarding its role in the saccadic acquisition of novel stimuli. Recording from single neurons in monkeys conditioned to make known eye movements, both groups have found similar discharge patterns; a simplified schematic summary of their results is presented in Fig. 7.

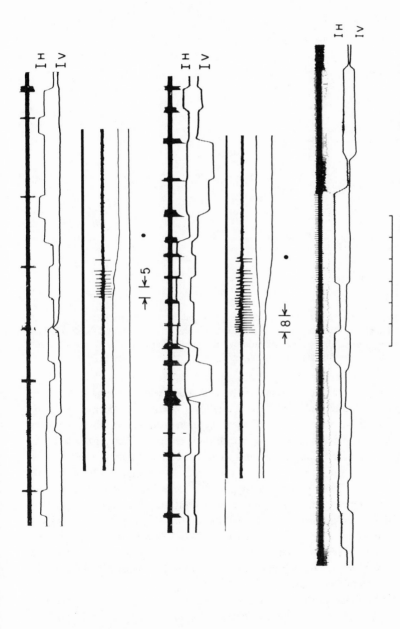
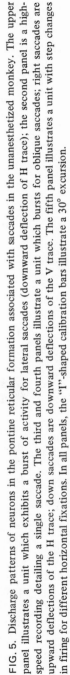

FIG. 5. Discharge patterns of neurons in the pontine reticular formation associated with saccades in the unanesthetized monkey. The upper panel illustrates a unit which exhibits a burst of activity for lateral saccades (downward deflection of H trace); the second panel is a high-speed recording detailing a single saccade. The third and fourth panels illustrate a unit which bursts for oblique saccades; right saccades are upward deflections of the H trace; down saccades are downward deflections of the V trace. The fifth panel illustrates a unit with step changes in firing for different horizontal fixations. In all panels, the "T"-shaped calibration bars illustrate a 30° excursion.

47

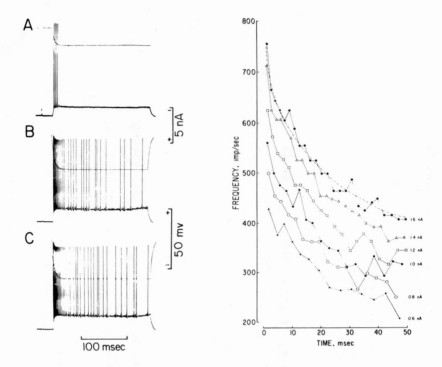

FIG. 6. Discharges in feline abducens neurons produced by the intracellular injection of current. Records A–C show the effects of increasing current strength on unit discharge. The right-hand graph shows the exponential decay of firing frequency after a step current injection of various amounts (after Barmack, 1974).

In the superficial or dorsal layers of the colliculus, which receive input from the contralateral visual field via both retinal and cortical projections, neurons have only visual sensitivity (Fig. 7, left column). Basically, these neurons respond to a changing visual stimulus within their receptive field, either to lights flashing on and off or to objects moving in any direction; furthermore, they are unconcerned about the size or shape of the object or whether it is light on dark or dark on light. These properties suggest that cells in the superficial layers detect the occurrence of novel stimuli or events within their receptive fields. In addition, Goldberg and Wurtz (1972b) showed that if the receptive field becomes the target of a prospective saccade, some of these neurons show an enhanced response (Fig. 7, left column, unit $\bar{c}$ atten.) suggesting that the increased attention paid to an important target (within a receptive field) facilitates the usual visual response evoked by that target.

In the intermediate and deeper layers, neurons have both visual and saccadic sensitivity (Fig. 7, middle column). These cells have receptive fields that are somewhat larger than those in the dorsal layers and, like the superficial cells, their fields can be mapped by jerking or moving objects in any direction. The visual properties of these cells are abolished by cooling the visual cortex (Schiller, Stryker, & Cyander, 1974). In addition, the same neuron will emit a burst of spikes for saccades but only for those saccades whose size and direction are appropriate to shift the direction of gaze to that location in visual space which contained the receptive field of the neuron (see Fig. 7, middle column). In other words, an object appearing within the receptive field of such a neuron first causes a transient visual response after 40–50 msec (Fig. 7, middle column). About 50 msec later, the unit again increases its activity, until 100 msec later a saccade occurs which slides the fovea (*f*) under the object of interest. Schiller feels that the accuracy of the saccade suggests that the colliculus participates in foveation of the target, whereas Wurtz and Goldberg feel that the colliculus deals

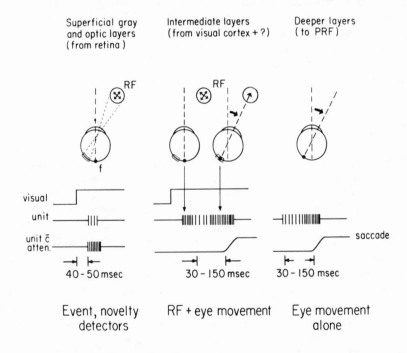

FIG. 7. Simplified schematic illustrating the neurons at various depths in the superior colliculus. The upper part of the illustration shows the spatial situation associated with locating receptive fields (RF) and sliding the fovea (*f*, dot on back of eyeball) under the receptive field after a saccade (thick arrow). The lower part of the illustration shows the correlation in time of the visual events (indicated by the step) with the resulting unit response and/or saccade.

with a grosser shift in visual attention which serves to redirect the eye to the general vicinity of a target.

In the deepest layers, neurons have only saccadic sensitivity. Once again, a burst of activity precedes only those saccades of a specific size and direction, a size and direction congruent with the location of the receptive fields of units lying just above in the intermediate layers. The deeper layers, then, project to the reticular areas involved with saccades (Kawamura, Brodal, & Hoddevik, 1974).

It is not possible simply to plug the collicular discharge into the pontine burst generator to complete the neural circuitry from the visual sensory event to the responding saccade. The collicular burst is rather constant and accompanies only saccades of a particular size and direction; therefore, the colliculus encodes retinal location in a spatial coordinate system. On the other hand, the units in the pons discharge for all saccades with a burst duration that increases with saccade size; therefore, the pontine reticular formation encodes saccade size with bursts of different duration in a temporal coordinate system. Hence, a spatial-to-temporal translation is still required between the colliculus and the burst neurons. Such a translator, which is obviously required whenever visual spatial receptive fields must be converted to an oculomotor output, is probably located in the pons.

DISCUSSION

STEINMAN: I have noticed in tracking small steps, by this I mean a degree or less, that individual subjects show quite idiosyncratic eye movement patterns. For example, I do what your monkeys are doing with their large steps. I make one saccade to the right, left, up, or down. It is not necessarily accurate, but it is one saccade, and it makes a clear record. But, for example, Haddad (of the University of Maryland), for some reason, always tracks left steps with a burst of 3 to 5 saccades made within a second. This is true when she tracks 6 min of arc steps as well as 25 min of arc steps. The records you have shown for the rhesus do not show such individual differences. Is this a species difference or do you, like me, prefer to show simple records, i.e., records that do not show that complicated programs may be used when saccades are used to make changes in the position of the eye?

ROBINSON: Why don't you bring Haddad up to our motility clinic?

STEINMAN: Skavenski does the same kind of thing as Haddad when he makes saccades on the vertical meridian. This was a nuisance when we were studying fixation of feeble targets (Steinman & Cunitz, 1968). We were supposed to make one jump up to make the target visible. Skavenski loves to make three jumps to go one degree and persisted in doing so even though he knew that it made it harder to collect records that were suitable for publication.

FUCHS: It is also normal in monkeys or humans to get a variety of patterns. But in a tutorial like this you try to get some salient features across, and I fully agree that there are a variety of responses.

ROBINSON: Does either of you have any ideas as to why?

STEINMAN: I think that, for some people, there may be a saccadic unit that makes these jumps some fraction of the distance to be traversed. Perhaps Haddad knows that she can only go $1/3$ or $1/5$ of the way and also that she is going to drift back after each saccade and just shoots off her burst in order to get where she wants to go.

FUCHS: You are suggesting that saccades are quantal in nature?

STEINMAN: Yes.

FUCHS: What is the quantum?

HALL: Quantum jump, really.

STEINMAN: Perhaps 5 or 6 min of arc—the smallest average voluntary saccade size (Haddad & Steinman, 1973). This is multiplied by some factor to traverse larger distances.

ROBINSON: I suppose different people have different quantum jump amplitudes in different directions.

FUCHS: A situation which makes a descriptive model for the effective saccadic stimulus impossible.

KOLERS: On this topic, but somewhat more complicated, there are enormous individual differences in people's regressive motions when they read a line of print. Some people typically undershoot the line; they take two or three saccades to get from the end of one line to the beginning of the next. Some people overshoot. Some people are on target.

YOUNG: I don't think there is any question that even though you can think of saccades as preprogramed, their control system must have a prior knowledge of the error that will be made by that saccade. Therefore, the corrective saccade is probably already programed and launched before the processing of the visual error of the first saccade.

ROBINSON: Here again, most models proposed for the saccadic system work on retinal sign alone and that is probably not very realistic. I would suspect that internal monitoring of eye position allows the brain to know that some programed saccade is not going to be adequate. By combining efference copy with retinal sign, it knows where the target position is in space and it can then devise one or a sequence of saccades to drive the eye to that position.

I think this would very nicely explain Hallett's observations which he will discuss later, that when a light is briefly flashed in the middle of a saccade and then it travels on some distance before it comes to rest, 200 msec later the eye can make a saccade correctly back to the position where the briefly flashed light was located. It is very difficult to make models based on retinal sign alone that can explain such behavior. But if you base them on the idea of recreating an internal knowledge of the position of that flash in space by taking millisecond-to-millisecond account of your own eye position, then, I think, this kind of behavior becomes very easy to explain.

YOUNG: Similarly, this applies for the double-step experiments that were popular some six or eight years ago. The response was a predictable and regular double jump of the eye. The error that would be made is taken into account even before the first erroneous saccade is made.

NODINE: These comments have taken on a great deal of significance for those of us who try to calibrate the subject. There have been a great number of experiments with subjects looking at a display that we are trying to calibrate; depending on how many times he's previously looked at that display and knows where the points are he is supposed to fixate, there is a tendency for him to look a little differently each time the display is presented for calibration.

It causes all kinds of problems. We think our equipment is not calibrated, something slipped, or whatever. This is apropos of Kolers' comment about regressive movements. Subjects do anticipate where the beginning of that sentence is before it is flashed on the screen and they make a very detailed series of orientation responses prior to the presentation of the display itself in anticipation of it.

I think one of the practical things that could come out of this kind of discussion is what is the best kind of calibration display and series of fixations on that display in order to eliminate some of these problems you are talking about. Is it better to present a novel display each time to calibrate? Is it better for the subject not to have to track a couple of points, but only look at one point versus multiple points, and so forth?

ROBINSON: As I understand it, if you ask a person to fixate a point for a reasonable length of time, e.g., 2 or 3 sec, and give him lots of time to make all the corrections he needs to get there, then he will settle down and stay within 6 min of arc of the target. I believe Steinman can tell us about this.

STEINMAN: In my lab, where subjects frequently serve for many years, we do calibrations over and over again. I find it convenient to use 10- to 20-sec fixation trials on a point and run 25 or 50 trials at different times to be sure of the scale of my eye-movement recording apparatus.

NODINE: This is a fixation on a single point?

STEINMAN: Yes, a single point that can be in different positions in space or in an otherwise dark field. The subjects know that it is going to be on the left (or right, up, or down) a degree or two as we usually do the calibrations. But it takes a number of consistent calibrations before I have any confidence in the calibration at all. I think that some of the high gains during smooth pursuit, particularly those done with the diffuse reflection technique, may have come from inadequate behavioral calibrations.

ROBINSON: Isn't there a contradiction here? I thought that those who study miniature eye movements tell us that if a human being fixates a target for 10 sec he won't drift more than about 6 min of arc away.

STEINMAN: The basis of making this kind of statement is on calibrations of the kind I have described, typically confirmed with some kind of physical measuring instrument as well, that displaces the recording beam through a known visual angle. However, B. J. Winterson is a nuisance to calibrate. If you ask her to shift a degree to a target and stay there, she will shift a degree and then change her mind about where the target is 10 sec later.

ANON: If the subjects are children, as Nodine often uses in his experiments, the six, seven, and eight-year olds, have enormous difficulty in holding even very brief fixations.

I.5

Oculomotor Control: The Vergence System[1]

Gerald Westheimer

University of California at Berkeley

The two eyes of the primate have extensively overlapping visual fields, but this would not require eye vergence changes if the visual apparatus did not exhibit the phenomenon of local signs. Stimulation of any small retinal region causes a sensation with a unique two-dimensional spatial signature. In order that a given external object have assigned to it identical spatial signatures in both eyes, it is necessary for the two eyes to assume a specific stance, namely the placing of the ocular images of the object on the retinal position of one eye which has an identical local sign as that on which the image is situated in the other eye. Such pairs of retinal positions in the two eyes are called corresponding points. In the normal subject, the two foveas are corresponding points.

At the outset we will restrict discussion to targets in the midsagittal plane.

Assume that a target is placed in the midsagittal plane at a distance x meters from the eyes. If the $1/2$ interocular distance is a meters, the *target vergence* may be defined as twice the angle whose tangent is a/x. A similar definition can be used for the description of eye vergence; thus if both eyes are fixating such a target, the eye vergence will equal the target vergence. The difference between target vergence and eye vergence is called *disparity*: a target nearer than the binocularly fixated point is said to be seen with convergent or crossed disparity, one farther with divergent or uncrossed disparity. It is seen that the visual stimulus to eye vergence responses is disparity. While there is such a thing as vertical disparity, it ordinarily does not correspond to real targets unless the eyes in their resting state are vertically diverging, or one eye is higher than the other

[1] This work was supported by the National Eye Institute under grant EY-00592.

and the object is not at infinity. Consequently, our capacity to make vertical vergence movements, while present, is rudimentary.

Complex problems of coordinates arise for corresponding points outside the foveas and they will not detain us here. Suffice it to say that there is also such a thing as cyclorotational vergence for which we have some capacity.

Before pursuing the discussion of the vergence control system, a few words about the sensory mechanism underlying it. Detection of the absolute level of eye vergence is not very good, but detection of disparity is exceptionally precise. Under the most ideal conditions it is just a few seconds of arc, but this small value depends on a variety of factors that may not always be satisfied. Exposure duration is one, but more important is the identification of the two component retinal patterns that are regarded as belonging together. We cannot, unfortunately, go into this fascinating aspect of the subject here, but as an example of what is meant, it may be pointed out that the random-dot stereo patterns of B. Julesz are usually presented with disparities about an order of magnitude above the stereo threshold. Even then, the sudden appearance of a global three-dimensional percept that is surprisingly stable speaks for the operation at higher perceptual levels, as also does the existence of hysteresis effects.[2] The subjective impression given by a target seen in disparity differs qualitatively with the degree of disparity. Disparities larger than half a degree or a degree give rise to the appearance of double vision, but it is probably not important to the response elicited by a disparate target whether or not it is seen in diplopia, provided, of course, the disparate images are received and processed by the two uniocular pathways. The important conclusion, however, is that there is ample capacity to detect disparity signals for ocular vergence responses.

What, then, are the characteristics of vergence eye movements? The most notable feature is that they are slow compared with the widely utilized saccades; the maximum velocity of a vergence change is likely to be 1/10 of that of an equivalent saccade. The reaction time is, however, about the same—somewhat less than .2 sec. A vergence response to a suddenly imposed disparity of 4°, i.e., the sudden appearance of a target at about 1 m when the eyes are parallel, will be substantially complete within about ¾ sec of the presentation of the stimulus. Figure 1 is a typical response to a 2° disparity which shows the slowness of the vergence change. There is also another fundamental difference between saccades and vergence responses. Saccades are ballistic in the sense that once initiated a saccade will be executed according to its original program, regardless of the changing need of visual perception. This is not the case for

---

[2] Random patterns observed in stabilized vision and fused to yield stereopsis retained three-dimensionality upon being further separated for many degrees even though vergence movements were impossible. The disparity was much greater than one would ordinarily expect a subject to be able to fuse. When stereopsis suddenly was lost, one could return them toward their original location and not recover stereopsis until they were virtually on corresponding points of the retinas. This would be a hysteresis phenomenon.

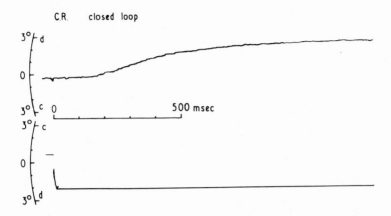

FIG. 1. Time course of a 2° convergence movement. Allowance should be made for the arc of the pen. Eye vergence: upper trace; target: lower trace. (After Rashbass & Westheimer, 1961.)

vergence responses. The simplest demonstration of this is contained in the series of responses to pulse stimuli of varying duration. About a reaction time after the occurrence of the return leg of the pulse stimulus there is always the beginning of the return of the response, regardless of the stage of completion of the beginning phase of the response. This can be seen quite clearly in Fig. 2.

This observation naturally leads to the question of the nature of the control or guidance system underlying such responses. Is the response directly and simply dependent on the stimulus, and what is the nature of the functional relationship? Rashbass and I (Rashbass & Westheimer, 1961) were able to demonstrate the rela-

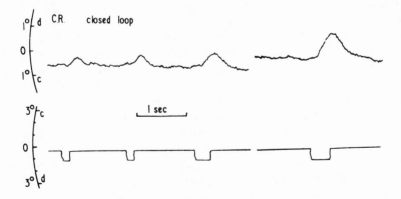

FIG. 2. Eye-vergence responses to 1° target-vergence pulses of various durations. (After Rashbass and Westheimer, 1961.)

C.R. open loop

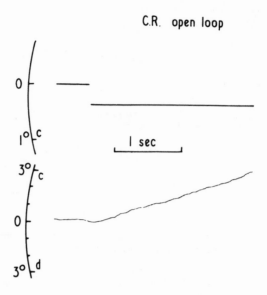

FIG. 3. Eye-vergence movement when a constant disparity is suddenly imposed and subsequently maintained, i.e., open-loop response. (After Rashbass & Westheimer, 1961.)

tionship by experimentally opening the loop between vergence input and the response. As Fig. 3 shows, there is a constant vergence rate produced by the constant disparity. As it turned out, a wide range of situations could be described by stating that the rate at which a subject was converging at any time was proportional to the error, i.e., the disparity, a reaction time earlier. In other words, as shown in Fig. 4, the velocity of convergence movements was a linear function of the imposed disparity: crossed disparity produces convergence and uncrossed disparity produces divergence. The implication of such a control system is that there is no steady-state error, for it would induce a constant convergence velocity. Good experiments by L. A. Riggs and E. W. Niehl with the contact lens method of recording eye movements have indeed shown that, contrary to the suggestions contained in earlier measurements, the eyes consummate the full convergence movement required by the stimulus. It should be pointed out, however, that the rather simple relationship between disparity and the time derivative of the convergence movement fails in a significant way when there are velocity and acceleration components in the disparity. Something akin to anticipation occurs then, as shown in Fig. 5, so that the disparity is *less* than would be expected from the results of the reduced experimental situation.

Vergence eye movements are ordinarily brought into operation by a normal observer when targets are closer than infinity. Since it is a rare occasion indeed in which the whole of the visual field is empty except for a single target, it

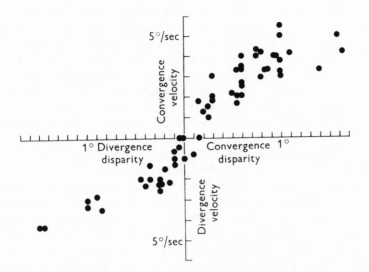

FIG. 4. Relationship between vergence velocity and open-loop disparity signal. Each point was obtained from a record such as that illustrated in Fig. 3. (After Rashbass & Westheimer 1961.)

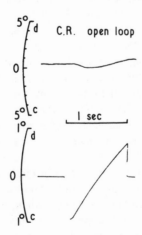

FIG. 5. Experiment illustrating anticipatory behavior of the disparity/eye-vergence system. The disparity program would not produce an inflexion of the response until one reaction time following the zero crossing, unless anticipation had occurred. (After Rashbass & Westheimer, 1961.)

follows that a certain amount of selection usually enters into the decision whether to make a vergence movement. True, under optometric testing procedures, the deliberate introduction of prisms will be used to force vergence and thus to uncover the range of capacity to make such movements. There is then a strong, compelling push toward completing whatever vergence movement is necessary to secure fusion of the two uniocular images, but it would be too simple to regard it as a visual reflex. There is a clear voluntary component here, shown also by the fact that it is not too difficult to inhibit voluntarily the fusion of a close-by object. We have already alluded to the significant perceptual aspect implied in the decision to regard certain often quite dissimilar retinal image patterns as making up a pair upon which to train convergence.

The need for vergence movements is accentuated in those individuals in whom, for anatomical or other reasons, there is a lack of alignment of the visual axes of the two eyes when they are at rest—patients with heterophoria and heterotropia. Experiences with retraining such patients have shown that considerable changes can be brought about in the amplitude of vergence movements and also, to some extent, in the position of the fusion-free position. Long-term tonic neural influences on the vergence position must be considered as a component of the vergence control system.

Easily the most far-reaching feature of the whole oculomotor system is a principle, first described by Hering, which now bears his name. It refers to the observation that ordinarily the two eyes move together as if they are yoked. While it is a functionally obvious coordination, it is not nearly so obvious if one remembers that the two orbits are mirror-symmetrical so that conjugate movements require quite complicated interplay between the twelve extra ocular muscles. All oculomotor responses discussed earlier in today's session obey Hering's laws and some of the neurological control mechanisms sketched are given substance by it. The big exception is the vergence system. In symmetrical convergence, for example, the two contracting muscles are the right and left medial recti, while in conjugate right movement, for example, they are the right lateral rectus and the left medial rectus muscles. It is not surprising, therefore, that the neural circuits subserving convergence movements are in major ways different from those subserving conjugate movements. This is underlined by two observations: (1) Donders' law does not hold during convergence, i.e., the cyclotorsional orientation of an eye may be different depending on whether it has reached a given eye position by a conjugate movement or by a combination of conjugate and vergence movements; and (2) when there is a certain neurological defect, the so-called MLF syndrome, an eye may not be able to get into a position by a conjugate movement and yet reach it by a vergence movement.

It should not be deduced from these differences that there is a separate muscle system subserving the conjugate and disjunctive eye movements. The evidence is strong that we merely have different inputs into a common motoneuron pool, which then serves as a final common pathway for all responses.

On the other hand, there is a strong linkage between convergence and other ocular functions that also participate in the response to a close-up object, namely, accommodation and pupil constriction. They have long been grouped together as a triad. Recent evidence from stimulation studies in the alert monkey has demonstrated the close neurological linkage of these three responses. Certain sites near the midline of the mesencephalon will release the complete Near Triad when stimulated with pulse trains of minute electrical current (a few micro-amps). These are identified in Fig. 6.

For a long time the clinical literature has made a lot of the distinction between accommodative convergence and fusional convergence. The former is named after the observation that a subject, when accommodating to a monocularly presented near target, will show not only accommodation in the other eye, but also a convergence of the visual axes, although the monocular presentation eliminates the need for convergence. Similarly, there is some convergent accom-modation, i.e., the association of increased accommodation with strong conver-

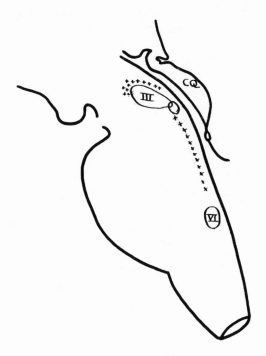

FIG. 6. Sites in midbrain in which low-current stimulation produces convergence responses in alert monkeys: +, convergence accompanied by accommodation and pupil constriction; X, convergence alone; CQ, corpora quadrigemina; III, VI, third and sixth cranial nucleus, respectively.

gence in response to abnormal fusional need. The primate stimulation experiments have given a neurological substrate to these clinical concepts—there is a common neural center for accommodation, convergence, and pupil constriction in the midbrain—and conversely, the possible nature of this neural center is illuminated by the clinical finding—the partial independence of accommodation, convergence, and pupil constriction precludes a single set of cells uniquely, directly, exclusively, and simultaneously serving to execute all three functions. The structures are schematized in Fig. 7.

Finally, Hering's law helps not only to delineate the neural circuits of vergence movements, but also to outline the mechanism of three-dimensional egocentric localization. The organization of our three-dimensional spatial environment into a cartesian 3-fold with three mutually orthogonal axes is a consequence of post-hoc analysis by geometricians. What we are given perceptually is something quite different. To study perception effectively we have to rid ourselves of centuries of prejudice dogmatically drummed into us by rigid representatives of the educational establishment. Instead we should look at eye-movement records. For example, let the stimulus be the famous situation named after the most important pioneers of stereoscopic vision, the so-called Panum–Wheatstone Grenzfall, in which a steadily fixated target is suddenly replaced by another one lying on the line of sight of one eye but not on that of the other. As a result of the interchange of targets, only one of the uniocular images is displaced from the fovea and it would seem simplest just to move that eye. But this is not what occurs. Each eye executes a complicated maneuver which, however, is quickly

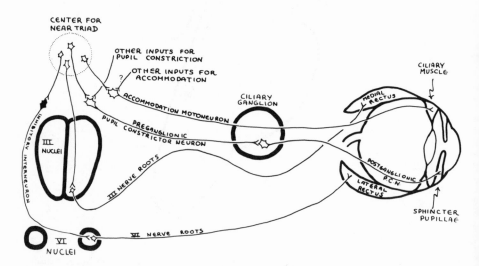

FIG. 7. Outline of motor pathways subserving accommodation, convergence, and pupil constriction. (After Westheimer & Blair, 1973a).

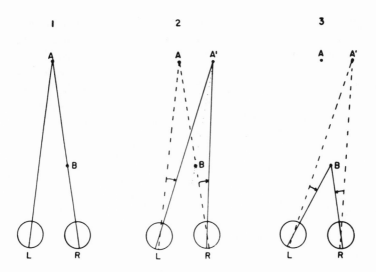

FIG. 8. Schematic diagrams illustrating the sequence of movements in changing fixation from A to B: step 1, binocular fixation of A; step 2, conjugate lateral movement to A' so that the bisector of the angle of convergence passes through B; and step 3, convergence movement from A' to B. Steps 2 and 3 are to some extent superimposed but are easily distinguished in view of their time characteristics. (After Westheimer & Mitchell, 1956.)

described in simple terms once it is realized that the stimulus has released both conjugate saccadic eye movements and a disjunctive convergence movement, also participated in by both eyes. These are shown in Fig. 8. The two movements have different latencies, but if one studies not the instantaneous positions of the two eyes but the mean of the position of the two eyes, this is found to have all the features of the saccades that were necessary—the target merely moved laterally while remaining at the same distance from the observer. On the other hand, the difference between the two eye positions follows exactly the same time course as if the target had merely been moved toward the observer on an unchanged bisector of the angle of convergence. The response to this particular target change, which incidentally is paradigmatic of all such changes, shows that for the purposes of making eye-movement responses the stimulus situation had been neatly dissected into two dimensions of angular coordinates, with a center somewhere near the midpoint of the two eyes, and a radial measurement of the target distance, using triangulation, disparity as the error, and convergence as the response. Such an organization of space at once places a whole series of aspects of ocular motor responses into perspective: (1) accommodation and convergence lose their separateness and can be regarded as joint responses to a near stimulus, subserved by a single neural center which has now been identified by stimulation studies; (2) the whole of the neural circuitry for saccadic pursuit and vestibular eye movements can, at a level above the distribution of the excitation to the twelve individual extraocular muscles, be regarded as binocular, and singular as far as the yoked pair of eyes is concerned, and thus directly relatable to associated functions such as head movements; and (3) a physiological basis has been established that ought to provide a more immediate substrate for the study of egocentric localization and visual perception than dry schemata invented by geometricians.

I.6

References

Allum, J., Tole, J., & Weiss, A. D. MITNYS: A digital program for on-line analysis of nystagmus. IEEE Transactions on Biomedical Engineering, 1975 *BME-22,* 196–202.

Angaut, P., & Brodal, A. The projection of the vestibulo-cerebellum onto the vestibular nuclei in the cat. *Archives Italiennes de Biologie,* 1967, **105,** 441–479.

Baker, R. G., Precht, W.; & Llinas, R. Cerebellar modulatory action on the vestibulo-trochlear pathway in the cat. *Experimental Brain Research,* 1973, **15,** 364.

Barmack, N. H. Saccadic discharges evoked by intracellular stimulation of extraocular motoneurons. *Journal of Neurophysiology,* 1974, **37,** 395–412.

Benson, A. J. Interactions between semicircular canals and gravireceptors. In D. E. Busby (Ed.), *Recent advances in aerospace medicine.* Dordrecht, Holland: D. Reidel, 1970. Pp. 249–261.

Benson, A. J., & Bodin, M. A. Interaction of linear and angular accelerations on vestibular receptors in man. *Aerospace Medicine,* 1966, **37,** 144–154.

Benson, A. J., Guedry, F. E., & Melvill Jones, G. Responses of semicircular canal dependent units in vestibular nuclei to rotation of a linear acceleration vector without angular acceleration. *Journal of Physiology,* 1970, **210,** 475.

Björk, A., & Kugelberg, E. The electrical activity of the muscles of the eye and eyelids in various positions and during movement. *Electroencephalography and Clinical Neurophysiology,* 1953, 5 595–602.

Brodal, A., & Torvik, A. Uber den Ursprung der sekundaren vestibulocerebellaren Fasern bei der Katze. Eine experimentell-anatomische Studie. *Archive fur Psychiatrie und Nervenkrankheiten,* 1957, **195,** 550–567.

Brooks, B. A. & Fuchs, A. F. Influence of stimulus parameters on visual sensitivity during saccadic eye movement. *Vision Research,* 1975, **15,** 1389–1398.

Carpenter, R. H. S. Cerebellectomy and the transfer function of the vestibulo-ocular reflex in the decerebrate cat. *Proceedings of the Royal Society of London, Series B,* 1972, **181,** 353–374.

Cheng, M. Y. N., & Outerbridge, J. S. Retinal contributions of optokinetic nystagmus. *Proceedings of the Association for Research in Vision and Ophthalmology,* Sarasota, Florida, 1973.

Cohen, B., & Henn, V. The origin of quick phases of nystagmus in the horizontal plane. *Bibliotheca Ophtalmologica,* 1972, **82,** 36–55.

Collewijn, H. An analog model of the rabbit's optokinetic system. *Brain Research*, 1972, **36**, 71–88.

Collewijn, H., & van der Mark, F. Ocular stability in variable visual feedback conditions in the rabbit. *Brain Research*, 1972, **36**, 47–57.

Correia, M. J., & Money, K. E. The effect of blockage of all six semicircular canal ducts on nystagmus produced by dynamic linear acceleration in the cat. *Acta Oto-Laryngologica*, 1970, **69**, 7–16.

Dichgans, J., & Brandt, T. Visual-vestibular interaction and motion perception. *Bibliotheca Ophthalmologica*, 1972, **82**, 327–338.

Dohlman, G. On the mechanism of transformation into nystagmus on stimulation of the semicircular canals. *Acta Oto-Laryngologica*, 1938, **26**, 425–442.

Fernandez, C., & Goldberg, J. M. Physiology of peripheral neurons innervating the semicircular canals of the squirrel monkey. II. The response to sinusoidal stimulation of the dynamics of the peripheral vestibular system. *Journal of Neurophysiology*, 1971, **34**, 661–675.

Fuchs, A. F. Saccadic and smooth pursuit eye movements in the monkey. *Journal of Physiology* 1967, **191**, 609–631.

Fuchs, A. F., & Luschei, E. Firing patterns of abducens neurons of alert monkeys in relationship to horizontal eye movement. *Journal of Neurophysiology*, 1970, **33**, 382–392.

Fuchs, A. F., & Ron, S. An analysis of the rapid eye movements of sleep in the monkey. *Electroencephalography and Clinical Neurophysiology*, 1968, **23**, 244–251.

Goebel, H., Komatsuzuki, A., Bender, M., & Cohen, B. Lesions in the pontine tegmentum and conjugate gaze paralysis. *Archives of Neurology*, 1971, **24**, 431–440.

Goldberg, M. E., & Wurtz, R. H. Activity of superior colliculus in behaving monkey. I. Visual receptive fields of single neurons. *Journal of Neurophysiology*, 1972, **35**, 542–559. (a)

Goldberg, M. E., & Wurtz, R. H. Activity of superior colliculus in behaving monkey. II. Effect of attention on neuronal responses. *Journal of Neurophysiology*, 1972, **35**, 560–574. (b)

Gonshor, A., & Melvill Jones, G. Changes of human vestibulo-ocular response induced by vision-reversal during head rotation. *Journal of Physiology*, 1973, **234**, 102P.

Gonshor, A., & Melvill Jones, G. Extreme vestibulo-ocular adaptation induced by prolonged optical reversal of vision. *Journal of Physiology*, 1976, in press.

Grüsser, O. J., & Grüsser-Cornehls, U. Interaction of vestibular and visual inputs in the visual system. In A. Brodal & O. Pompeiano (Eds.), *Progress in brain research* Vol. 37. Amsterdam: Elsevier Publishing, 1972.

Guedry, F. E. Orientation of the rotation-axis relative to gravity: Its influence on nystagmus and the sensation of rotation. *Acta Oto-Laryngologica*, 1965, **60**, 30–48.

Haddad, G. M., & Steinman, R. M. The smallest voluntary saccade. Implications for fixation. *Vision Research*, 1973, **13**, 1075–1086.

Henn, V., Young, L. R., & Finley, C. Vestibular nucleus units in alert monkeys are also influenced by moving visual fields. *Brain Research*, 1974, **71**, 144–149.

Heywood, S., & Churcher, J. H. Eye movements and the afterimage. I: Tracking the afterimage. *Vision Research*, 1971, **11**, 1163–1168.

Heywood, S., & Churcher, J. H. Eye movements and the afterimage. II: The effects of foveal and nonfoveal afterimages on saccadic behavior. *Vision Research*, 1972, **12**, 1033–1043.

Hwang, J. C., Poon, W. F., & Cheung, Y. M. Electrophysiological studies on the projections of saccules to the Deiter's nuclei and the Group Y cells in cats. Paper presented at the

26th International Congress, New Delhi, *Abstracts of Volunteer Papers,* 1974, **682,** 228.

Ito, M. Inhibitory and excitatory relay neurons for the vestibuloocular reflexes. In A. Brodal & O. Pompeiano (Eds.), *Basic aspects of central vestibular Mechanisms.* Amsterdam/London/New York: Elsevier Publishing, 1972. Pp. 543–544.

Ito, M., Nisimaru, N., & Yamamoto, M. The neural pathways mediating reflex contraction of extraocular muscles during semicircular canal stimulation in rabbits. *Brain Research,* 1973, **55,** 183–188. (a)

Ito, M., Nisimaru, N., & Yamamoto, M. The neural pathways relaying reflex inhibition from semicircular canals to extraocular muscles of rabbits. *Brain Research,* 1973, **55,** 189–193. (b)

Ito, M., Shiida, T., Yagi, N., & Yamamoto, M. Visual influence on rabbit horizontal vestibulo-ocular reflex presumably effected via the cerebellar flocculus. *Brain Research,* 1974, **65,** 170–174.

Jones, G. M., & Milsum, J. H. Spatial and dynamic aspects of visual fixation. *IEEE Transactions on Biomedical Engineering,* 1965, **12,** 54–62.

Jones, G. M., & Spells, K. E. A theoretical and comparative study of the functional dependence of the semicircular canal upon its physical dimensions. *Proceedings of the Royal Society of London, Series B,* 1963, **157,** 403–419.

Jongkees, L. B. W. On the otoliths: Their function and the way to test them. *Third symposium on the role of the vestibular organs in space exploration.* Pensacola, Florida, 1967, p. 307–330 (NASA SP-152).

Kawamura, K., Brodal, A., & Hoddevik, G. The projection of the superior colliculus onto the reticular formation of the brainstem. An experimental anatomical study in the cat. *Experimental Brain Research,* 1974, **19,** 1–19.

Keller, E. L., & Robinson, D. A. Absence of a stretch reflex in extraocular muscles of the monkey. *Journal of Neurophysiology,* 1971, **34,** 908–919.

Koerner, F., & Schiller, P. H. The optokinetic response under open and closed loop conditions in the monkey. *Experimental Brain Research,* 1972, **14,** 318–330.

Kommerell, G., & Klein, U. Über die visuelle Regelung der Okulomotorik: die optomotorische Wirking exzentrischer Nachbilder. *Vision Research,* 1971, **11,** 905–920.

Kommerell, G., & Taumer, R. Investigations of the eye tracking system through stabilized retinal images. *Bibliotheca Ophthalmologica,* 1972, **82,** 280–287.

Komoda, M. K., Festinger, L., Phillips, L. J., Duckman, R. H., & Young, R. A. Some observations concerning saccadic eye movements. *Vision Research,* 1973, **13,** 1009–1020.

Lightstone, A. D. Visual stimuli for saccadic and smooth pursuit eye movements. Doctoral dissertation, University of Toronto, 1973.

Lorente de Nó, R. Ausgewahlte Kapitel ausder vergleichenden Physiologie des Labyrinthes. Die Augenmuskelreflexe beim Kanichen und ihre Grundlagen. *Ergebnisse der Physiologie, Biologischen Chemie und Experimentellen Pharmakologie,* 1931, **32,** 73–242.

Lorente de Nó, R. Vestibulo-ocular reflex. *Archives of Neurology and Psychiatry,* 1933, **30,** 245–291.

Luschei, E., & Fuchs, A. F. Activity of brain stem neurons during eye movements of alert monkeys. *Journal of Neurophysiology,* 1972, **35,** 445–461.

Maekawa, K., & Simpson, J. I. Climbing fiber activation of Purkinje cells in the flocculus by impulses transfered through the visual pathway. *Brain Research,* 1972, **39,** 245–251.

Maekawa, K., & Simpson, J. I. Climbing fiber responses evoked in the vestibulo-cerebellum of rabbit from the visual system. *Journal of Neurophysiology,* 1973, **36,** 649–665.

Malcolm, R. C., & Melvill Jones, G. A quantitative study of vestibular adaptation in humans. *Acta Oto-Laryngologica,* 1970, **70,** 126.

Melvill Jones, G. Ocular nystagmus recorded simultaneously in three orthogonal planes. *Acta Oto-Laryngologica*, 1964, **56**, 619–631.

Melvill Jones, G. Vestibulo-ocular disorganization in the aerodynamic spin. *Aerospace Medicine*, 1965, **36**, 976–983.

Melvill Jones, G. Interactions between optokinetic and vestibulo-ocular responses during head rotation in various planes. *Aerospace Medicine*, 1966, **37**, 172–177.

Melvill Jones, G. Neural reflection of vestibular mechanics. *Third Symposium on the Role of the Vestibular Organs in Space*. Pensacola, Florida, 1967, 169–180 (NASA SP-152).

Melvill Jones, G. Origin significance and amelioration of coriolis illusions from the semicircular canals: a nonmathematical appraisal. *Aerospace Medicine*, 1970, **41**, 483–490.

Melvill Jones, G., Downing, D., & Rolf, R. Human subjective and reflex responses to sinusoidal vertical acceleration. Ames Progress Report, NASA, Mountain View, Calif. 1973.

Melvill Jones, G., & Gonshor, A. Extreme vestibular habituation to long-term reversal of vision during natural head movements. *Proceedings of the Annual Science Meeting, Aerospace Medical Association*, Bal Harbour, Florida, 1972.

Melvill Jones, G., & Gonshor, A. Goal-directed flexibility in the vestibulo-ocular reflex arc. In G. Lennerstrand and P. Bach-y-rita (Eds.), *Basic mechanisms of ocular motility and their clinical implications.* Oxford/New York: Pergamon Press, 1975. Pp. 227–245.

Melvill Jones, G., & Milsum, J. H. Neural response of the vestibular system to translational acceleration. *Symposium on Systems Analysis Approach to Neurophysiological Problems.* Brainherd, Minnesota, 1969, 105–117.

Melvill Jones, G., & Milsum, J. H. Characteristics of neural transmission from the semicircular canal to the vestibular nuclei of cats. *Journal of Physiology*, 1970, **209**, 295–316.

Melvill Jones, G., & Milsum, J. H. Frequency response analysis of central vestibular unit activity resulting from rotational stimulation of the semicircular canals. *Journal of Physiology*, 1971, **219**, 191–215.

Miller, E. F. Counter rolling of the human eyes produced by head-tilt with respect to gravity. *Acta Oto-Laryngologica*, 1962, **54**, 479.

Miller, E. F., & Graybiel, A. The effect of gravitational force on ocular counter rolling. *Journal of Applied Physiology*, 1971, **31**, 697.

Murphy, B. J., & Kowler, E. To pursue or not to pursue. . . . Paper presented at the Association for Research in Vision and Ophthalmology, Sarasota, Florida, May 1974.

Niven, J. I., Hixson, W. C., & Correia, M. J. Elicitation of horizontal nystagmus by periodic linear acceleration. *Acta Oto-Laryngologica*, 1966, **62**, 429.

Oman, C. M., & Young, L. R. Physiological range of pressure difference and cupula deflections in the human semicircular canal: Theoretical considerations. In A. Brodal & O. Pompeiano (Eds.), *Basic aspects of central vestibular mechanisms.* Amsterdam/London/New York: Elsevier Publishing, 1972. Pp. 529–539.

Oyster, C. W., Takahashi, E., & Collewijn, H. Direction-selective retinal ganglion cells and control of optokinetic nystagmus in the rabbit. *Vision Research*, 1972, **12**, 183–193.

Pompeiano, O., & Morrison, A. R. Vestibular influences during sleep. I. Abolition of the rapid eye movements during desynchronized sleep following vestibular lesions. *Archives Italiennes de Biologie*, 1965, **103**, 569–595.

Precht, W. Vestibular and cerebellar control of oculomotor functions. *Bibliotheca Ophthalmologica*, 1972, **82**, 71–88.

Precht, W., & Baker, R. G. Synaptic organization of the vestibulo-trochlear pathway. *Experimental Brain Research*, 1972, **14**, 158–184.

Precht, W., & Llinas, R. Functional organization of the vestibular afferents to the cerebellar cortex of frog and cat. *Experimental Brain Research*, 1969, **9**, 30–52.

Rashbass, C. The relationship between saccadic and smooth tracking eye movements. *Journal of Physiology* 1961, **159**, 326–338.

Rashbass, C., & Westheimer, G. H. Disjunctive eye movements. *Journal of Physiology* 1961, **159**, 149–170.

Robinson, D. A. The mechanics of human saccadic eye movement. *Journal of Physiology* 1964, **174**, 245–264.

Robinson, D. A. The oculomotor system, a review. *Proceedings of the IEEE,* 1968, **56**, 1032–1049.

Robinson, D. A. Oculomotor control signal. In G. Lennerstrand and P. Bach-y-rita (Eds.), *Basic mechanisms of ocular motility and their clinical implications.* Oxford/New York: Pergamon Press, 1975. Pp. 337–374.

Robinson, D. A., & Keller, E. L. The behavior of eye movement motoneurons in the alert monkey. *Bibliotheca Ophthalmologica,* 1972, **82**, 7–16.

Ron, S., Robinson, D. A., & Skavenski, A. A. Saccades and the quick phase of nystagmus. *Vision Research,* 1972, **12**, 2015–2022.

Schiller, P. H., & Koerner, F. Discharge characteristics of single units in the superior colliculus of the alert monkey. *Journal of Neurophysiology,* 1971, **34**, 920–936.

Schiller, P. H., & Stryker, M. Single-unit recording and stimulation in superior colliculus of the alert rhesus monkey. *Journal of Neurophysiology,* 1972, **35**, 915–924.

Schiller, P. H., Stryker, M., Cyander, M., & Berman, N. Response characteristics of single cells in the monkey superior colliculus following ablation or cooling of visual cortex. *Journal of Neurophysiology,* 1974, **37**, 181–194.

Schwindt, P. C., Richter, A., & Precht, W. Short latency utricular and canal input to ipsilateral abducens motoneurons. *Brain Research,* 1973, **60**, 259–262.

Shimazu, H., & Precht, W. Tonic and kinetic responses of cat's vestibular neurons to horizontal angular acceleration. *Journal of Neurophysiology,* 1965, **28**, 991–1013.

Shimazu, H., & Precht, W. Inhibition of central vestibular neurons from the contralateral labyrinth and its mediating pathway. *Journal of Neurophysiology,* 1966, **29**, 467–492.

Skavenski, A. A., Haddad, G. M., & Steinman, R. M. The extraretinal signal for the visual perception of direction. *Perception and Psychophysics,* 1972, **11**, 287–290.

Skavenski, A. A., & Robinson, D. A. Role of abducens neurones in vestibulo-ocular reflex. *Journal of Neurophysiology,* 1973, **36**, 724–738.

Stark, L., Vossius, G., & Young, L. R. Predictive control of eye tracking movements. *IRE Transactions, Human Factors in Electronics,* 1962, *HFE-3* 52–56.

Steinbach, M. J. Eye tracking of self-moved targets: The role of efference. *Journal of Experimental Psychology,* 1969, **82**, 366–376.

Steinbach, M. J., & Held, R. Eye tracking of observer-generated target movements. *Science,* 1968, **161**, 187–188.

Steinman, R. M., & Cunitz, R. J. Fixation of targets near the absolute foveal threshold. *Vision Research,* 1968, **2**, 277–286.

Steinman, R. M., Haddad, G. M., Skavenski, A. A., & Wyman, D. Miniature eye movement. *Science,* 1973, **181**, 810–819.

Steinman, R. M., Skavenski, A. A., & Sansbury, R. V. Voluntary control of smooth pursuit velocity. *Vision Research,* 1969, **9**, 1167–1171.

Sterling, P., & Wickelgren, B. G. Visual receptive fields in the superior colliculus of the cat. *Journal of Neurophysiology,* 1969, **32**, 1–15.

Stone, J., & Fukuda, Y. Properties of cat retinal ganglion cells: A comparison of W-cells with X- and Y-cells. *Journal of Neurophysiology,* 1974, **37**, 722–748.

Szentágothai, J. The elementary vestibulo-ocular reflex arc. *Journal of Neurophysiology,* 1950, **13**, 395–407.

ter Braak, J. W. G., Schenk, V. W. D., & van Vliet, A. G. M. Visual reactions in a case of long-lasting cortical blindness. *Journal of Neurology, Neurosurgery and Psychiatry*, 1971, **34**, 140–147.

Tole, J., & Young, L. R. MITNYS: A hybrid program for on-line analysis of nystagmus. *Aerospace Medicine*, 1971, **42**, 508–511.

Volkmann, F. C., Schick, A. M. L., and Riggs, L. A. Time course of visual inhibition during voluntary saccades. *Journal of the Optical Society of America*, 1968, **58**, 562–569.

Westheimer, G. H., & Blair, S. M. Parasympathetic pathways to internal eye muscles. *Investigative Ophthalmology*, 1973, **12**, 193–197. (a)

Westheimer, G. H., & Blair, S. M. Oculomotor defects in cerebellectomized monkeys. *Investigative Ophthalmology*, 1973, **12**, 618–621. (b)

Westheimer, G. H., & Blair, S. M. Unit activity in accessory optic system in alert monkeys. *Investigative Ophthalmology*, 1974, **13**, 533–534.

Westheimer, G. H., & Mitchell, A. M. Eye movement responses to convergence stimuli. *Archives of Ophthalmology*, 1956, **55**, 848–856.

Wheeless, L., Boynton, R. M., & Cohen, G. Eye-movement responses to step and pulse-step stimuli. *Journal of the Optical Society of America*, 1966, **56**, 956–960.

Wurtz, R. H., & Goldberg, M. E. Activity of superior colliculus in behaving monkey. III. Cells discharging before eye movements. *Journal of Neurophysiology*, 1972, **35**, 575–586. (a)

Wurtz, R. H., & Goldberg, M. E. Activity of superior colliculus in behaving monkey. IV. Effects of lesions on eye movements. *Journal of Neurophysiology*, 1972, **35**, 587–596. (b)

Yasui, S. Nystagmus generation, oculomotor tracking, and visual motion perception Doctoral dissertation, Massachusetts Institute of Technology, Department of Aeronautics and Astronautics, 1974.

Yasui, S., & Young, L. R. Perceived visual motion as effective stimulus to pursuit eye movements, *Science*, 1975, **190**, 906–908.

Young, L. R. The dead zone to saccadic eye movements. *Proceedings of the Symposium on Biomedical Engineering*, Milwaukee, 1966, **1**, 360–362.

Young, L. R. Pursuit eye tracking movements. In P. Bach-y-rita and C. Collins (Eds.), *Control of eye movements*. New York: Academic Press, 1971.

Zuber, B. L., Stark, L., & Cook, G. Microsaccades and the velocity–amplitude relationship for saccadic eye movements. *Science*, 1965, **150**, 1459–1460.

Part II

THE ROLE OF EYE MOVEMENTS IN VISION AND IN THE MAINTENANCE OF VISION

The normal interplay of ocular motion and perception has been investigated for many purposes. This session dealt with questions in three areas important to this topic.

1. How is vision affected by saccadic eye movements? Under what conditions does saccadic suppression, or the decreased efficiency of vision during saccades, occur? Is suppression related predominantly to peripheral factors such as smear of the image on the retina or shearing forces in the retina, or is it necessary to postulate a central inhibitory effect? Is the suppression really saccadic at all, or is it related instead to properties of the stimulus field? Is it a useful concept?

2. How is vision maintained during normal fixation? What are the roles of various categories of small eye movements (flicks, drift, tremor)? Techniques of producing stabilized images on the retina have been useful in delineating important variables in the maintenance of vision during fixation, and have raised additional questions: What are the temporal properties of image disappearance with stabilization; what variables affect image reappearance? What are the organizational properties of image disappearance and reappearance, and what is the possible relevance of this organization for models of feature detection?

3. What varieties of data and of theoretical positions are available which examine the role of eye movements in the maintenance of a phenomenally clear and stable visual world?

The Chairperson of this session was Dr. Frances C. Volkmann of Smith College.

II.1

Saccadic Suppression:
A Brief Review[1]

Frances C. Volkmann

Smith College

It is a common observation that the visual world remains phenomenally clear and stable in spite of the frequent and rapid saccadic eye movements that we make in looking from one object to another in the visual field. Visual perception seems to extend continuously through long intervals of time, even though a complete relocation of the visual field must take place every time we make a saccade. The stability and clarity of the scene in the face of retinal image motion during saccades is to be distinguished from the related problem of stability in the face of changes in position on the retina, or local sign, of images which are viewed in the successive fixational pauses between saccades. These two aspects of phenomenal stability may or may not be accomplished by the same mechanisms. This question will be discussed below by Dr. Ethel Matin, and later on by the contributors to Part IV.

Now, however, I want to review very briefly some major lines of evidence and theoretical positions related to the apparent neglect or suppression of vision during saccadic eye movements in awake human subjects. The question may be phrased as follows: If there is a neural mechanism that compensates for saccadic movements, and allows us to perceive the world as stable, does the same neural mechanism inhibit or suppress vision at the time of the eye movement? Does a central neural suppression constitute, in fact, a part of the means by which the stationary rather than the moving signals reaching the brain are given priority?

The finding is well documented that under most normal conditions of every-day viewing, we simply do not notice the blurred images that sweep across our retinas during saccades. This phenomenon was pointed out by early investigators (Holt, 1903; Dodge, 1905; Woodworth, 1906; and later Ditchburn, 1955) and

[1] The preparation of this manuscript was supported in part by Grant No. 41103 from the National Science Foundation to Frances C. Volkmann and Lorrin A. Riggs.

has subsequently been quantified and extended (Latour, 1962; Volkmann, 1962; Zuber & Stark, 1966; Beeler, 1967; Volkmann, Schick, & Riggs, 1968; Starr, Angel, & Yeates, 1969; Mitrani, Mateeff, & Yakimoff, 1970b). The present question, then, is not whether visual performance is decreased during saccades, but rather why this decrease occurs and what the mechanisms of suppression might be (see also E. Matin, 1974).

Four major types of explanations for visual suppression have been offered: retinal smear, central inhibition, shearing forces in the retina, and visual masking.

1. Retinal smear. Stimuli which arrive at the retina during a saccade are swept rapidly across the receptors, decreasing the duration of stimulation on each of them and decreasing, in turn, the probability that the stimulus will be noticed. Furthermore, the duration of a typical saccade is so short that it may be compared to that of a photographic snapshot. Moving the camera or the eye during the snapshot will result in a blurred picture because each point on the image is smeared over a finite distance depending on velocity and exposure time. In normal vision retinal smear must indeed play an important role in saccadic attenuation (see also Mitrani, Mateeff, & Yakimoff, 1970a); some early investigators such as Dodge (1905) believed that smear could account entirely for the phenomenon.

Two sorts of evidence cast doubt on the smear explanation, however.

1. Even when the stimuli presented to the moving eye are made closely comparable to the stimuli presented to the fixating eye (i.e., retinal smear is minimized), visual attenuation during saccades is not eliminated. Figure 1, taken from some of our early work, shows detection thresholds for the moving and for the fixating eye when smear is minimized by presenting the stimuli to the fovea in very brief (20 μsec) flashes. Specifically, the threshold for detection of a flash of added brightness superposed on a steady light fixation field was found to be raised by the equivalent of about .5 log unit of relative luminance for the moving eye as opposed to that for the fixating eye. A difference of .5 log unit is substantial, and under certain conditions it can signify that the same stimuli that are seen almost all the time by the stationary eye are very seldom seen at the time of a saccade. It is not a dramatic difference, however. The term "blanking out of vision during saccades" and the currently fashionable term "saccadic suppression" overstate the case. Nevertheless, vision is attenuated during voluntary saccades even when retinal smear is minimized.

2. Other evidence that image smear on the moving retina is an inadequate explanation for saccadic attenuation came from experiments designed to map the time course of the inhibitory effect. Figure 2 shows two examples of these results: the top curve comes from Latour's work (Latour, 1962) and the lower curves from work in the Brown laboratory, plotted on the same time scale (Volkmann et al., 1968). In general, the attenuation effect begins with test flashes coming as long as 40 msec before the onset of a saccade and persists for

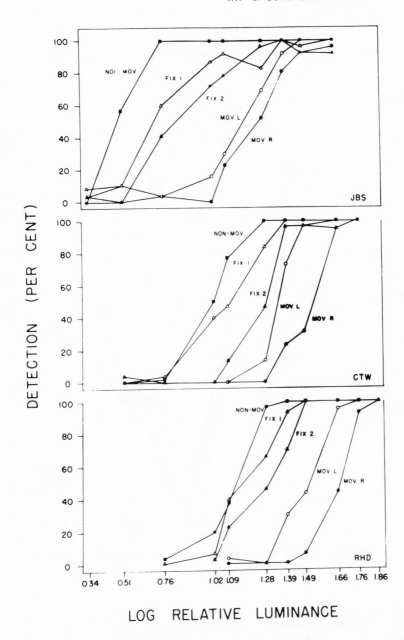

FIG. 1. Percentage of light flashes detected, as a function of the log relative luminance of the flash for each of three subjects. Experimental conditions included presentation of the flash to the eye when it was fixating steadily (NON-MOV), just before a saccade (FIX 1), just after a saccade (FIX 2), and during a saccade to the left (MOV L) or to the right (MOV R). (After Volkmann, 1962.)

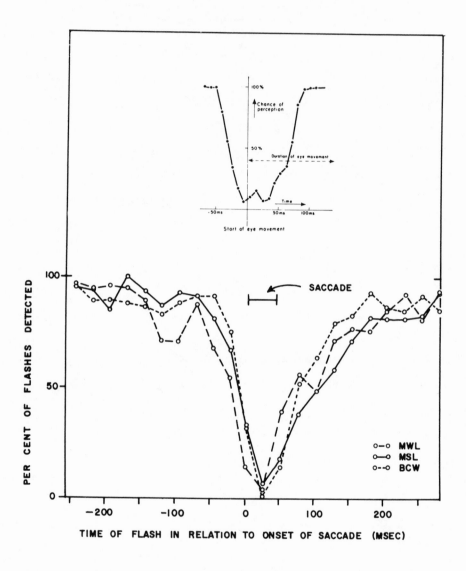

FIG. 2. Top: Latour's (1962) curve of visual threshold during eye movements; bottom: curves replotted from Volkmann et al. (1968) to match the scale of Latour's curve. Percentage of flashes detected is plotted as a function of the time at which the flash occurred in relation to the onset of a saccade, for three subjects. Average durations of saccades in each experiment are indicated on the appropriate graph.

some time, occasionally showing up on test flashes given as late as 100 msec after the saccade has ended. Table 1 shows a summary of several such time-course experiments. Given the very wide range of values of experimental variables used in these experiments (size of saccade, retinal location of stimulation, adaptation of the eye, luminance and spectral characteristics of the background field and of the test flash, etc.), it is perhaps surprising that the duration and range of inhibition are not more variable than they are from study to study.

The psychophysical data have been supported also by the results of several electrophysiological studies that investigated cortical evoked potentials during saccades. Figure 3 presents, for example, some results of Chase and Kalil (1972) which show attenuation of summated visual evoked responses (VER) to test flashes of low luminance presented during saccades. Other related experiments come from Gross, Vaughan, and Valenstein (1967), and Michael and Stark (1967). Figure 4, from Duffy and Lombroso (1968), shows their curve of the time

TABLE 1
Summary of Some Major Findings of Eight Experiments on the Time
Course of Saccadic Suppression (After Volkmann et al., 1968)

Author	Size of saccade	Adaptation	Retinal location	Duration of inhibition, msec	Range of inhibition, msec[a]
Zuber, Michael, Stark, 1966	20°	Dark	Variable	70–80	−60 to +20
Latour, 1962	15°?	?	?	90–100	−30 to +60 or 70
Latour, 1966[b]	15°	Dark	Variable but not foveal	60	−40 to +20
Lederberg[c], 1970	7°	Light	Foveal	100	−30 to +70
Volkmann, Schick, Riggs, 1968	6°	Light	Foveal	90–100	−20 to +75
Zuber, Crider, Stark, 1966	Involuntary flicks	Dark	Probably foveal	50	−25 to +25, roughly
Krauskopf, Graf, Gaarder, 1966	Involuntary flicks	Dark	Foveal		No inhibition found
Beeler, 1967	Involuntary flicks	Light	Foveal	130	−65 to +65, averaged

[a]Range of inhibition is defined as the interval by which a flash preceded (minus values) or followed (plus values) the onset of the saccade.

[b]This is but one example, chosen to agree with Latour's own summary. Latour has noted many parameters of this effect and presents a variety of results in several different forms. The interested reader should consult Latour's thesis directly.

[c]The results here are average ones; durations and ranges of inhibition were found to differ with the wavelength and the luminance of the stimulus flashes.

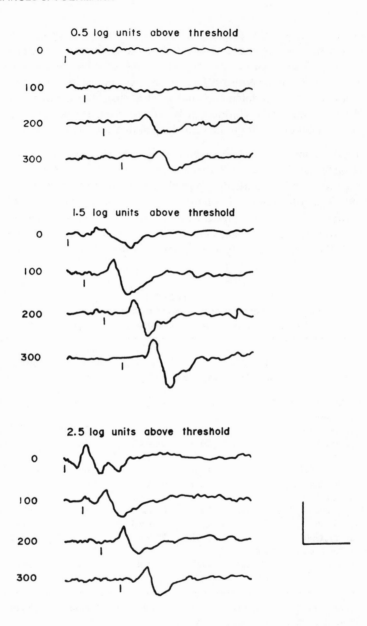

FIG. 3. Summated visual evoked responses (VER) to 100 flashes presented at three intensities. Traces begin at the onset of eye movement. Numbers to the left give test flash (TF) delay in msec. The TF occurs at the point indicated by a marker below each trace. Positivity at the occipital electrode is recorded in the upward direction. The calibration is 70 μvolt on the ordinate, 250 msec on the abscissa. (After Chase & Kalil, 1972.)

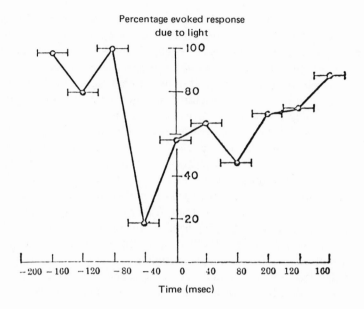

FIG. 4. Percentage of average energy of the evoked response attributable to light plotted against time where T^0 corresponds to the beginning of eye movement. (After Duffy & Lombroso, 1968.)

course of saccadic attenuation at the cortex. The model of image smear on the retina cannot readily account for any of these data.

2. Central inhibition. For a number of us, an attractive alternative has been the notion that the visual and oculomotor systems act together during saccades in a kind of feed-forward loop in which visual performance is actively inhibited somewhere in the central visual system by the neural signals given to the oculomotor system to execute a saccade. A large proportion of the data presented above support the idea of central inhibition without actually ruling out some other possibilities.

3. Shearing forces in the retina. Richards (1968, 1969) has offered an ingenious and very different explanation of saccadic attenuation. He suggests that a saccade has an effect on the eyeball of rapidly rotating a bowl of jelly; different parts of the intraocular materials, including the layers of the retina, accelerate and decelerate at different relative velocities. Thus mechanical shearing forces are set up which may disrupt neural signals in the retina. Even stimuli that arrive as early as 40 msec before the onset of a saccade might be less effective if the neural signals resulting from those stimuli were still being processed in the retina when the saccade began. These time relations are possible ones. Richards supports his model with data on visual suppression during passive eye movement, the Stiles–Crawford effect during saccades, the effects of background luminance, and retinal delay. Figure 5 shows his curve of the Stiles–Crawford effect measured during the dead time between two saccades executed as rapidly as possible (the eye jumped from one fixation point to a second point and then back again; the flash occurred 40 msec after the onset of the first saccade). Not only is relative sensitivity poorer at this time than during steady fixation, but also the curve is shifted slightly in the direction opposite the first saccade. If this notion is correct, the amount of suppression should vary importantly with saccade size. Richards did not investigate this variable. Looking at the experiments summarized in Fig. 3 might lead us to infer that the magnitude of the effect does not depend importantly on saccade size. On the other hand, Latour (1966) and Mitrani, Yakimoff, and Mateeff (1970) have reported a positive relation. Existing data on this variable are, in fact, not clear.

Figure 6 presents Richards' (1969) data on the effect of background luminance on suppression. He argues that the finding of a decrease in the suppression effect at low levels of background luminance supports a retinal rather than a central site for the effect; Fig. 6, of course, shows minimal suppression at low

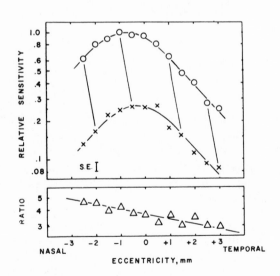

FIG. 5. The change of the Stiles–Crawford effect following a saccade. The circles (o) show the customary attenuation vs. eccentric entry; the crosses (×) show the new sensitivities 40 msec following the beginning of a 5° saccade. Note the slight temporal displacement of the curve, as well as the reduced sensitivity. This shift of the curve is also shown more clearly by the declining ratios between the crosses and circles, plotted below with triangles (△). (After Richards, 1969.)

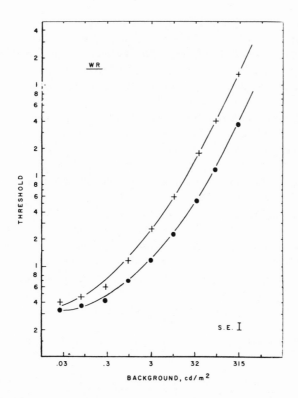

FIG. 6. Thresholds obtained for a 1° foveal test flash for steady fixation (●) and for fixation 40 msec following the beginning of a 5° saccade (×). As the background luminance is decreased, the effect of the preceding saccade on the threshold is reduced. However, the change of the logarithm of the equivalent background luminance following the saccade appears to be independent of the luminance level (Observer WR). (After Richards, 1969.)

luminances. The question of whether suppression occurs in darkness is clearly an important one; Riggs will present additional data on this point. Richards summarizes additional experiments to support his peripheral model of suppression, but we must move on to a last and related set of models that I want to mention, namely, those concerned with visual masking.

4. Visual masking. The sources of possible masking effects in experiments on saccadic suppression are many (see, for examples, Alpern, 1969; Bridgeman, 1971; Brooks & Fuchs, in preparation; Davidson, Fox, & Dick, 1973; MacKay, 1970; E. Matin, 1974; E. Matin, Clymer & L. Matin, 1972; E. Matin, L. Matin, Pola, & Kowal, 1969; L. Matin, 1972; Weisstein, 1972). Although different types of masking effects may interact in a given experimental situation, analyses have emphasized either the temporal or the spatial features of possible masking phenomena.

Alpern (1969, p. 98) emphasized the temporal features: he suggested that saccadic suppression might be accounted for by postulating that "the effect of excitation of the retina at some time after movement was completed, acted (retroactively) to wipe out the effects of prior retinal excitation, particularly those occurring before, during and immediately after the movement." This is, of course, a description of metacontrast. Figure 7 shows Alpern's presentation of one of his metacontrast curves superposed on one of our time course curves. Experimental support for this type of model has come from E. Matin and some of her co-workers (see E. Matin, below).

MacKay (1970), on the other hand, emphasized the possible lateral masking effects of contours on the retina or in physical space in a spatial analysis of masking. He presented stimulus flashes to the fixating eye during a saccadic-like motion of a background field, and found that the percentage of flashes detected fell approximately to zero over a time course similar to that reported for voluntary saccades. He concluded that "the displacement of the retinal image during a saccade can in some cases produce a suppressive effect without any assistance by postulated corollaries of the activation of eye muscles or mechanical shearing of the retina" (MacKay, 1970, p. 91). MacKay thus accounts for what we think of as saccadic suppression by the rapid displacement on the retina of a contour-bearing field, whether the motion is produced by the eye or by displacement of the field itself. Riggs and Johnstone (in preparation), however,

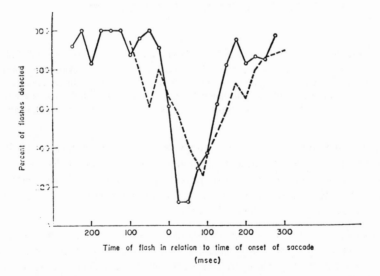

FIG. 7.   The frequency of detection of a foveal flash as a function of the time of onset of a saccadic eye movement lasting about 40 msec, according to Volkmann et al. (1968) (open circles). The dotted line represents the reduction of the brightness of a flash of light in one eye produced by an adjacent asynchronous flash to the other eye under conditions of steady fixation. The abscissa in this case represents flash asynchrony. (After Alpern, 1969.)

have repeated the MacKay experiment and found less evidence than had MacKay for an impairment due to image displacement without eye movements.

If contour is indeed a critical feature of a masking stimulus, then suppression would not be expected to occur during saccades executed in total darkness. Experimental results are not in agreement on this point. A decrease in saccadic suppression accompanying a decrease in background luminance has been reported by Richards (1969), Mitrani, Mateeff, and Yakimoff (1971) and Brooks and Fuchs (in preparation). Latour (1966), on the other hand, found a maximal rise in threshold during saccades in darkness. Zuber, Michael, and Stark, and Zuber, Crider, and Stark (see Zuber, Stark, & Lorber, 1966) also found saccadic suppression for stimuli flashed against a dark field. These workers apparently used dim fixation marks, however, thus providing some oppoertunity for masking by contours. In a recent series of experiments, Riggs, Merton, and Morton (1974) found some suppression of electrically produced phosphenes flashed during saccades in complete darkness, when no contour at all was present in the field. Dr. Riggs will address himself to these experiments today.

Needless to say, the temporal and spatial characteristics of masking interact importantly, but the ways in which they interact to produce all or a part of saccadic suppression are not yet clear. Most experiments on saccadic suppression present complex conditions of visual masking. The question is whether the "suppressive" or "masking" effect depends entirely on the temporal, spatial, and intensive relations on the retina, or whether a component of the effect is attributable to the visual effects of saccades per se.

II.2

Saccadic Suppression of Phosphenes: Evidence of a Neural Basis for Saccadic Suppression

Lorrin A. Riggs

Brown University

First, I'd like to go a little further with the point Volkmann just raised about possible masking effects of the visual scene as it moves across the retina.

Figure 1 shows the field of view in one of her experiments (Volkmann, Schick, & Riggs, 1968) on the partial suppression of vision that occurs during saccades. The subject was instructed to fixate on the gap between the two vertical lines on the left; and then, on signal, to make a rapid saccade from that gap over to the corresponding one on the right.

The dots are not present except for one instant of time when they are delivered by a strobe flash. The dots are the test stimulus; their luminance is progressively reduced until a threshold is reached where they are barely detectable by the subject. Volkmann plotted ogive curves, showing that as luminance is reduced, the probability of detection goes down. Remember that the ogive curves reveal a low threshold (high sensitivity) under the stationary-eye condition and a high threshold (low sensitivity) under the moving-eye conditions. Two important features of all of the experiments that have been done under like conditions (Volkmann, 1962; Volkmann et al., 1968; Lederberg, 1970) are (1) that no black fixation marks are present in the foveal region, and (2) that the test field is large enough so that a portion of it always falls on the foveal region.

Quite a different testing situation was used in the observations described by MacKay (1970). He posed the question whether the suppression or loss of vision that others have attributed to eye movements might occur just as well when the

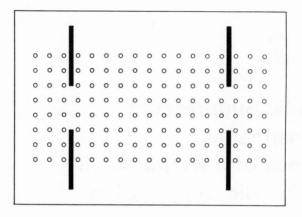

FIG. 1.   Stimulus field used by Volkmann et al. (1968).

eye was stationary all the time and the movement of the field across the retina was actuated by the stimulus apparatus instead of the eye movement.

In the MacKay situation, a 10° bright background field was deflected 3.2° horizontally, and the threshold was tested for a 2° test spot during that jump of the visual field even though the eye was fixating at all times on a black dot a quarter of a degree in diameter. MacKay reported that under these conditions his subject did show a partial loss of vision; something that could be seen as a short flash at other times was not likely to be seen if it were delivered during this rapid jump of the background field.

Johnstone and I (Riggs & Johnstone, in preparation) repeated the MacKay experiments in the Physiological Laboratory at Cambridge, England. We also measured thresholds, which MacKay had not done. He had merely measured the percentage of detection of targets during this rapid excursion of the field. We found a mean elevation of threshold of .21 log unit for three subjects as a result of this jump. In comparison with threshold elevations of .5 log unit or more that have been reported by Fran Volkmann and a number of other people with stroboscopic flashes during real eye movements, the above change in threshold is considerably smaller.

Johnstone and I, therefore, question whether one can account for the entire amount of suppression on the basis of any masking paradigm. In fact, MacKay does not claim that he had accounted for it. He just raised that as a possibility, without having actually determined thresholds. Our own conclusion is that, while there is indeed a slight elevation of threshold due to the masking that is produced by movement of the bright background field, there is a considerably larger elevation of threshold that accompanies real saccadic eye movements.

I will now describe another set of experiments that I was able to do in Professor W. A. Cobb's laboratory in the National Hospital at Queens Square in London. I was very fortunate to be able to work there with Merton of the Physiology Department at Cambridge and with Morton, who is a wizard at setting up equipment for doing experiments. The three of us (Riggs, Merton, & Morton, 1974) decided that we would get together and eliminate the optical factors that had been so bothersome and controversial in some of these experiments. We did this by putting the subject into total darkness. Not only was the room dark, but we covered him with a sort of tent of black cloth and made sure that under the real conditions of the experiment he could not see a thing.

You may well ask how we can test vision under conditions where there is not any light. The answer we came up with was to deliver a pulse of electric stimulation to the eyeball and, in other words, to elicit a phosphene and use that for a visual stimulus.

For any one of you who has done this, you will recognize that this really is a visual stimulus; you cannot tell the difference between seeing a phosphene generated by a little quick pulse of current and seeing a flash of light over a Ganzfeld. In either case you experience a very dim sort of film of light at threshold.

Our procedure was to ask the subject, in total darkness, to make horizontal saccades between two imaginary fixation points that were about $10°$ apart. The electro-oculogram (EOG) resulting from these saccades could be used to actuate a loudspeaker, producing a weak but clearly audible click whenever the saccade was of proper amplitude. Thus the subject could use the clicks to monitor his eye movements in the absence of any visual controls.

A psychophysical procedure of forced choice was used to measure phosphene thresholds. The subject was asked to make two saccades in succession, each of which produced the audible click. With one of the clicks we did deliver an electric pulse to the eye, with the other one we did not, and there was a randomizing circuit in the apparatus so that neither the experimenter nor the subject knew ahead of time whether there was to be a current passed through the eye at time 1 or time 2.

The subject's response, if he did detect a phosphene, was to tell us whether it came at time 1 or time 2. If no phosphene was detected he was to guess. You will recognize this as a typical forced-choice procedure in which there is a 50% chance of success without any current delivered to the eye. As the current intensity grows, the success rate runs up to 100%. So much for the general manner of the experiment.

Figure 2 shows the equipment that was needed for this purpose, and Merton and I were very much indebted to Morton for putting all this together very successfully for the experiment. You can see the happy subject with an electrode above and below one eye through which a pulse of current could be delivered by

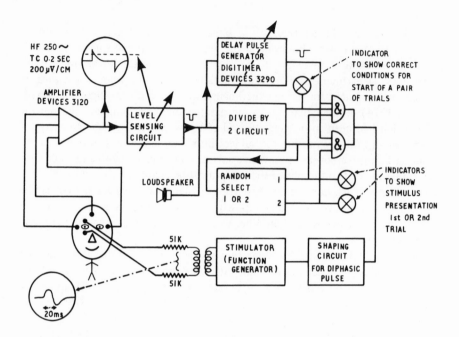

FIG. 2. Block diagram showing arrangements for stimulating the eye with electric pulses. (After Riggs et al., 1974.)

the function generator in the system. He also had EOG electrodes to the left and right of the eyes so that we could monitor the saccade.

The subject was actually trained in the light to make a saccade between two fixation points separated by $10°$, and then he was trained to do it with very dim illumination and very tiny fixation points. Then, in the last stage, he was put into total darkness and told to imagine that the fixation points were still present and to make the same kind of saccade.

We did have to scold the subject occasionally. He would make saccades bigger and bigger or smaller and smaller as the case might be, so that we did keep after him and kept the saccades within a rather narrow range of amplitude in the dark. Also shown in Fig. 2 is the loudspeaker that acted as the signal for the two intervals of time, and a delay circuit that was built in so that it was possible to trigger the phosphene instantaneously with the saccade or to delay its delivery for as long as we wished after the saccade had been made. The rest of the diagram shows the monitoring and measuring arrangements that are necessary for this kind of experiment.

Now for the results that were obtained. As I said, we scored the subject correct or incorrect on each judgment of which click was accompanied by a stimulus pulse. Figure 3 is a plot of percent correct as a function of current strength. The first line at the left is a plot on probability graph paper, as you see, running from 50% success up to a very high percentage of success. The open circles refer to the stationary-eye condition when the pulses of current were delivered to the eye without any saccade. All the other symbols refer to moving-eye conditions with various amounts of delay.

I will call your attention particularly to the last line at the right, which represents the solid square symbols. This is for a 40-msec delay such that the saccade triggered the delay circuit and 40 msec later the pulse of current was delivered to the eye. Notice that this one, being farthest to the right, seems to represent the largest elevation of threshold. There is no overlap between the stationary-eye data and the data obtained with a moving eye, especially for favorable times such as the 40 msec delay.

Figure 4 shows samples of our time-course data for three different subjects. The ordinate is log elevation of threshold determined on the basis of curves such as those shown in Fig. 3. We defined threshold as 75% success and measured the amount of elevation of threshold for pulses delivered after different amounts of delay in the experiment, running from zero time delay to 80 msec. In other experiments we had a considerably larger range of delays and found that the amount of elevation came down to zero after a second or so.

KOLERS: Is that time after the onset of the saccade or after the end?

RIGGS: It is time from the onset of the EOG trigger. The trigger occurred rather early in the course of the saccade. The saccade also has a rather small time course of 20 or 25 msec so that the total time through which the eye was moving was up to about 20 msec on the baseline of Fig. 4.

Now, there are several questions that arise at this point. One is the question of why there should be a 40-msec delay for the most depressed vision, and another

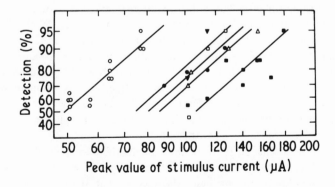

FIG. 3. Sample of results for detection of a phosphene under stationary- and moving-eye conditions. See text for details. (After Riggs et al., 1974.)

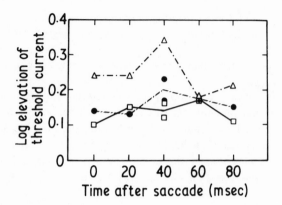

FIG. 4. Samples of curves showing elevation of threshold as a function of delay time after a saccade. (After Riggs et al., 1974.)

is the question of the amount of this depression which, in terms of log units of current, is not very large.

We did a great many experiments and the median amount of elevation of threshold in units of microamps came out to be about .2 log unit. Compare that with the .5 log unit that we just heard about for the visual experiments and it sounds rather low. I would like to make some comments about both of those points.

Let us first talk about the amounts of threshold elevation and the question of how the electrical test compares with a test using real light flashes. To get information on this we put half a ping-pong ball over the eye of the subject. We still worked in complete darkness, except that this time we allowed a brief flash of real light to hit the ping-pong ball in one of two test intervals. Thus we determined thresholds for the real light by the same forced-choice method that we had used with phosphenes, but with the stationary-eye condition only.

Figure 5 shows four samples of results. As the luminance of the light is increased, of course, we get better and better success in our forced-choice procedure, and we get the lines showing the relationship between percent correct and log of the intensity, this time of flashes of light. Now, the solid lines have slopes that are in the range characteristic of all threshold experiments with a Ganzfeld. Notice the slope of the dashed lines on the same graph. This is the slope that we get for the average experiment with the phosphenes. It is more than twice as steep as those we get with light.

Perhaps this makes sense in terms of the fact that here we are scaling current; if we were scaling current squared or power or energy, then it would be more like the light condition. In any case, the fact is that there is a more than two-to-one relationship of the slope of the phosphene function to that of the real light functions. In other words we can go down from nearly 100% success to nearly chance success with a very small shift of current as compared to a somewhat larger shift, more than twice as large a shift, in energy of light.

In order to reinforce that conclusion, we did another experiment which is shown in Fig. 6. Here we went slightly above threshold, and we simply asked the subject to look at two dim flashes, one of which was elicited by the electric pulse as a phosphene and the other by light. The current pulse was simply varied until the subject reported that the phosphene was of the same brightness as the light. We then raised the light intensity to a higher level and repeated the matching procedure. Each line of Fig. 6 represents an experiment in which the subject matched phosphene to light. The broken line has a slope of .5 for reference. Thus we see again that there is approximately a two-to-one relation of log intensity of light to log intensity of current. This led us to conclude that if we had done our experiments with real light instead of electric pulses our .2 log unit median elevation of threshold might instead have come out to be a little over .4 log unit.

With regard to the time aspect, we might now consult Fig. 7, from an earlier paper by Volkmann et al. (1968). In this diagram we pretend that we know when the suppression occurs. This, of course, is not true because only with some microelectrode kind of method would we be able to determine when the actual suppression occurs inside the head. But this is a diagram that was put together a

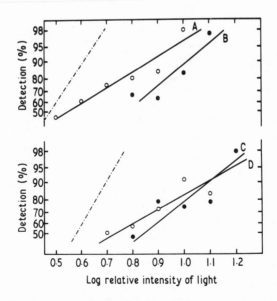

FIG. 5.   Samples of detection curves for flashes of light. (After Riggs et al., 1974.)

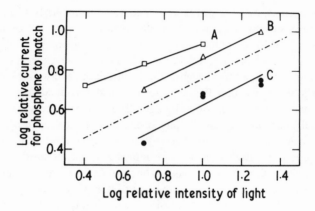

FIG. 6. Samples of current and light matches. (After Riggs et al., 1974.)

few years ago by Volkmann, Schick, and myself, to try to account for the time relations of some of these phenomena.

If we imagine that the suppression effect is shown by the dashed lines in relation to the saccade which takes the eye from one place to another, then we realize that any stimulus flash that is used as a test of suppression must come in

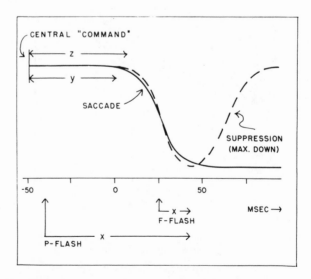

FIG. 7. Diagrammatic representation of the possible time course of some central mechanism for saccadic suppression, showing the unknown physiological latencies x, y, and z. Specification of these latencies would appear to be required for an accurate description of the actual time course of suppression. (After Volkmann et al., 1968.)

ahead of the time of the greatest suppression if it is to have a maximum neural effect. This is because there is a latent time x between the flash itself and the effect that it produces upon this locus in the head wherever it may be.

For a very weak flash of light delivered to the periphery in the Ganzfeld situation, that must be a very long latency, whereas using the tiny dots in the foveal situation, the latency can be shorter because of the known shorter latency of the fovea in responding to relatively bright spots of light.

Now, what about the phosphene? In that case we are bypassing not only the optics but also the photochemical events in the retina, and our best guess is that the phosphene is produced by activation of bipolars or other neural structures of the retina. That means that we can put in the electric pulse later than we could put in any light pulse and get a similar effect.

In fact, looking at this diagram, we see that the 40-msec time is about right for hitting the suppression mechanism if we assume that a very short latency indeed is present when electric pulses are delivered as compared to pulses of light.

In summary, then, I think what we have found is that a depression of vision occurring in total darkness is very nearly, if not quite, as large as the one that has been obtained with the stroboscopic light experiments of the kind Volkmann just reported; and that the time relations of this make pretty good sense in terms of known properties of the latency of this kind of stimulus. Whatever the origin of saccadic suppression, we think that there is a truly neural suppression that is linked to saccadic eye movements. In our phosphene experiments no retinal events are produced by motion of the visual field across the retina. We feel that if this masking occurred at all in the earlier experiments of Volkmann and others, it contributed only a small amount of the total suppression effect that was measured.

I am not speaking now of the optical smearing that occurs in real life when the images of objects are carried across the receptors during a saccade. In the laboratory conditions that I have just been telling about, neither the stroboscopic flash nor the phosphene can produce any appreciable amount of retinal smear. In ordinary vision the elevation of threshold due to smearing of the image may well be greater than that due to neural suppression per se.

DISCUSSION

FUCHS: As you already know, B. A. Brooks and I have been doing some similar saccadic suppression experiments at the University of Washington. We have two basic points that don't quite agree with your data. I was wondering if you'd like to comment on them.

First of all, we actually tested visual sensitivity during saccades in complete darkness in a psychophysical situation either to a small point stimulus of light or to a full field flash (otherwise complete darkness), and found, as you did in your phosphene experiment, a very modest one-tenth to two-tenths of a log unit suppression under those conditions. That speaks against, I think, a corollary discharge, at least a motor-linked event in that sense.

Second, we also repeated some of the experiments that MacKay has done with slightly different conditions in which we both had saccades made across structured visual fields and moved the structured visual field in saccadelike fashion and looked at visual sensitivity and found we were completely able to reproduce the saccadic suppression phenomena, including the temporal characteristics, that is, the decrease in sensitivity before the saccade, by simply jerking the background at saccadic speeds.

We conclude from those kind of data that it is more likely to be a visual masking phenomenon than a motor effect.

RIGGS: First I'd like to comment on the first point you raised, namely how much of a change there is in darkness using a light type of stimulus. This is something I haven't done myself. However, I would guess on the basis of my Fig. 7 that you would have to deliver your weak test flash not during the saccade but about 40 msec earlier to get the maximum effect.

The amounts of suppression reported by Latour (1966) and by Zuber and Stark (1966) have ranged between half a log unit and one log unit, which seem like very large amounts to me. I have never seen them quite as large myself. I really can't say why there should be the discrepancy between your results and theirs, except for the stimulus time that I have mentioned.

E. MATIN: Dr. Riggs, I'd like to make a suggestion about a possible reason for the discrepancy between the work of Zuber and Stark (1966) and the work that Dr. Fuchs has been describing. In Zuber and Stark's experiment there were two fixation dots, as I remember it, and the target that was being used to test for sensitivity appeared between them.

We did this once quite by accident in the course of doing another experiment. I was the subject for the experiment and was sitting in a dark room with a contact lens on, triggering a flash of light. The flash was located between the two fixation points as it was in Zuber and Stark's experiment.

I kept missing the flashes, but my husband, who was outside of the experimental booth and had a light in series with the lamp that I was supposed to be seeing, kept seeing the flashes. Finally, we found out what was happening. The flash was being masked by the two fixation targets. After we moved it up so that it wasn't in the line of fire between those two fixation targets, we could see it and proceed with our business.

We weren't measuring thresholds, but I think our experience suggests a possible reason why Zuber and Stark got such enormous figures while other people working under different conditions have much more modest ones.

RIGGS: Yes, I am very glad that you mentioned that because I think it is a very important point, that some investigators have used rather large dots that were very prominent in their experiments, and I think this is unfortunate. I am glad that Dr. Volkmann in her experiments always used a gap between lines as a guide for fixation. The alternative you mentioned seems like a very reasonable one, to have the test object out of line with the two fixation marks.

E. MATIN: I think if it is out of line with the course of the two fixation marks, then it is not going to be as badly masked. You don't get around the problem completely because lateral masking can be involved. That really is a kind of dilemma. It is difficult to do the experiment in such a way that you can be sure there is no masking at all. However, I think in Zuber and Stark's experiment there really must have been a great deal of visual masking.

VOLKMANN: I believe that Latour, on the other hand, put his flash 4° above the line of the two fixation marks, and got a good deal of saccadic suppression in the dark. So again the issue is not quite clear.

E. MATIN: Did Latour get figures like a log unit, and one and a half log units, or were his results more like yours?

VOLKMANN: He claimed three log units at one point. But most of the time he didn't measure the effect in terms of luminance changes. Mostly he chose one stimulus luminance which could always be seen by the fixating eye and then presented that in various relations to saccades to get a time course for the inhibitory effect.

E. MATIN: I'd like to make another point about Latour's experiments. I think he presented flashes to different retinal loci, a procedure that might result in very substantial differences in threshold that have nothing to do with saccadic suppression at all.

On the other hand, I think the more modest increases of threshold that have been reported in some experiments might well point to something other than visual masking. You say you still end up with .1 log unit, Dr. Fuchs?

FUCHS: A tenth to .2.

E. MATIN: You more or less categorically said that has nothing to do. . .

FUCHS: Quite clearly that is the remnant, if you will, of a motor effect. That is what we feel must be left.

E. MATIN: It doesn't have to be a motor effect.

FUCHS: Right.

E. MATIN: There is something other than what you are prepared to attribute to visual masking, perhaps.

FUCHS: Right.

E. MATIN: But it is another step to say it has to be a motor effect. It could be the Richards (1969) effect that Volkmann pointed to. And then there is another theory which people have forgotten about, the one proposed by Holt (1903). I think we would now call that theory intersensory masking. That is, Holt didn't think that the suppression, the "central anesthesia" that he was talking about, was due to outflowing impulses in the way that I think you do, Dr. Volkmann. He thought that the proprioceptive impulses coming back after the eye movement was initiated were responsible for the inhibition effect. And I think it is fair to say that this is another one of the set of possible alternatives to an outflow theory.

There is very little evidence for masking by proprioceptive stimuli per se. On the other hand, when you make an eye movement, there are movements of the conjunctiva, movements of the retrobulbar tissues, and so on, all of which could contribute to an intersensory effect. I might add I don't want this to be known as Matin's theory; it is strictly Holt's theory. Nonetheless, I don't think we can rule it out of the set of possibilities. In a study of intersensory effects published by Novak (1965), an interaction between vision and the somesthetic system was described. This interaction has an extended time course of the kind you find in visual masking and in saccadic suppression—so temporal factors per se don't rule out Holt's theory.

RIGGS: My own feeling is that the time is all wrong for that, that it would take so long for any feedback from the eye movement structures to get there, that one wouldn't get this kind of a time relation.

E. MATIN: I would have hesitated to mention Holt's idea at all. He based it on incorrect information. That is, he believed that the suppression didn't begin until the eye movement was under way and, therefore, he explicitly rejected the outflow idea. He said it couldn't be due to "feelings of innervation" because it started too late.

And as you say, my first feeling would have been to say the time course isn't right. But when I look at Novak's experiments, there are temporally backward effects in intersensory interactions just as there are in visual masking. So Holt's theory is not necessarily excluded, any more than the Richards possibility is excluded, or, of course, the outflow theory. The unfortunate thing is, we have a mess of variables to contend with.

RIGGS: Yes, that's for sure.

E. MATIN: It's going to be very hard to disentangle them.

RIGGS: Maybe before we wander off too far, I should answer the second of Dr. Fuchs' question as best I can. I am afraid I can't really answer it clearly because there is quite a disagreement among the various experimenters on what is the depression that occurs with the stationery eye when one jumps the field across.

I think it does depend very much on the kinds of fixation points that are present in the field and the total amount of the background field that has jumped across, the luminance of the field, and all those variables.

I think to do a good experiment of that kind it is important to cut down those variables as much as one can. For example, one might use a very large background field and avoid the use of fixation points in the fovea whenever the test is delivered to the fovea. To the extent that I was able to do that in the Cambridge lab with Ray Johnstone, we did find this very minimal amount of elevation of threshold in comparison with what had been found with real eye movements.

But I don't really have an explanation of why others have found larger effects. I might just ask whether you did measure threshold or it was just a percent diminution of *yes* judgments that were measured.

FUCHS: We varied the neutral density filters in front of the test flash in an ascending and descending series until the subject could not perceive objects.

We measured the visual threshold both during fixation and, under the exact same conditions, during either movements of the eye or movements of the background stimulus.

RIGGS: On that one point I would like just to mention that I think that people ought now to use the forced-choice method whenever possible because I think that it contributes a good deal to the stability of the experiment and tends to avoid changes of criteria and things of that kind that can creep in.

I don't mean to say that the old data are wrong because they didn't do this. I think most of them are quite carefully controlled and the subjects were quite well instructed and cooperative, so that I think the old data are okay. But signal detection theorists have shown us the advantages of finding a discrimination index (d') value that is fairly immune to shifts of criterion and bias. Forced-choice procedures that distinguish between signal plus noise and noise alone would seem to be a good idea for future experiments.

VOLKMANN: It's an important point.

HALLETT: Dr. Volkmann, there is an ordinary everyday condition where you can see the smear of your retinal image. If one goes out at night, the faintest street lights, whether they are bright or dim I wouldn't say, certainly are streaked during saccades. So there is a common situation where one sees retinal smear.

With regard to the discussions of Dr. Volkmann and Dr. Riggs, it was my impression when I reviewed the literature on saccadic suppression some years ago that a great many workers did their experiments in such a way that the test light fell at different retinal positions. Since the threshold of the dark-adapted eye varies very strongly with position, this is an uncontrolled factor.

Visual threshold can be elevated (sometimes considerably elevated) by many factors extraneous to the object of the experiment, (e.g., Hallett, 1969), but cannot normally be lowered by much more than about .2 log without an obvious increase in guessing. It is therefore appropriate to give special stress to data in which "saccadic suppression" is slight or absent.

VOLKMANN: Yes, there are two points here: one regarding our ability to see retinal smear, and another regarding the variation in threshold with retinal location of stimulation.

It makes sense to me that we can see blurred or smeared images of street lights at night. The lights would have to be bright enough to be above threshold for the moving eye, that is, bright enough to stimulate the individual receptors during the very brief time that it reaches each of them as the eye sweeps past the light. Once that condition is met, we should see the light as smeared since the duration of stimulation is long and many receptors are successively stimulated. In fact, I suppose the data would lead us to expect that we should see any sufficiently bright, high-contrast, long-duration stimulus as smeared if we saccade across it in an otherwise contour-free field, such as in the dark.

I think Dr. Hallett's point (and Dr. Matin's earlier one) about retinal location of stimulation is especially important. Many of the experiments on saccadic suppression have not taken care to always present the stimulus flash to the same retinal location (see, for example, Table 1 of my paper). Since threshold varies importantly with retinal location, it is difficult to interpret experiments in which it is not controlled. I don't know of any good experiment in which the retinal position of a stimulus flash presented to the moving eye was systematically varied to assess the relative thresholds of different retinal sites during saccades, although there is a paper related to this point by Mitrani, Mateeff, and Yakimoff (1970b).

In our own work we have tried to avoid the problem. We used a light-adapted eye and, as Dr. Riggs showed you, the dot field in the stimulus flash was made to cover an area which was larger than the distance between the two fixation marks. So, regardless of where the eye might be in executing a saccade, the stimulus always came to the fovea.

HALL: I'd like to ask if rapid eye movement just by itself will produce a phosphene. I may be aging or something, but I notice it in the morning. I am wondering whether the mechanism involved here might not be just the process which gets rid of this as a noise factor and that really what we are looking at is a system which gets rid of the mechanical stimulation of the receptors.

RIGGS: That's a very interesting idea to me because I first noticed the phosphenes that you mentioned only a few months ago.

KOLERS: Some of us haven't seen them yet.

RIGGS: I filed it away in my little checklist of things I must ask my ophthalmologist about.

HALL: They don't know.

RIGGS: So, I don't know either, and I suppose that it may indeed go back to the fact that one of the consequences of not being quite so young any more is that the vitreous humor becomes more aqueous, and it is much less of a support to the retina and detachments occur. I hope this isn't the first step toward a detachment for you and me.

In any case, I confirm your observation. It is an interesting point that stimuli of that kind can result from saccades and the possibility that they may indeed be somewhat suppressed by the mechanisms that we have been talking about. I have noticed this particularly on getting up in the morning. I don't know whether that is your experience.

HALL: Same observation.

RIGGS: Evidently a quiescent time of quite a long duration followed by new movements of the eyes is what leads up to it. Are there any ophthalmologists that can tell us about these things?

BISHOFF: I have a brief question about Fig. 7, Dr. Riggs.

RIGGS: It's a diagram of the time course.

BISHOFF: Right. The dashed line shows the suppression. There are two questions. First, how serious can it really be taken, for the present, that there is a maximum about 40 msec after the onset of the saccade? The second question is about the saccade which just lasted 20 msec, which was briefer than the one depicted. Does this mean that the timing of the suppression is independent of the timing of the saccade?

RIGGS: In answer to your first question, I tried to make it clear that no one knows when the suppression occurs and we will not know until we have electrodes in there to tell us when it occurs. So it is purely imaginary that it would have this particular timing and the only reason we drew it in with that time is that it made it easier to conceptualize the latencies of flashes that were photopic flashes in one case and scotopic ones delivered to the periphery in the other case. In other words, nobody knows where this thing is, but it is somewhere in here in relation to the eye movement.

The duration of the eye movement is also a little hard to specify. If you think of the major components of it as being the part when it is going quite rapidly, then it may be 20 msec, whereas if you try to include the entire time course from the starting steady state to the final steady state it will be a very much longer time of perhaps 50 msec.

STEINMAN: I noticed in the summary of the prior experiments that there is some disagreement as to whether or not an elevation effect occurs with microsaccades. There is an experiment that shows none, and two that show it. Does anyone have a belief, opinion, or knowledge of the status of that phenomenon?

VOLKMANN: The experiments that I can think of are those of Beeler (1967) who found a suppression during involuntary flicks (if we can call them that any more) and those of Krauskopf, Graf, and Gaarder (1966) who did not find suppression during such flicks (which I think occurred around a fixation point in the dark).

As far as I know, those two sets of experiments have not been reconciled. I don't know what the differences in experimental conditions were, but I doubt that they account for the differences in the results. Does anyone know? Apparently no one does.

ANLIKER: I hate to bring up the subject of brain waves in which we looked at the phase-contingent time of arrival of a flash in relation to the alpha rhythm. That is, if you consider a typical visual evoked response, the flash was delivered without respect to the incident phase of the alpha. However, one can go back and reclassify the data. In our case, we do it in a somewhat elaborate way: we either define the alpha period in terms of time, or we do it in terms of quadrature analysis so that we can define the entire phase series for particular series of responses.

We then reclassify the visual evoked response on the basis of the incident phase of the alpha rhythm at the time the flash arrives. Then if you look at the subset of phase-classified data of the submeans, instead of the grand means of the visual evoked response, you get a very interesting phase-contingent relation which is a very orderly process.

But that is not the critical part of it. What you see in all these contingent means is that the major part of the evoked response, no matter what the initial phase, is at a fixed place that agrees with the grand mean. In order to accomplish this, the brain must be phase shifting its response to bring this about at the appropriate time.

The contribution of the different phased components to the grand mean, then, is variable in a series, but orderly with the successive set of means. Then by determining the signal-to-noise relationship between the submean and the grand mean to try to determine which phase contingency contributes the most to the response, we get a phase contingency cycle in terms of responsiveness of the evoked response to the time, i.e. the phase of arrival of the flash.

Now, it could well be that in saccadic suppression studies the saccades do not occur at random, but are timed in relation to some central nervous timing cycle. In that case, one would expect that there would be a raising and lowering of the threshold in relation to the saccade if the saccade is departing from the central timing cycle in a more or less fixed phasic relationship. That possibility will some day have to be taken into account in this type of experiment.

RIGGS: I don't have any particular comment except to say this might well enter into any neural process that may account for the things that we have been describing. Since my experiment was done in Prof. Cobb's lab, we were also interested in the evoked potential aspects, which I didn't speak about, but which we will publish along with our other results.

One thing that you might be interested in is that the so-called lambda wave that people have spoken of as a component of eye-movement effect became less and less as we went to dimmer and dimmer situations. It finally was absent in the total-darkness experiments. Whereas some people have thought that the lambda wave might be contingent upon corollary discharge or some other of these hypothetical mechanisms that would result in suppression, in our experiments we were able to measure suppression under conditions where the lambda wave didn't show itself.

II.3

The Role of Eye Movements in Maintenance of Vision

Ulker Tulunay-Keesey

University of Wisconsin

In this contribution, I would like to concentrate on the micromovements of the eye which occur during fixation and their role in the maintenance of vision. Figure 1, taken from Riggs and Ratliff (1951), is a sample recording that shows clearly the different components of eye movements, namely the saccades, the drift, and the tremor motions. The calibration mark is 100 sec of arc. Among the three types of movement, the saccades and the drifts are the larger, each with an average amplitude of 5 min of arc and an irregular rate of occurrence. The saccades are fast with an average duration of 25 msec, the drift is slow having a duration of 100 msec or longer. The tremor motion is small and fast with an average amplitude of 20 sec of arc, and a rate of occurrence up to 100 times per sec. These spontaneous movements of the eye result in displacements of the image in relation to the retina. It is calculated that in a typical fixation period of 4 sec the image remains in the fovea but travels back and forth across 30–50 receptors. Therefore, many cone receptors receive stimulation with a frequency and amplitude that depend on both the characteristics of the motion and the spatial contrast properties of the image. It is reasonable to assume that such a rich variety of stimulation supplied by eye movements amplifies the response of the receptor or receptor groups, eventually aiding visual function. Indeed, for a long time after their discovery these fixational eye movements were regarded as the mechanism subserving acuity and contrast discrimination. Acuity is the sensitivity of the human visual system to the size of spatial detail in the stimulus; contrast sensitivity refers to the just discriminable level of contrast, regardless of the size of the detail.

One of the first concentrated efforts to examine the role of eye movements in acuity was made by Ratliff (1952). He recorded eye movements occurring

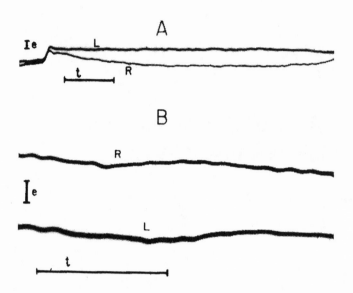

FIG. 1. Sample records of eye movements: A shows saccades, slow drifts, and minute tremor; B shows an enlarged view of the tremor movements. In each record L is the trace for the left eye and R for the right eye, t represents .1 sec of time, and e represents 100 sec of angular rotation of the eye. From Riggs and Ratliff (1951).

during a very brief, 74 msec, presentation of a flash that contained a grating. Both the size of light and dark bars and their orientation were varied until the subject could no longer discriminate a horizontal grating from a vertical one. The results indicated that acuity was better, i.e., finer gratings could be correctly identified, when the eyes were relatively still.

The role of eye movements in acuity could be evaluated better if acuity were to be measured under conditions when the effect of eye movements was eliminated, i.e., when no motions of the retinal image were allowed. The technique for stabilizing the retinal image developed from such a concern.

As is well known, this is an optical (or electronic) technique which in essence monitors movements of the eye and enables the target to move as much as the eye does. Thus, the image of the target remains stationary in relation to the retina. There are three major studies (Riggs, Ratliff, Cornsweet, & Cornsweet, 1953; Keesey, 1960; Fender & Nye, 1962) that utilized the stabilized-image technique to examine acuity systematically. In two of these studies the exposure duration of the target was chosen so that the whole range of image motions could occur, yet it was short enough to prevent disappearance of the image, a characteristic of prolonged stabilized vision. In the other study the target was viewed for longer periods; attempts were made to alleviate disappearance by flickering the stabilized target.

Figure 2 shows the results of the experiment in which short-exposure durations were used. The target was a single dark line superimposed on a bright background. The width of the line was manipulated to obtain thresholds of detectability. The independent variable was exposure duration, ranging from about 10 msec to 1.2 sec. The stabilized-image condition, which we called the stopped image at that time, is depicted by the solid line, and the dashed line represents the normal unstabilized viewing condition.

It is clear that under both of these viewing conditions acuity improved to a maximum value within 200 msec. Only a slight improvement was indicated for longer exposures of the target. Same results were obtained with vernier and grating targets. The general conclusion was that the mechanisms subserving acuity were dependent on exposure duration but independent of image motion.

All investigators who have used the stabilized-image method agree that a target whose image is stationary on the retina gradually fades after a few seconds of viewing; the field loses contrast and eventually the whole target disappears. The same target under the same prolonged fixation conditions stays sharply in view if it is not stabilized. It would seem, therefore, that the type of stimulation supplied by image motion, while immaterial in determining maximum levels of acuity, is essential in maintaining clear visibility of targets. The question becomes then the dimension of the motion necessary for sustaining continuous visibility.

To obtain an approximate answer to this question, we set up our apparatus so that we could compensate for known percentages of image motion (Riggs & Tulunay, 1959).

In Fig. 3, the zero point on the abscissa refers to the perfect alignment of the optical paths so that presumably 100% of all the eye movements are rendered ineffective. That is, the eye and the image move through the same angle, and the retinal image motion is zero. (Subsequent calibrations showed that a residual movement of about 1 min of arc remained due to a combination of factors including the slippage of the contact lens the subject has to wear.) The plus values indicate that the image moves more than does the eye in the same direction. At 1, the image goes through twice the angular rotation of the eye. The negative values indicate a condition when the image moves less than the eye, again in the same direction.

The data suggest that at point zero where image motion is minimum, visibility of the image is also minimal. (Visibility is defined as the length of time the subject reports that the target is seen clearly in a given period of time.) This minimum is not sharply defined, however. Eye movements that are 10% effective (when a 5-min-of-arc rotation of the eye causes an image motion of 30 sec of arc) succeed in increasing visibility only by 10%. In order to achieve close to continuous visibility, about 60% of the eye movement had to be effective, e.g., an eye movement of 5 min of arc had to produce an image excursion of 3 min of

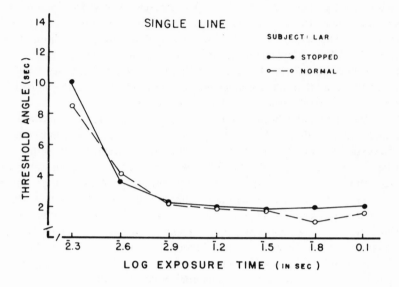

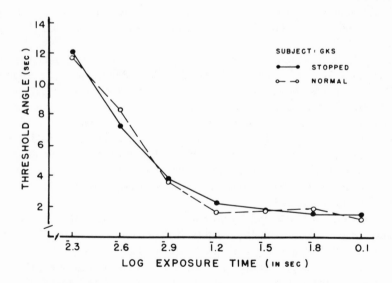

FIG. 2. Threshold curves for the detection of single black lines as a function of log exposure time under stopped and normal viewing conditions.

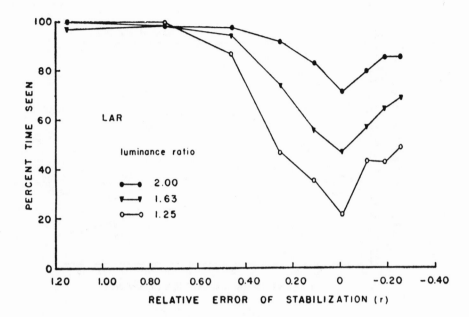

FIG. 3. Mean percent time that the test object was seen as a function of r, relative error of stabilization. Each mean represents six runs obtained over three days.

arc. This figure also shows that visibility under stabilized vision depends on the contrast of the target. The target in this case was a bipartite field. The interaction between image motion and the luminance ratio between the two halves of the field was such that visibility was determined by contrast alone when the image is motionless on the retina.

The next attempt was concentrated on delineating the component of eye motion most important in supporting the continuous visibility of the target (Keesey & Riggs, 1962). We stabilized the image and imposed on it motions of known amount and amplitude approximating motions that would have been caused by the normal eye movement. The results (Fig. 4) showed that the target, in this case a Mach band, was clearly discernable for 15 sec under the unstabilized conditions. It disappeared readily within a few seconds when it was stabilized, and when sinusoidal motions of about 1 min of arc were imposed on the stabilized image, visibility did not increase appreciably. The extent of image motion had to exceed 1 min of arc to sustain visibility at the levels achieved with unstabilized vision. Frequency of motion was critical: the faster motions of 8 and 13 Hz did not succeed in lengthening the visibility of the stabilized image regardless of the magnitude of image displacement.

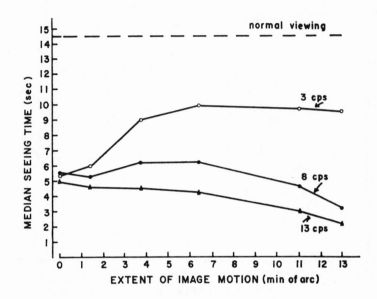

FIG. 4. Average time (median of 8 observations) to the first disappearance of the bright Mach band as a function of peak-to-peak amplitude of sinusoidal motions of the retinal image.

The conclusion to be reached from these data is that the component of eye movement essential for the maintenance of vision is the drift motion causing slow large movements of the image. The tremor with frequencies higher than 10 Hz was judged to be ineffective. We could not speculate on the role of the saccades because the motions we imposed on the stabilized image did not contain any of the features of a saccade.

There were other experiments that were concerned with the same questions. Among them the studies of Gerrits and his colleagues, Gerrits & Vendrik (1974) in Holland, were unique in that in these studies the stabilized target was rotated; waveform characteristics closely duplicated the image motion that would have been caused by the normal motions of the eye. There was general agreement on the main conclusion. Vision was sustained by the slow and continuous motion of the image resulting from the drift component of eye movements, rather than from the tremor and the saccadic motions that contain high-frequency components.

The next question is whether a displacement of the image across the retina is necessary, or whether a local temporal variation of luminance is sufficient to maintain vision.

To answer this question we stabilized the image and simply modulated its intensity in time. The target was a bright line superimposed on a dimmer background. It flickered sinusoidally around a constant mean luminance. The ratio of the average line luminance to the background, the amplitude of flicker, was one of the variables in addition to the frequency of luminance variation. The dimmer background was always steadily illuminated. Visibility was once more defined as the duration of time that the edges of the bright line stayed in clear view.

The main result here, as shown in Fig. 5, was that flicker at rates less than 5 Hz sustained visibility almost continuously. Between 5 Hz and 15 Hz, visibility declined linearly until at 15 Hz it was down to the level achieved with a nonflickering stabilized image. The higher rates of flicker did not enhance visibility.

The importance of contrast is demonstrated in Fig. 6. There appeared to be three ranges of frequency by which visibility of targets of any contrast could be manipulated. The most effective rates for all contrast targets were between .4 and 4 Hz. Low-contrast targets interact with flicker frequency—e.g., a stabilised bar containing .3 contrast which initially is visible for 5 sec will be seen for 40 sec if it is flickered at a rate of 3 Hz, or if its contrast is increased to 1 and flickered at a higher rate of 6 Hz. At 9-Hz flicker and at flicker rates greater than 15 Hz, contrast is the sole determinant of visibility. But visibility never reached the levels achieved when the image flickered at slow rates.

The main point of these experiments is that the effectiveness of the drift motion of the eye in maintaining visibility is due to the variations in temporal

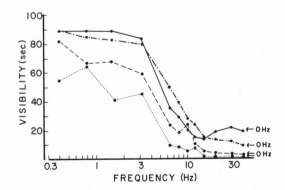

FIG. 5. Visibility of a bright bar as a function of sine-wave flicker frequency for selected contrast ratios: dotted line for .06; dashes for .25; dash-dot for 1; and solid line for 10. Each point is an average of 10 judgments. Visibility of the bar when it was steady (0 Hz) is indicated with arrows along appropriate contrast functions. Viewing is stabilized.

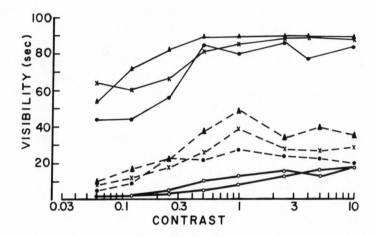

FIG. 6. Visibility of a bar as a function of contrast ratio for frequencies of sine-wave flicker: for .4, solid triangle, solid line; for .8, X, solid line; for 3.2, solid circle, solid line; for 6.4, solid triangle, dash line; for 8.0, X, dash line; for 10, solid circle, dash line; and for 20 and 40 Hz, circle, solid line. Only representative selected frequencies are shown. Each point is an average of 10 judgments, with stabilized viewing, and the author (UTK) as subject.

luminance it supplies to the receptors; an excursion over several receptors is of secondary importance in sustaining vision.

DISCUSSION

VOLKMANN: Dr. Cornsweet has requested considerably less than equal time to raise what he considers to be a serious and perplexing problem, relating to the perception of stabilized visual stimuli, for which he believes no immediate solution is at hand.

CORNSWEET: I just want to point out, very briefly, a problem having to do with eye movements and perception that I believe is very important. When a large luminous disk on a dark background is stabilized on the retina, it disappears, but if it is then moved across the retina just a minute of arc, the whole disk reappears. The only parts of the retina that are receiving changing stimulation are two narrow crescents, one at the leading and the other at the trailing edge, but the whole area of the disk seems to brighten. The same phenomenon can be observed without a stabilized image. If you look steadily at a luminous disk, the middle should darken because your normal eye movements only affect the edges of the image. Why don't we see bright and dark crescents at the edges of all large areas all of the time?

There are two aspects to this question. First of all, is it a legitimate question? Does the center of a large luminous disk really look brighter than its dark background? That's not as easy to tell as you might think. There have been very few good measurements bearing on this question, but the ones that exist (Davidson & Whiteside, 1971) indicate that the center does look brighter (although much less bright than the inner edges of the disk). Second, if the phenomenon does exist, how can it be explained? The literature contains a few theories, but none of those really is very convincing to me. I am not saying they are wrong, but just that they are not complete enough to be convincing to me. If we can develop an understanding of this phenomenon that is as close as is our understanding of the inhibitory interactions that underlie contrast effects, I believe we will have mastered the relationship between luminance and brightness.

HALL: I'd like to comment on the retinal blood vessel method because at one time I used that to study stabilized images. It is a destabilizing of a previously stabilized image, in a sense. One of the things that is sort of interesting is the rate at which these retinal blood vessels disappear once you stop a light that was moving across the sclera.

You can do this with a penlight and I am sure you have all done it. If you stop the movement of that light, the blood vessel images disappear almost instantaneously. It seems to me a similar phenomenon occurs in afterimages. For example, if you put an afterimage in the eye at the same time that you are looking at your retinal blood vessels and move a light source across the sclera, you will sustain that afterimage for long periods of time, much longer than you would in normal vision.

The thing that I am thinking about here is, there is some kind of an active process that is getting rid of all these afterimages so we can get new information coming into the system. In other words, perhaps there is some kind of an active suppression process that gets rid of afterimages and other high-contrast items in the retina, so we can pick up new information as it comes in.

CORNSWEET: I think the active process is inhibition.

ANLIKER: To me it seems likely that it is a hysteresis phenomenon arising from the use of the method of limits. It's been observed again and again, but it is usually factored out in the graphic displays that come out of the data. If a subject is trying to distinguish pairs of flashes that are made closer and closer together in time, he becomes increasingly uncertain and finally decides that the flash pairs have fused. One might then think that it would be possible to back up a step or two, increasing the interval between the pair of flashes, and see two again.

In fact, one has to separate the signals by a much larger amount. The same thing is true each time you reverse the direction. There is an old study by Paul Schiller (1932), Peter Schiller's father, in which he showed many years ago that if you compare a visual flicker and tactile flicker (by rotating a disk under the fingertips with a series of radiating bumps on it) you find a most impressive intersensory effect. If you produced both visual and tactile threshold fusion, then by producing either visual or tactile flicker by a small reduction in frequency you would also observe flicker in the other modality.

So there may be a general neurological process which has to do with the problem of finding the thing that is to be discriminated.

My point is that it could well apply to tracking back and forth onto and off from a spot.

TULUNAY-KEESEY: This may not be completely relevant to your comment nor, surely, will it answer any of the questions you raised, but it may help. If we look at data for a situation where there is a high-contrast flickering target well above threshold level, we find that it is clearly visible when it is first presented to the retina under stabilized conditions. There are two important components; there is a spatial-change component which is generated by the edges, and a temporal-change component which arises from the flicker. What happens is that from some very low frequency of flicker to about 4 Hz or thereabout, the target is visible. That is, something that one calls a *line* has *edges* whose brightness changes under stabilized conditions. At a higher frequency, one can no longer see the edges but there is an awareness of the sensation of flicker. It is as if in the human visual system there are two separate subsystems that carry information on temporal and on spatial aspects of a stimulus. What seems to disappear first is the spatial aspect, as if the transmission lines have different shorter time characteristics for the spatial than for the temporal aspect transmitters. Also relevant to this is that many of us have shown that visually evoked potentials resulting from flickering stabilized targets are just as large as those elicited by a target viewed under the unstabilized condition. In other words, the potentials that are evoked by a nondisappearing normally viewed target are the same as those evoked by a target that is stable on the retina and flickering. So presumably, the signal that we're picking up does not arise from those particular channels that lose their output when the stimulus is stable on the retina and which apparently process spatial stimulus aspects.

NAKAYAMA: I wanted to ask Dr. Tulunay-Keesey whether or not there is a qualitative difference between the disappearance of afterimages and that of stabilized images. It is my experience that afterimages are quite persistent if you use very bright targets. Is it just the fact that they have greater contrast?

TULUNAY-KEESEY: Yes, afterimages take more time to disappear than stabilized images. Further, afterimages that are produced by stabilized images are much more persistant than afterimages that are produced by nonstabilized images.

I don't know what to make of all this. We have some very casual observations, which we hope to quantify soon, that the thresholds we take on an afterimage that is produced by a stabilized adapting light are about .6 log unit larger at the start of the data taking than the threshold on an afterimage produced by a nonstabilized adapting light.

So there is, I think, a little bit of a difference between the photochemistry and electrophysiology of stabilized images and afterimages.

CORNSWEET: Can I share in that answer? Most afterimages in fact have enormous contrasts compared with most targets that are used as stabilized images. The highest contrast Tulunay-Keesey used in her stabilization experiments is still much lower than the typical contrast in an afterimage experiment. If you observe carefully, you can see afterimages from patterns with normal contrast and they disappear very quickly. If you flick your eye from one place to another, you see afterimages very briefly. They look just like stabilized images to me.

AREND: With respect to the last comment, I believe that Yarbus (1967) in the USSR used extremely high-contrast stabilized objects and still found very rapid disappearance. In fact, he even stabilized the image of a lamp filament on the retina and found a disappearance time of something like 3 to 5 sec.

I am not sure that contrast is what is involved in that time difference. On the same topic, I'd like to say that is not the only problem of latency of disappearance we seem to have. Many people now tend to believe that lateral inhibitory feedback is responsible and the consequent loss of spiking in units is perhaps related to the disappearance of stabilized retinal images. However, the disappearance in activity in most of the units that are involved is much more rapid than the disappearance of the stabilized retinal images. I am less sure about the disappearance of brightness and color in the Ganzfield situation. If a subject looks at a homogeneous display where there are no contours to generate temporal changes on the retina as the eye moves, you would imagine that he would get some kind of fading similar to the fading of stabilized retinal images. This experiment does produce fading after what seems to be a very long period of time, perhaps as much as 30 sec. It seems to me that there are several phenomena that should be related to the time course of fading that don't seem to correspond very well under these circumstances.

E. MATIN: It is also interesting to note that in the case of saccadic suppression there is a phenomenon that you would think would be related to it, that is, the suppression of afterimages. And that has a time course which is of an entirely different order of magnitude. That is, it goes into seconds whereas the saccadic suppression which Dr. Volkmann and others have studied has a time course of the order of a few hundred milliseconds.

FARLEY: I wish to comment on Cornsweet's problem which, as I understand it, is how small movements of less than a degree can maintain an image that is much bigger than that. I propose that the perceptual input from the eye to the perceptual system is actually only an indication of the locations and features of discontinuity of stimulation on the retina.

The extent and types of features would differ with locations on the retina. Hubel and Wiesel (1968) have shown that the receptive field of primates seems to react to a stimulation surrounded by an area of no stimulation. In other words, a discontinuity in the field is created, causing the ganglion representing that receptive field to fire.

Actually, what is happening when you show a white disk is that you receive a white circle input with no discontinuity signal in the middle so you perceive that as a white disk. Then, from what we have heard thus far, it is clear that these discontinuities must themselves be discontinuously applied to the retina to create a new perceptual field activity.

Thus, when you have a small movement, you have actually completely translated that white circle on the retina and now you see the white circle again. Now consider the problem of a stabilized red circle around a stabilized white disk. If you move the red circle you have actually recreated the red circle, and since you have received no discontinuity signal from the inside of the circle you now perceive the whole thing as a red disk.

CORNSWEET: If you take that approach, and I certainly agree that that is going in the right direction, you have to account for the crucial data. It appears to be true that a disk, for example, when it is first turned on, looks the same as when it's been stabilized and disappeared and then shifted a little bit sideways.

I don't know whether those two things really look the same, but superficially they do. However, I can't think of a model that would give you the same excitation from the center of the disk under those two conditions. Something like what you are describing may be able to be developed to the point that it would say that, but you haven't been explicit enough to convince me.

FARLEY: I guess I am actually saying that there is no excitation occurring in the middle of that disk. You are getting a picture of a white contour with no discontinuity inside.

CORNSWEET: I hear you. Then you are committed to explaining why the sudden onset of light on a whole bunch of receptors in the center of the disk doesn't do anything. That's easy to explain if you have the right kind of inhibition. You are committed to explaining that the output is the same under those conditions as when shifting the edges.

Maybe you can do that, but it is not clear to me. You will have to do it in detail.

VOLKMANN: I apologize for closing this discussion so abruptly, but we must go on. We will next be concerned with the varieties of data and of theoretical positions available which examine the role of eye movements in the maintenance of a phenomonally clear and stable visual world.

II.4

Saccadic Suppression and the Stable World

Ethel Matin[1]

Columbia University

Earlier we discussed the causes of saccadic suppression. Now we are going to consider its function. Specifically, I want to comment on the relation between suppression and the fact that the visual (perceived) direction of an object doesn't change when the location of its image on the retina changes as a result of a voluntary saccade. Although there isn't much historical precedent for doing so, I'll refer to this latter phenomenon as the "constancy of visual direction." My purpose in so doing is to emphasize its formal similarity to such effects as color, size, and brightness constancy which also involve a more or less invariant relation between perception and the physical stimulus despite a change in the retinal stimulus.

The Extraretinal Signal and Saccadic Suppression: A Dual-Mechanism Approach to Direction Constancy

From the outset, let me say that it seems logically self evident that even a complete blanking out of vision during saccadic eye movements could not per se explain direction constancy. Unless some other mechanism were also operating, we would expect the world to appear displaced after the suppression ends. If it does not appear displaced, there is a change in the visual or perceived direction that is associated with a given retinal locus. I will refer to this change as a shift of the mapping of *retinal space into visual space*. This latter shift compensates, in effect, for the shift in the mapping of *physical space into retinal space* that results from the eye movement. Assume, for example, that a given object in the

---

[1] Now at C. W. Post College, Greenvale, N. Y.

environment stimulates the central fovea prior to a $2°$ saccade. After the saccade, this same object stimulates a retinal area $2°$ in the periphery. If no perceived displacement of the object occurs, it must be the case that the particular visual direction seen when the central fovea is stimulated before the saccade is seen when a stimulus is delivered $2°$ in the periphery after the saccade. This shift in the mapping of retinal space into perceived space is the essential fact to be explained, and, as I noted above, saccadic suppression cannot logically be the primary factor in the explanation.

Nonetheless, we have concluded that suppression plays an important, albeit secondary role, in maintaining direction constancy (Matin, 1972; Matin & Matin, 1972; Matin, 1974). Essentially, we have argued that the stable world is achieved through a dual mechanism.

First, an *extraretinal signal* (information about eye position or change in eye position other than that which can be derived from retinal stimulation) produces a shift in the mapping of retinal space into perceived space that is in the direction required to compensate for the movement of the eye.[2] This extraretinal compensation works reasonably well for the final ocular displacement. However, it is grossly imperfect for the information that impinges on the retina in the transient period shortly before, during, and shortly after the saccade, during much of which the eye is moving at very great and rapidly changing velocities.

The second aspect of the dual mechanism is saccadic suppression. This contributes to stability by preventing the perception of stimulation received in the transient period during which the extraretinal compensation is poor.

Given the earlier discussion about the magnitude of suppression (see the papers by Drs. Volkmann and Riggs), this conclusion may well be surprising. What seems to be required for our purpose is something close to a blanking out of the information received during a saccade, not a modest suppression of the order of .1–.5 log units. Note, however, that these estimates of the magnitude of suppression have come from studies designed specifically to determine if a suppression exists other than that which can be ascribed to saccadic retinal stimulation. (By the latter I mean the characteristic, very complex shifting of the retinal image that results from a saccadic eye movement, including the stimulation received in the immediate pre- and postsaccadic periods.) These studies have been designed, in effect, to determine if some extraretinal process is involved in suppression. In accordance with this purpose, experimenters have sought to minimize, if possible to eliminate, those suppression factors that are related to

---

[2] We use the noncommittal expression, extraretinal signal, to avoid any premature conclusions about the source of this information. This source might be related to, or corollary to, the motor discharge that initiates the eye movement. However, the evidence does not preclude other possibilities. Information about the extraretinal signal has been summarized in the references cited above; it is also considered in Part IV by Leonard Matin and Jordan Pola.

saccadic retinal stimulation. They have, for example, presented stimuli on relatively unstructured backgrounds. In addition, very brief flashes have been used to minimize the possibility that "blurring" could be causing the suppression that is being measured. However, when we make saccades under ordinary conditions of viewing and report that "things stay put," these factors are not eliminated, and a much larger amount of saccadic suppression can be expected— large enough, I think, to fulfill the functional role we are suggesting.

Saccadic Retinal Stimulation and Suppression

The fact that saccadic retinal stimulation plays a part in the suppression found under ordinary conditions of viewing has been recognized since this phenomenon was first described (Dodge, 1900, 1905; Woodworth, 1906, 1938). Woodworth, for example, reported that he obtained suppression when he held his eye still and moved his surroundings rapidly with a mirror. However, there has been very little experimental study of the effects of this complex stimulus. Indeed, there is a "flavor" to most of the literature, both classical and modern, which seems to suggest that suppression due to it is somehow trivial and unworthy of study in its own right. An example of this kind of thinking can be found in Dodge's criticism of the "central anesthesia" theory of suppression (Dodge, 1900, 1905). With his usual elegant prose and clear thinking, Dodge made an excellent beginning to the analysis of what I am herein calling saccadic retinal stimulation. In addition to recognizing the significance of "blur," he anticipated the suggestions by several recent authors that backward visual masking is a factor in the suppression effect (see Matin, 1974, for the relevant quotations from Dodge and for references to the recent literature). He closed his discussion, however, with the following comment: "I feel that these explanations rob the problem of most of its mystery, but I think they have some advantage in the direction of probability" (Dodge, 1905, p. 199).

With all due respect for this great scientist, I do not share this opinion. It seems to me that the saccadic retinal stimulation is itself a mysterious object and that Nature may well reward us with some delightful surprises if we explore it as such and do not regard it primarily as an artifact.

Needless to say, I have no quarrel with experiments that are concerned specifically with the relation between suppression and some extraretinal process. In such experiments, retinal stimulation quite obviously *is* an artifact and it's important to eliminate it. From a larger point of view, however, that "artifact" contains what are probably quantitatively the most powerful factors in the overall suppression effect. Some refocusing of our attention to recognize that fact explicitly is, I think, desirable. What, in fact, *are* the visual consequences when the retinal image leaves one location, is accelerated rapidly to very great speeds, and then comes to a screeching halt at a new location? What reductions can we make in the overwhelmingly complex stimulus situation that is "ordinary" viewing to permit an analysis of the various suppression factors that might be involved? What bridges can we find between suppression and the general psychology and physiology of the visual system that might give us some hints about how to proceed in the most fruitful way?

An example of such a bridge can be seen in the suggestions linking suppression to the psychological literature on visual masking. My co-workers and I had a hand in exploring this bridge in a study of suppression effects that we attributed to metacontrast masking (Matin, Clymer, & Matin, 1972). In this experiment, we illuminated a suprathreshold vertical slit of light on a dark background as the eye traversed the 1° position in the course of a 4° horizontal saccade. The time during which the slit was illuminated varied from trial to trial. On trials for which the slit was extinguished before the saccade ended, the saccadic retinal stimulation appeared simply as a horizontally extended smear, the length of which depended on the duration of the flash. On trials for which the flash extended sufficiently far into the period after the saccade, a sharp image was seen at one end of the smear. To this point, the results I've described are pretty much what we might have expected simply from the spatial distribution of light on the retina. However, on trials with flashes of still longer durations (i.e., with the slit illuminated well into the postsaccadic period), pronounced suppression of the saccadic smear was observed. To explain this suppression, we suggested that temporally backward and spatially lateral masking (metacontrast) occurs when the duration of the flash is long enough to permit the development of a mask through temporal integration of illumination in the postsaccadic period.

In the experiment I've just described, the saccadic retinal stimulation was severely reduced. Despite that fact, the observed suppression effects were very pronounced. Even larger backward masking effects could be expected, however, if the stimuli employed permitted "overlapping" effects (i.e., a mask that falls directly over the smear that is being suppressed, rather than lateral to it). To my knowledge, that case of backward masking has not yet been formally studied in the context of saccadic suppression.

Needless to say, there is no reason why the bridge that links suppression to masking should permit traffic in only one direction; while masking may help us to understand suppression, the converse could also be true. As an example of the possibilities here, we might note that the rapidly developing literature on backward masking contains almost no considerations about the functional significance of the phenomenon per se (as apart from its significance as an analytic tool in studying the temporal processing of visual information). Indeed, one author has even suggested that metacontrast is an inadvertent and undesirable by-product of lateral inhibitory mechanisms that function primarily in light adaptation and for the enhancement of contours (Bridgeman, 1971, p. 538). What I have said above, however, suggests a very different possibility: If metacontrast masking contributes to saccadic suppression, the neural "hardware" for it might well have developed in the evolutionary context of saccadic eye movements, i.e., rather than being an epiphenomenon relative to suppression, metacontrast might have evolved *because* of its survival value in producing saccadic suppression. This in turn suggests that masking, as it is ordinarily studied, is only a limiting (and limited) case of a more general process and that we should look to the images generated on the retina by the saccading eye for suggestions about how to broaden the class of stimuli that are studied in masking experiments.

To close this talk, I'd like to mention what I think might be another two-way bridge between suppression and general visual science. This one leads to the physiological literature, specifically to the recent intensive study at several levels in the visual nervous system, of cells that have been variously labelled X and Y (Enroth-Cugell & Robson, 1966) sustained and transient (Cleland, Dubin, & Levick, 1971), or type I and type II (Fukada, 1971). It has been suggested that the X (sustained) cells function primarily in the perception of form and contrast while the Y (transient) cells are specialized for the perception of movement (Fukada, 1971, among others).

At least some of the transient cells, however, have a property which suggests that they might be involved in saccadic suppression. This property is a sensitivity to stimuli moving at high velocities—more than 100°/sec (e.g., Cleland, Dubin, & Levick, 1971, p. 481). In the human observer, such velocities do not elicit the sensation of movement. They are, however, quite routinely generated on the retina during saccadic eye movements. Since we know that some of the cells in the Y group are able to detect this saccade-generated movement, it would be interesting to explore the possibility that these cells are involved in the suppression process, perhaps participating in the psychophysically studied masking phenomenon.

DISCUSSION

VOLKMANN: Is it your feeling then that saccadic suppression is mediated in fact by retinal stimulation during saccades?

E. MATIN: Largely, although not entirely. I'm persuaded by the research on this question, culminating in the study that Dr. Riggs described earlier, that something is involved in suppression other than saccadic retinal stimulation. Whether that other something is a corollary discharge, however, I think is still very much an open question.

VOLKMANN: I'd like to have Dr. Wurtz comment on this also.

WURTZ: I will comment on specific experiments on monkeys later but I could comment on the physiology which might be related to Professor Riggs' ingenious experiment. In experiments on cells in the monkey cortex I saw cells that gave very different responses following rapid-eye or -stimulus movements across a background from those following slow-stimulus movements. Recent experiments in cats suggest that the Y cells in the geniculate (loosely speaking, those with phasic discharge and higher conduction velocities) respond preferentially during eye movements made across a background. There is even the possibility that the Y cells are activated during eye movements across patterns, and the impulses from these cells arrive at the geniculate to inhibit the slower X-cell system. The relevance of these observations here is that when we stimulate the retina directly, cells that are not normally activated together are activated at the same time; the effect of ordered interactions of the visual system cells following visual stimulation might be nullified. Provided the phosphene is produced in the dark, what remains seems likely to be a good estimate of the extraretinal input. Since this remainder appears small to me, I am not at all sure that the effect would be easily seen using single-unit recording techniques.

E. MATIN: Dr. Wurtz, you have described cells in the striate cortex and the colliculus that respond to velocities of several hundred degrees per second. Could these cells be related to the Y cells of Enroth-Cugell and Robson (1966)?

WURTZ: Unfortunately, the X and Y system has not been clearly identified in the visual system of monkeys. There is some indication in the retinal ganglion cells that P. Gouras studied that showed it. An X and Y system may be present in the monkeys but at present our extrapolations to monkeys is generous. The X and Y concept is based mainly on experiments in cats with a little information from rat and rabbit.

E. MATIN: There is also a study in the goat, if I may just add another species.

WURTZ: And bring it closer to man.

E. MATIN: You are, I think, speaking about the cells Gouras (1969) has called "phasic" and "tonic"? I looked into that, hoping there would be information in the primate that would be useful to us. Since his experiments were done primarily with color theory in mind, however, I really wasn't sure. It seems, though, that his "phasic" cells might prove similar to the Y cells if investigated with appropriate stimuli.

WURTZ: It's possible. There are also cells in the cortex which could be placed in one category or the other. But the physiological designation of X and Y is much more exact than just categorization by response properties.

SENDERS: If I understood what you said earlier, you suggested that in the real world, as opposed to the laboratory, something to do with the complexity of the visual field might lead to complete saccadic suppression rather than the partial (half or two-tenths log unit) threshold elevation that is found in the laboratory.

In the days when aircraft had propellers, I spent many minutes observing the propellers of aircraft in flight by the simple expedient of making saccades and then choosing the radius at which I would direct my gaze. I found that not only could I see the propeller perfectly well, but also read the fine print on it when I was seated reasonably close.

This means that under these very complex visual circumstances there is not complete suppression. In fact, I remember once being rather concerned about the fact that I was reading an article about saccadic suppression while flying an airplane and looking at the propeller from time to time to amuse myself and convince myself that it wasn't quite true.

VOLKMANN: In fact, Prof. Senders, I think the situation you just mentioned is probably not at all like that encountered in the normal everyday average eye movement. Perhaps the reason you can see the fine print on the propeller is that you aren't getting smear on your retina from the propeller under those conditions. It is only the surround that is smeared.

SENDERS: Of course.

E. MATIN: You are, I think, saying that according to my earlier suggestions the background might be expected to suppress the "stabilized image" of the propeller through metacontrast masking. The fact that no masking occurred that was large enough to completely suppress your view of the propeller is really not surprising, though. Metacontrast is a highly form-specific phenomenon. Uttal (1970) has found, for example, that even relatively minor differences between the shape of a target and a mask can result in very significant decreases in masking. Under ordinary viewing conditions, each stimulus provides its own mask when a saccade occurs—and form specificity is more or less assured. That is not the case, however, in the situation you've described. The shapes in your background were presumably quite different from the shape of the propeller and we might expect masking effects, if any, to be minimal.

Afterthoughts

Since this paper was given, two articles have appeared in which some of the suggestions presented above are further elaborated (Matin, 1974, 1975).

II.5

Role of Eye Movements in Maintaining a Phenomenally Clear and Stable World[1]

Robert M. Steinman

University of Maryland

Five weeks ago I received a letter from Dr. Volkmann (whom I had not yet met at that time) asking me to address myself to the question of the role of eye movements in the maintenance of a phenomenally clear and stable world. That letter came as a shock. I am not sure that the answer to this question is known to God (Jones, 1966); perhaps only to Leon Festinger (Marquis, 1972). I had not yet met either of these distinguished persons and knew no one to whom I could turn. But after a few weeks of thinking about the question and discussing it with several young collaborators, who had both ideas and the energy to do new experiments, I am ready to attempt a tentative answer. Before answering, however, I must make a few observations about human eye movements—these observations have influenced the answer that I will give.

Perhaps the most striking aspect of human oculomotor performance is its independence from stimulus variables. By this I mean that a normal human adult can look about in his visual world and attend whatever region catches his fancy undisturbed by the distribution of light on his retina, or, in perceptual terms, the way the visual world looks at a particular moment.

[1] I thank my colleagues G. Haddad, E. Kowler, P. McGrath, B. Murphy, and B. Winterson for many valuable suggestions as well as their reassurances during the weeks of terror following receipt of the assigned topic.

This report and the research on human oculomotor performance were supported by Grant No. 00325 from the National Eye Institute. The research on head rotations was done in collaboration with David A. Robinson whose laboratory is supported by Grant No. 00598 from the National Eye Institute.

Such independence is very useful. It permits the human being considerable freedom in directing his attention to any region without regard to the color, brightness, shape, or motion of objects within it. The freedom we each have as individuals, however, makes problems for those of us who wish not only to use our eyes to look around, but who also try to model the oculomotor system—a system whose output is determined by a large variety of inputs, including many that are in the mind's eye and, therefore, rarely under control of the unsuspecting experimenter. The human oculomotor system is not entirely without constraints imposed by visual input, but I will reserve comment about what is constrained until after I have presented some support for what some of you may feel is a presumptuous declaration of oculomotor independence.

I got my first hint of such independence more than 10 years ago when I did my very first eye-movement experiment (Steinman, 1965). At the time it was disheartening. I had examined the effects of size, luminance, and color on characteristics of maintained fixation, hoping to induce oculomotor characteristics from the orderly variations one usually finds in the visual system when such variables are manipulated. Instead, I found that variations in the luminance, size, and color of the fixation target had statistically reliable but quite trivial effects on mean fixation position and stability—effects not larger than 3 or 4 min of arc.

Now, this result was a disappointment. It was also a disappointment abroad where it provoked considerable activity in R. W. Ditchburn's laboratory. First, Boyce (1967) reexamined the effects of luminance and color on fixation, confirming my results and extending the work over a larger range of stimulus values. Next, Rattle (1969) looked at the effects of the size of the stimulus display and also found "unexpected fixation stability" when subjects maintained the line of sight at the imagined center of targets as large as 240 min of arc.

Murphy, Haddad, and Steinman (1974), in the most recent extension of this line of work, found that the line of sight can be maintained anywhere within or at the edges of simple forms without any influence of the form on mean fixation position or stability. Here I will run through some of the data because it not only supports the notion of oculomotor independence, it also has bearing on topics that will be discussed in other sessions.

Figure 1 shows the variety of simple forms and fixation positions studied. The subject's task was to keep his line of sight on the specified positions within or on the boundary of each of these simple forms while his two-dimensional eye movements were recorded [see Haddad & Steinman (1973) for a description of the recording apparatus whose position sensitivity was about 3 sec arc as used in these experiments].

Fixation trials were run in blocks. First, the subject would be asked to place a point in one of the specified positions on or within one of the forms. He then fixated the point and started the trial. When he started the trial, the form would disappear and he would maintain fixation on the point for 5 sec. At the end of

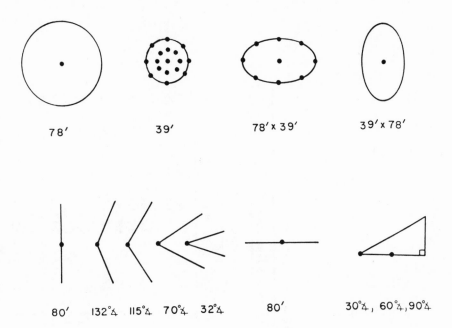

FIG. 1. The stimuli (shapes) and fixation positions (filled circles) used in the experiments on the fixation of forms. Each point represents one of the fixation positions studied. Subjects fixated either one of the specified regions within each of the forms or a small point in the same physical position in the absence of the form. (After Murphy et al., 1974.)

that time the trial ended, the form reappeared; he repositioned his eye on the point, and started the next trial. But this time the point disappeared and he maintained fixation at the specified position within or on the boundary of the form for 5 sec. Many such alternating trials were run for each position shown in Fig. 1.

The results of the experiment are shown in Tables 1, 2, and 3. Table 4 summarizes the main result for those who prefer prepackaged information.

I take these data to mean that, at least when the form is confined to the foveal floor [Polyak's (1941) designation], the oculomotor system is capable of maintaining the line of sight in whatever region a subject is required to fixate free from stimulus constraints. For those not impressed by standard deviations, I can say that the differences in mean fixation positions (constant errors) averaged only 3 min of arc and were not systematically related to the form or fixation position required. Human beings may have preferences to orient the line of sight to particular places within such forms, but these preferences are not imposed by oculomotor system control characteristics. This is contrary to a conclusion drawn by Kaufman and Richards (1969) a few years ago from the fixation behavior of naive subjects.

TABLE 1

Inverse Fixation Stability of Subject GH[a]

Stimulus conditions	Mean standard deviations, $\overline{SD}$ (min. arc)[b]						Trials[d]	
	On horizontal meridian			On vertical meridian				
	$\overline{SD}_F$	$\overline{SD}_P$	Δ^c	$\overline{SD}_F$	$\overline{SD}_P$	Δ^c	N_F	N_P
Circle (78') center	7.4 (.0)[e]	7.4 (.0)[e]	.0	6.1 (.0)[e]	6.1 (.0)[e]	.0	8	9
Circle (39') center	4.5 (1.4)	3.2 (.9)	1.3	3.0 (1.8)	3.0 (1.1)	.0	36	39
Edges:								
Horizontal	3.2 (.9)	3.4 (1.1)	−.2	2.8 (.5)	2.8 (.6)	.0	30	32
Vertical	3.6 (.9)	3.2 (.7)	.4	2.9 (.7)	3.1 (1.1)	−.2	29	30
Right oblique	3.5 (1.1)	3.3 (.7)	.2	3.3 (.9)	3.3 (.8)	.0	31	31
Left oblique	3.7 (1.2)	3.6 (1.3)	.1	3.4 (1.1)	3.1 (1.1)	.3	30	33
Halfway to edge:								
Horizontal	4.2 (1.5)	3.0 (.8)	1.2	3.2 (.9)	3.0 (.7)	.2	30	33
Vertical	3.9 (1.3)	2.9 (.5)	1.0	2.7 (.7)	2.7 (.6)	.0	29	31
Right oblique	3.7 (1.1)	3.2 (.5)	.5	3.8 (1.8)	3.7 (1.3)	.1	30	32
Left oblique	3.6 (1.4)	3.0 (.7)	.6	3.2 (1.1)	3.5 (.8)	−.3	29	33
Vertical ellipse (78' × 39') center	4.6 (1.5)	2.5 (.7)	2.1	3.2 (1.1)	3.1 (.8)	.1	31	31
Horizontal ellipse (39' × 78') center	5.6 (2.1)	3.2 (1.0)	2.4	2.2 (.6)	2.5 (.6)	−.3	29	30

Edges:								
Horizontal	4.0 (1.3)	3.5 (.8)	.5	2.7 (.8)	2.9 (.9)	-.2	33	35
Vertical	4.1 (1.4)	3.2 (.7)	.9	2.9 (.8)	2.9 (.6)	.0	30	30
Oblique	4.0 (1.6)	3.0 (1.4)	1.0	2.9 (.9)	2.9 (1.3)	.0	57	59
Horizontal line (78') center	5.4 (1.6)	3.5 (1.1)	1.9	3.0 (.7)	2.9 (.6)	.1	35	33
Vertical line (78') center	3.7 (.6)	4.1 (.8)	-.4	4.8 (1.1)	4.0 (1.0)	.8	31	33
Angle at vertex								
115°	5.1 (1.2)	4.4 (.9)	.7	4.4 (1.2)	3.9 (.7)	.5	36	36
70°	2.9 (.6)	2.6 (.6)	.3	2.0 (.4)	2.3 (.4)	-.3	32	32
32°	3.7 (1.4)	2.9 (.8)	.8	2.2 (.5)	2.6 (.8)	-.4	32	33
Triangle								
At 30° corner	3.7 (.8)	3.3 (.6)	.4	3.4 (1.0)	3.8 (.9)	-.4	30	30
Center of line between 30° and 90° angles	4.1 (1.7)	3.4 (.8)	.7	3.2 (1.0)	4.1 (1.2)	-.9	30	30

[a]Fixation maintained at selected positions within a variety of forms F or at a point P in the same physical position in the absence of the form.

[b]Inverse fixation stability is summarized as mean standard deviations $\overline{SD}$ in min. of arc on horizontal and vertical meridians.

[c]Differences $\Delta = \overline{SD}_F - \overline{SD}_P$.

[d]Number of trials run for form (N_F) and point (N_P).

[e]The standard deviations of the standard deviations are given in parentheses.

TABLE 2
Inverse Fixation Stability of Subject RS[a]

Stimulus conditions	Mean standard deviations, $\overline{SD}$ (min. arc)[b]						Trials[d]	
	On horizontal meridian			On vertical meridian				
	$\overline{SD}_F$	$\overline{SD}_P$	Δ^c	$\overline{SD}_F$	$\overline{SD}_P$	Δ^c	N_F	N_P
Circle (78') center	4.3 (1.3)	4.6 (1.3)	−.3	2.8 (.8)	3.3 (.9)	−.5	29	29
Circle (39') center	3.6 (1.3)	4.5 (1.7)	−.9	2.6 (1.1)	3.3 (1.1)	−.7	32	29
Edges:								
Horizontal	4.6 (2.0)	2.5 (.6)	2.1	4.7 (1.7)	3.4 (1.2)	1.3	31	33
Vertical	3.8 (.8)	4.2 (1.6)	−.4	2.8 (.8)	3.5 (1.2)	−.7	32	32
Right oblique	4.9 (1.9)	5.0 (2.0)	−.1	2.6 (.9)	3.7 (1.2)	−.3	35	31
Left oblique	4.2 (1.4)	4.2 (1.3)	.0	2.4 (.8)	3.5 (1.1)	−1.1	30	31
Halfway to edge:								
Horizontal	3.4 (1.5)	4.1 (1.9)	−.7	2.0 (1.5)	3.4 (1.3)	−1.4	30	31
Vertical	3.1 (1.1)	4.1 (1.6)	−1.0	2.3 (.8)	3.2 (1.2)	−.9	32	34
Right oblique	3.4 (1.5)	3.9 (1.7)	−.5	2.1 (1.5)	3.0 (1.1)	−.9	32	32
Left oblique	3.3 (1.2)	3.9 (1.3)	−.6	2.1 (1.2)	3.2 (1.1)	−1.1	31	31
Vertical ellipse (78' N 39') center	4.0 (1.1)	4.4 (1.6)	−.4	3.1 (1.2)	3.7 (.9)	−.6	31	31

Horizontal ellipse (39' × 78') center	4.3 (1.4)	4.3 (1.4)	.0	2.8 (0.6)	3.3 (.8)	−.5	36	42
Edges:							
Horizontal	4.4 (1.3)	5.0 (2.0)	−.6	3.0 (.8)	3.7 (1.4)	−.7	28	32
Vertical	4.2 (1.4)	5.0 (2.0)	−.8	3.1 (1.2)	4.1 (1.3)	−1.0	33	33
Oblique	4.3 (1.5)	5.4 (2.2)	−1.1	3.7 (1.5)	5.0 (1.6)	−1.3	57	47
Horizontal line (78') center	5.0 (1.6)	5.8 (2.6)	−.8	3.9 (.8)	5.6 (1.6)	−1.7	27	27
Vertical line (78') center	4.2 (1.4)	5.3 (2.1)	−1.1	3.9 (.9)	4.6 (1.4)	−.7	25	25
Angle at vertex							
132°	5.7 (1.7)	6.1 (2.2)	−.4	4.3 (1.2)	5.0 (1.2)	−.7	22	24
70°	4.7 (2.0)	4.8 (2.0)	−.1	3.4 (1.2)	3.9 (1.5)	−.5	27	28
32°	3.9 (0.8)	4.4 (1.1)	−.5	3.1 (.8)	3.3 (.8)	−.2	27	26
Triangle							
At 30° corner	4.5 (1.5)	5.1 (1.7)	−.6	2.8 (.7)	3.8 (.7)	−1.0	26	26
Center of line between 30° and 90° angles	3.7 (1.0)	4.5 (1.4)	−.7	2.6 (.5)	4.5 (1.2)	−1.9	25	25

[a]Fixation maintained at selected positions within a variety of forms F or at a point P in the same physical position in the absence of the form.

[b]Inverse fixation stability is summarized as mean standard deviations $\overline{SD}$ in min. of arc on horizontal and vertical meridians.

[c]Differences $\Delta = \overline{SD}_F - \overline{SD}_P$.

[d]Number of trials run for form (N_F) and point (N_P).

[e]The standard deviations of the standard deviations are given in parentheses.

TABLE 3

Inverse Fixation Stability of Subject RS[a]

| | Mean standard deviations, $\overline{SD}$ (min. arc)[b] | | | | | | Trials[d] | |
| | On horizontal meridian | | | On vertical meridian | | | | |
Stimulus conditions	$\overline{SD}_F$	$\overline{SD}_P$	Δ[c]	$\overline{SD}_F$	$\overline{SD}_P$	Δ[c]	N_F	N_P
Circle (78') center	2.8 (1.8)	3.2 (2.1)	−.3	2.4 (1.2)	2.1 (.7)	.3	27	27
Vertical ellipse (78' × 39') center	3.8 (1.9)	4.1 (2.0)	−.3	2.6 (1.0)	2.8 (1.7)	−.2	29	29
Horizontal ellipse (39' × 78') center	4.0 (1.7)	4.3 (2.2)	−.3	2.2 (.9)	2.2 (1.1)	.0	31	32
Edges:								
Horizontal	3.8 (2.1)	4.1 (2.3)	−.3	2.5 (1.4)	2.8 (1.7)	−.3	33	33
Vertical	4.0 (2.7)	4.0 (2.1)	.0	3.1 (1.8)	3.4 (2.6)	−.3	32	34
Oblique	4.2 (2.0)	3.6 (1.2)	.6	3.0 (1.5)	3.7 (2.0)	−.7	44	43
Horizontal line (78') center	4.2 (1.7)	3.9 (2.2)	.3	2.6 (1.1)	3.2 (2.1)	−.6	27	27
Vertical line (78') center	3.7 (2.1)	3.5 (2.1)	.2	3.0 (1.7)	2.7 (1.8)	.3	25	25
Angle at vertex								
132°	4.0 (2.2)	4.2 (2.1)	−.2	2.5 (1.0)	3.2 (1.4)	−.7	25	24
70°	4.8 (2.9)	4.9 (2.5)	−.1	3.0 (1.6)	2.7 (1.3)	.3	28	28
32°	3.0 (1.0)	3.1 (1.7)	−.1	2.3 (.7)	1.7 (.5)	.6	28	28
Triangle								
At 30° corner	3.8 (1.9)	2.6 (1.4)	1.2	1.8 (.6)	1.8 (.9)	.0	30	31
Center of line between 30° and 90° angles	2.6 (1.5)	2.8 (1.6)	−.2	1.7 (.7)	1.9 (1.5)	−.2	27	26

[a]Subject uses slow control exclusively to hold his eye at selected positions within a variety of forms F or at a point P in the same physical position in the absence of the form.

[b]Inverse fixation stability is summarized as mean standard deviations $\overline{SD}$ in min. of arc on horizontal and vertical meridians.

[c]Differences $\Delta = \overline{SD}_F - \overline{SD}_P$.

[d]Number of trials run for form (N_F) and point (N_P).

[e]The standard deviations of the standard deviations are given in parentheses.

128

TABLE 4
The Take Home Message

	Horizontal $\mid\overline{\Delta}\mid^a$ in min arc	Vertical $\mid\overline{\Delta}\mid^a$ in min arc	Number of trials
Subject GH	.80 (.65)	.23 (.25)	1463
Subject RS	.62 (.46)	.90 (.43)	1357

[a]Differences in fluctuations of the line of sight are less than 1 min of arc regardless of where or what you are fixating.

Subjects also have the option of maintaining the line of sight on an attended target without jumping about (making saccades). This is a long story and I will not attempt to review it in detail (see Steinman, Haddad, Skavenski, & Wyman, 1973) but the basic finding is summarized in Fig. 2. A typical fixation pattern is shown in the record on the left. The typical slow control pattern is shown at the right. The difference between the two conditions is simply a matter of instructions. The subject has been told not to make saccades in the record on the right. Standard deviations of eye position are typically only 2 to 3 min of arc under slow control and 4 to 6 min of arc during fixation. Saccades can be suppressed with a variety of targets, e.g̈., a point, a disk, a foveal annulus, and annulus in the periphery regardless of whether they are steadily illuminated or flickering (Haddad & Winterson, 1975). Slow control is best and saccade suppression easiest with a steadily illuminated foveal disk about .5° in diameter.

Subjects also can use these different oculomotor options while tracking a moving point. This is shown in Fig. 3. In the bottom record a subject is shown tracking a ramp stimulus with pure slow movement. In the top record the same subject is making many small saccades while tracking. The stimulus was the same in both cases, again only the instruction changed. There were no step-ramps or other engineering tricks. The subject was just told to do one thing or to do the other.

We have also found that subjects can adjust the velocity of their smooth pursuits to specified fractions of the velocity of the target as is shown in Fig. 4 and summarized in Fig. 5.

We also know that the subject has the option of not tracking as long as he looks at a stationary detail in the visual field. Robinson made reference to this option earlier. This option is illustrated in Fig. 6 which is taken from a recent series of experiments reported by Murphy and Kowler (1974) and by Murphy, Kowler, and Steinman (1975). The performance of two subjects is shown in Fig. 6: BW, running in her first eye-movement experiment without any prior tracking experience, and myself (RS). I have been doing this kind of thing for many

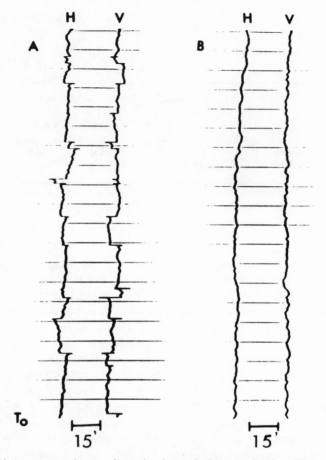

FIG. 2. (A) A representative two-dimensional record of human fixation. (B) A representative two-dimensional record of human slow control. Both records begin at the bottom (T_0); repetitive horizontal lines show 1-sec periods of time and the bars show 15 min of arc on both horizontal (H) and vertical (V) meridians. (After Steinman et al., 1973.)

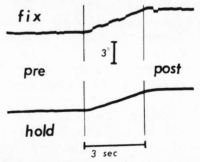

FIG. 3. Selected recordings for subject RS fixating (fix) and holding (hold) before (pre), during, and after (post) a constant velocity (60 min arc/sec) displacement of the target. The onset of target motion is shown by a thin dark line to the left of center in the figure and the end of target motion if shown by a similar dark line to the right of center. The target moved to the right on these trials (upward in the recorded trace). (After Puckett & Steinman, 1969.)

130

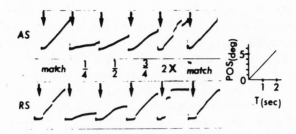

FIG. 4. Horizontal eye-movement recordings of the subjects AS and RS tracking a horizontal constant-velocity target moving at 172 min arc sec to the left (upward) through an angle of 6°. The record for each subject shows six consecutive trials run under the following sequence of instructions: on the first trial (shown at the left of the figure) subjects tried to match velocity with the target, on the subsequent four trials they tried to pursue at ¼, ½, ¾, or twice (2X) the velocity of the target. This sequence was followed by a final attempt to match the velocity of the eye to the velocity of the target. The arrows point to a faint dark line that marked the time of appearance of the moving target on the film. (After Steinman, Skavenski, & Sansbury, 1969.)

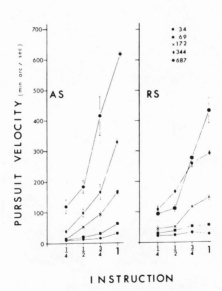

INSTRUCTION

FIG. 5. Mean smooth pursuit velocities for subjects AS and RS tracking constant-velocity targets under instructions to smoothly pursue at ¼, ½, ¾, or 1, the velocity of the moving target. The symbols in the upper right of the figure refer to velocities (min arc/sec) of the five targets used in this experiment. Error bars show one standard deviation above and below the mean pursuit velocity for those cases where variability exceeded the size of the symbols used to make this graph. (After Steinman et al., 1969.)

131

years. We both performed in the same way. The stimulus was a point of light seen superimposed on a high-contrast foveal square-wave grating (4° arc diam). The subject's instruction in the particular experiment illustrated in this figure was to use slow control to stay on the point while the grating moved to the left. The velocity of the grating was 5 min arc/sec, 48 min arc/sec, or 480 min arc/sec—a range that extends from a velocity near the normal drift of the eye with a stationary target up to a velocity that the engineers consider brisk enough to be a good input for smooth pursuit (Robinson, 1965). Figure 6 shows the average result. There was virtually no effect of the moving high-contrast grating on slow control. Smooth pursuit and slow control can be activated voluntarily. These subjects tracked these stimuli quite well once they were told to track rather than to stay in place.

Figure 7 summarizes one of the results of Wyman and Steinman (1973a). It shows that a subject can track very small target steps. I put this material in because Fuchs suggested that I would say something about such small voluntary movements. It seemed quite reasonable to do so since these tiny saccades are

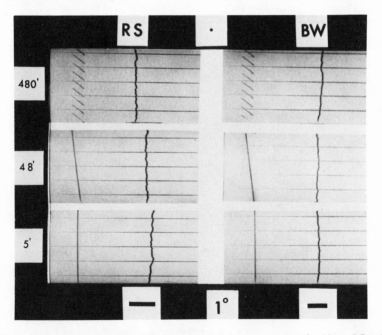

FIG. 6. Three representative records of horizontal eye movements of subjects RS and BW using slow control to maintain a steady line of sight on a stationary point superimposed on a leftward moving grating whose velocity was 5, 48, or 480 min arc/sec. Records are read from bottom to top. Horizontal lines are 1-sec time markers. The eye trace is at the right of each record. Grating velocity is proportional to the slope of the trace at the left of each record. The bar below each subject's records represents a 1° arc rotation. (After Murphy & Kowler, 1974.)

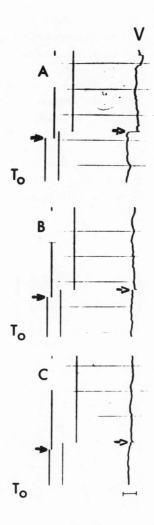

FIG. 7.   (A) A representative record of small-step tracking on the vertical (V) meridian. The
record begins at the bottom (T_0) and the filled black arrow points to the time a small point
target moved downward 15 min of arc. The open black arrow points to the saccade made to
follow the instantaneous displacement of the target. (B) A similar record of the saccade
made in response to a downward target step of 7 min of arc. (C) A similar record of the
saccade made in response to a downward step of 3.5 min of arc. Repetitive horizontal lines
in all records show 1-sec periods of time and the black bar at the bottom indicates 15 min of
arc. The event marker to the left of the eye position analog shows the operation of a trigger
that monitored the eye-position channel and stopped a timer that was started when the
target stepped, permitting us to measure the reaction time for small-step saccadic tracking.
(After Steinman *et al.*, 1973.)

among our many oculomotor options. Both Haddad and I did equally well in this kind of task despite the fact that at the time she was beginning in the eye-movement game and ran as a totally inexperienced subject. We both found this task easy, tracking 98–99% of unpredictable target steps that were 3.5 min of arc or larger.

Figure 8 shows that we could also make microsaccades down in the 5–6 min of arc ball park without any change in the position of the stimulus (Haddad & Steinman, 1973). The stimulus was a stationary point of light seen in an otherwise completely dark environment. When a tone sounded, the subject's task was to make the smallest possible saccade in a randomly chosen direction specified before the trial by the experimenter. We found that the smallest average voluntary saccade was the same size as the average fixation microsaccade (5.6′, S.D.<3) which shows that we have the option of looking away from a

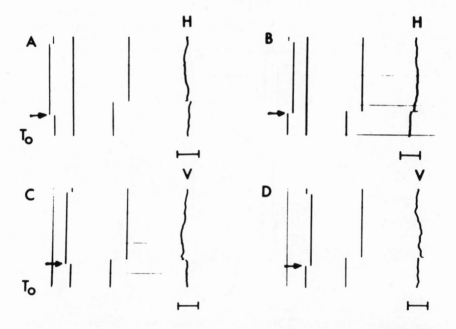

FIG. 8. (A) A record of the eye-movement pattern on the horizontal (H) meridian when the subject was asked to make one small voluntary saccade to the left while looking at a point that remained stationary throughout the trial. The record begins at the bottom (T_0). The black arrow indicates when an auditory signal told the subject to make his smallest possible saccade to the left. The eye-position trace shows that a small saccade was made to the left after the signal was given. The size of this small voluntary saccade can be estimated from the black bar (15 min of arc). The event marker to the left of the eye-position analog shows the operation of the trigger which stopped a reaction timer when the saccade was made. The other three records show small voluntary saccades made in the other directions: (B) to the right, (C) up, and (D) down. (After Steinman et al., 1973.)

stationary fixation point in any direction. We can do this with the same precision with which we can correct small eye-position errors produced by drifts of the eye or changes in the position of the fixation target.

Now let me say a word about constraints on the oculomotor system that otherwise seems to allow the human being to move his eye in any way that he pleases. First, it is well known that smooth pursuit without a moving target is extremely difficult. It is easy when a vivid afterimage is provided, as Robinson and Young have demonstrated at this symposium. But this exception, although very important in our understanding of the oculomotor system, requires a vivid afterimage which is rarely encountered in ordinary visual search. There is another constraint on what you can do with your eyeball. It is well known that it is hard to maintain eye position if there is no visual input. Skavenski & Steinman (1970) found that the line of sight can only be maintained within $\frac{3}{4}°$ over periods of 40 sec in the dark and only within 3° or 4° over 7.5-min periods (Skavenski, 1972). Your eye is also constrained by the luminance of the fixation target. Everything I have said about oculomotor independence applies only to the operation of the oculomotor system under photopic illumination. If targets are too feeble to be seen when they fall on the fovea, a good deal of voluntary control is lost and a maladaptive eye-movement pattern ensues. A feeble target, placed in the near periphery where it can be seen, will be returned to the central fovea where it disappears (Steinman & Cunitz, 1968).

Finally, I must emphasize that I have been talking about human oculomotor capacity, what an individual can do, not what he will choose to do if you flash a light at him or have something dance about in his visual world without telling him what you want him to do. Observing these capacities requires explicit instructions to the subject who does best when provided with feedback about his success. Once he is instructed and told how he is doing, a large degree of independence from stimulus variables and a wide range of oculomotor options can be demonstrated in ordinary adults.

Given such voluntary control of the way in which the eye can be moved or kept in place in the presence of a wide range of perturbations in the visual scene, all kinds of possibilities open up for using this motor skill for information processing. This motor skill is most highly developed in man where it is perhaps second only to control of the larynx in importance. This skill might be very significant for maintaining a phenomenally clear and perceptually stable environment. It could, in addition, provide a useful tool for the measurement of such things as distances and velocities in visual space.

However, recently I have come to doubt that the human oculomotor system is ever used, outside the laboratory, in the ways that I have described. My doubts were provoked by Winterson who insisted that I could not answer the question at issue without some idea of what the eye does when the head is not held rigidly in place on a bite board (the way we study small eye movements in the laboratory). So, having spent a good deal of time extolling free will and describing oculomotor options, I would like next to consider the conditions

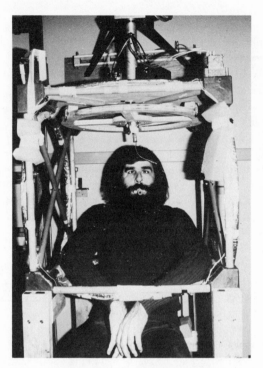

FIG. 9. Murphy in position for two-dimensional recording of rotations of his head by means of the magnetic-field search-coil technique. The head search coil is mounted on a dental bite plate. The field coils can be seen surrounding the subject.

under which man might be able to use these options when his head is not stabilized by artificial means.

Our first experiment on this problem is illustrated in Fig. 9. Figure 9 is not what it appears to be. It is not a photograph of a Druid sitting on an ancient Celtic throne, but rather Brian Murphy sitting comfortably in Robinson's magnetic-field search-coil recording apparatus. Clenched between his teeth is an acrylic bite board. Attached to the front of the acrylic bite board is a little coil of wire whose twisted lead is carried up above the head on the way to a phase-lock amplifier. Murphy is surrounded by large coils of wire that (by means of magic understood best by a small group of people who have worked with magnetic phonograph cartridges) make it possible to detect the orientation of the moving coil attached to his bite board with respect to the stationary magnetic field in which he is immersed. Murphy has been asked to be as still as possible for 40 sec while the rotational components of his head movements are recorded.[2] Let me emphasize that Murphy is committed, obviously very serious, and obviously relaxed. He is fully prepared to try to be as still as possible while

_____

[2] The head movement trials were 40 sec in length to conform with a suggestion by Ditchburn and Foley-Fisher (1967) who proposed that we all adopt 40 sec as the interna-

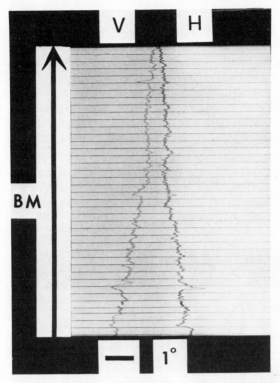

FIG. 10. A representative two-dimensional head-rotation record of the least stable subject. The record begins at the bottom and the repetitive horizontal lines indicate 1-sec periods of time. The bar beneath the record shows 1° arc rotation on both horizontal (H) and vertical (V) meridians.

he uses normal human postural supports to keep his head in place. Five subjects participated in this series of experiments. The typical performances of the worst and the best subjects are shown in Figs. 10 and 11.

We have not had time to do a power spectrum on these head-movement records but it is quite clear that there are appreciable oscillations at about 2–3 Hz that have a peak-to-peak amplitude of about 15 to 20 min of arc. There also seems to be a relatively large .2 to .4 Hz component and a large d-c component as well. These movements are very large in the worst subject (Fig. 10) but appreciable even in the best subject (Fig. 11) where we can also see rotations on

tional fixation duration. They hoped that we could develop some normative oculomotor data and ignore individual differences by standardizing conditions. I think that it would be better to find out why these differences are observed, but we used the recommended duration and formally propose that we all use 40-sec trials to study head rotation in the future. If we agree to do this, it might lead to an International Commission for the Evaluation of the Fixation Duration that could meet annually in Paris.

the horizontal meridian that probably reflect the human pulse. The pulselike
rotations occur about once each second and move the head through about 12
min of arc. We did not do the control experiment—stopping the heart to
guarantee that these rotations are really caused by the heartbeat. But regardless
of their origin they would produce appreciable displacements of the retinal
image of the fixation target as would the other rotations that seem to have
frequency characteristics like slow oculomotor control. They differ mainly by a
scale factor—the head rotating roughly through ten times the angle shown by the
eye when the head is supported on a bite board. Figures 10 and 11 show what
the head does when we try very hard to be still. Let me emphasize that these are
just rotations. I can say nothing about head translations at the moment. We have
not recorded them. They have only been measured once to my knowledge by
Findlay (1969) who did not measure translations with the head completely free.
He used a variety of bite boards and a chin rest.

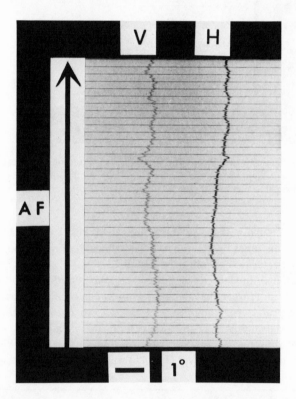

FIG. 11.   A representative two-dimensional head-rotation record of the most stable subject.
The record begins at the bottom and the repetitive horizontal lines indicate 1-sec periods of
time. The bar beneath the record shows 1° arc rotation on both horizontal (H) and vertical
(V) meridians.

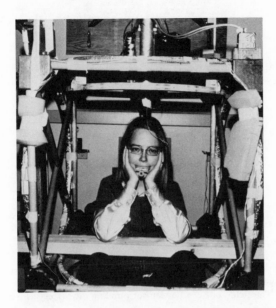

FIG. 12. Winterson in position for two-dimensional recording of rotations of her head by means of the magnetic-field search-coil technique. The head search coil is mounted on a dental bite plate. The field coils can be seen surrounding the subject who is using her hands to support her head.

Next, an attempt was made to see whether our subjects could improve matters by using special but natural supports to hold the head in place. How this was done is shown in Figs. 12 and 13 where you can see Winterson (who got this whole thing going) holding her head while its rotations are recorded. This kind of posture is natural and frequently used outside the laboratory. It is, however, subject to individual differences as can be seen in Fig. 13 which shows Kowler ready to run. The results of this experiment with a stabilized head are shown, once again, for the worst and the best subjects in Figs. 14 and 15.

We are beginning to get something resembling a stable platform—the d-c level shift is much reduced but there is still a large low-frequency a-c component. This proved to be caused by breathing as can be seen in Figs. 16 and 17 which show the best and the worst performances when the head was supported and the breath held.[3]

[3] I call the reader's attention to a new biological phenomenon in the horizontal trace in the 12th second in Fig. 14. I call such small high-velocity rotations of the head "head" flicks. Another example can be seen in the horizontal trace in the 32nd second of Fig. 17. These are not electrical artifacts. Skavenski (private communication) subsequently observed such head flicks in his laboratory. I cannot imagine what the significance of these strange movements might be but I call them to your attention because they are seen from time to time in the records of all the subjects.

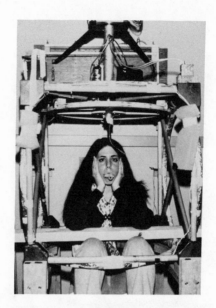

FIG. 13. Kowler in position for two-dimensional recording of rotations of her head by means of the magnetic-field search-coil technique. The head search coil is mounted on a dental bite plate. The field coils can be seen surrounding the subject who is using her hands to support her head.

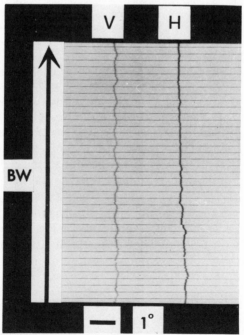

FIG. 14. A representative two-dimensional head-rotation recording of the least stable subject when the head was supported. The record begins at the bottom and the repetitive horizontal lines indicate 1-sec periods of time. The bar beneath the record shows 1° arc rotation on both horizontal (H) and vertical (V) meridians.

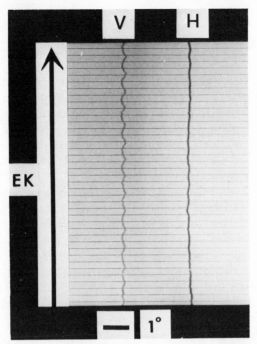

FIG. 15. A representative two-dimensional head-rotation recording of the most stable subject when the head was supported. The record begins at the bottom and the repetitive horizontal lines indicate 1-sec periods of time. The bar beneath the record shows 1° arc rotation on both horizontal (H) and vertical (V) meridians.

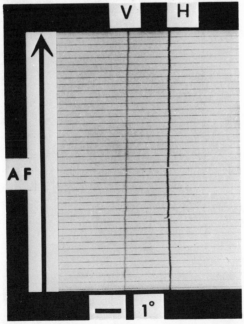

FIG. 16. A representative two-dimensional head-rotation recording of the least stable subject when the head was supported and the breath held. The record begins at the bottom and the repetitive horizontal lines indicate 1-sec periods of time. The bar beneath the record shows 1° arc rotation on both horizontal (H) and vertical (V) meridians.

141

Holding the breath while supporting the head can be helpful, but not always. The worst subject (Fig. 17) showed a systematic drift that became very large by the end of the 40-sec trial. It looks as though he is about to keel over by the end of the trial. This kind of stressful experiment should probably not be undertaken by emphysemic middle-aged men regardless of their scientific dedication. The subject is shown (at the beginning of the trial) in Fig. 18 and the results of these experiments are summarized in Table 5.

In conclusion, I still believe that the human oculomotor system is largely free from stimulus constraints. This is a very nice thing. It allows you to pick, and choose, and operate on visual input in any manner that seems suitable to the task at hand. However, these options may only be available after you stabilize your head and hold your breath. Of course, we may find that the vestibuloocular reflex is effective enough to provide the stable platform that would allow the oculomotor options that we have noted when the head is stabilized on a bite board. I do not believe that this is known, which has encouraged us to prepare to do simultaneous recordings of eye and head movements.

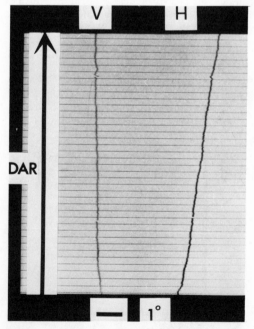

FIG. 17. A representative two-dimensional head rotation recording of the most stable subject when the head was supported and the breath held. The record begins at the bottom and the repetitive horizontal lines indicate 1-sec periods of time. The bar beneath the record shows 1° arc rotation on both horizontal (H) and vertical (V) meridians.

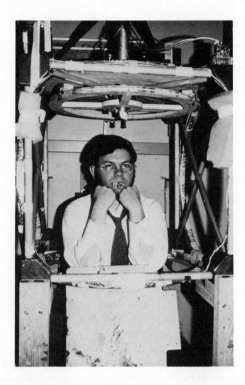

FIG. 18. Robinson in position for two-dimensional recording of rotations of his head by means of the magnetic-field search-coil technique. The head search coil is mounted on a dental bite plate. The field coils can be seen surrounding the subject who is using his hands to support his head.

As matters now stand, I must end on a note of gloom. I think there is a very good possibility that our oculomotor system is completely committed to and very busy compensating for movements of our bodies. Whether this system has any time left to do other things remains to be seen. My answer, then, to the question posed by our Chairperson is that eye movements are essential to maintaining a phenomenally clear and stable world. They serve to stabilize image motion produced by our normal bodily activities. It seems unlikely to me that the eye moves to keep images from fading because of stabilization.[4] Of great

[4]We now have good reason to believe that the eye moves to stabilize retinal image motion produced by normal bodily movements. The gain of the slow compensatory oculomotor subsystem does not exceed .8–.9 over the frequency range of .1–10 Hz when both vestibular and visual imputs are provided. This means that there is a great deal of retinal image motion when the head is not supported on a bite board. Now we must find out why the visual world looks stable and why visual acuity is excellent in everyday life. See Steinman (1975) and Winterson *et al.* (1975) for details of our experiments that report characteristics the "Minivor" (the miniature vestibuloocular response) and "natural" retinal image motion.

TABLE 5
Mean Error and Inverse Head Stability for
Five Subjects

Subject	Error (min. arc)	Inverse head stability[b] SD (min. arc)		Bivariate area (min. arc)^2
		H	V	
		Naturally^c		
AF	25 (10)^e	9 (3.6)^e	10 (2.9)^e	530 (206.9)^e
EK	41 (23)	8 (1.8)	19 (5.6)	802 (229.4)
BM	80 (26)	18 (8.2)	20 (7.3)	1407 (428.0)
DR	89 (16)	22 (8.3)	29 (16)	2271 (971.9)
BW	86 (29)	24 (9.3)	21 (9.5)	2003 (924.2)
Mean	64 (29)	16 (7)	20 (7)	1403 (748)
		Supported, breath held^d		
AF	18 (7)	3 (.1)	7 (1.6)	90 (50.0)
EK	19 (8)	6 (3.8)	4 (2.5)	186 (216.6)
BM	30 (18)	9 (4.8)	8 (3.5)	338 (182.2)
DR	63 (25)	18 (9.4)	9 (6.3)	340 (215.6)
BW	37 (22)	7 (3.5)	12 (6.9)	262 (146.1)
Mean	33 (18)	9 (6)	8 (3)	243 (107)
Noise^f	0	4	.4	1.4

[a]Absolute distance between median head position during the first 5 sec of a trial and median head position during the last 5 sec.
[b]Mean bivariate contour ellipse areas and mean standard deviations SD.
[c]Maintaining head position naturally.
[d]Head was supported by the arm and hand for 40 sec. while the breath was held.
[e]Standard deviations are given in parentheses.
[f]The noise level of the recording and digitizing apparatus.

interest is a report by a physician whose vestibular mechanism became effectively functionally destroyed through clinically administered streptomycin. He reports (C., 1952) that even the pulse beat in his head while reading made the letters on a page jump and blur, and that walking destroyed his ability to read signs and recognize faces. The loss of the vestibulooculomotor control system apparently led to a wide range of bizarre and distressing experiences. I recommend the article for those who would like a naturalistic view of the real meaning of the vestibuloocular control system.

However, since much of this symposium is devoted to the role of the oculomotor system in human perception and cognitive processes, I close by reassuring you that there are circumstances during which the head is stabilized and there is no pulse or breath—circumstances in which a human being may be able to tap the wide range of oculomotor skills he has evolved. This is shown in Fig. 19.

DISCUSSION

FUCHS: You said that for the small target steps of 6 min of arc or so that 98 to 99% of the microsaccades were in the right direction. Were they also the right size?

STEINMAN: Their accuracy depends on the subject, the direction, and the experiment. For example, Haddad typically tracks target steps that go to the left

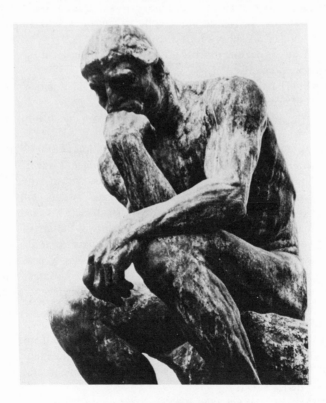

FIG. 19. Rodin's Thinker.

with a burst of 3 to 5 saccades. This is true even when the steps are as small as 6.9'. In all other directions Haddad tends to follow a target step with a single saccade that is reasonably accurate. I tend to make a single saccade that ends near the new target position. [See Wyman & Steinman (1973a) for the details of this work.] However, in a prior experiment (Timberlake, Wyman, Skavenski, & Steinman, 1972) both Skavenski and I went only half way to the target position when the target stepped from 5' to 180'. We had no idea that we were doing this while the data were collected. I suspect that for some mysterious reason we both decided that overshooting was a bad thing and erred in the other direction just to be sure that we did not go too far. People show similar quirks when they play tennis or golf, which requires quite similar motor skills.

In my opinion the only way to find out about the actual accuracy and precision of saccades is to give the subject feedback about the size of his off-set error and run him until performance is asymptotic. This should make it possible to estimate the limits of the high-velocity subsystem's operation. Until now we and everyone else have been studying various individuals' styles and preferences when they use saccades to reduce position errors in a particular experiment. I know of no data on saccade accuracy collected in an experiment designed to measure the limits of the subsystem's performance.

FUCHS: In all those microsaccades, an overshoot made up a considerable portion of the response.

STEINMAN: That is my characteristic response. Haddad and Winterson, for example, do not usually show such overshoots.

BROWN: Why, do you think, was Rashbass (1961) unable to show these microsaccades?

STEINMAN: I do not know the answer to the question. Rashbass' result never made any sense to me or to Cornsweet or Nachmias when it was first published. Nachmias showed me his correspondence with Rashbass in which Nachmias asked Rashbass how he reconciled his "dead zone" results with Nachmias' (1959) and Cornsweet's (1956) finding that very small saccades can be corrective during maintained fixation. Rashbass could not answer the question. I cannot answer the counterquestion. Our result, unlike Rashbass', is at least consistent with other well-known aspects of the use of microsaccades. I have run in many tracking experiments and I am convinced that if I can see a target move, I can track it. I am as certain of this as I am certain that if an engineer sees something move, he will model it.

HALLETT: Do you have to follow small steps?

STEINMAN: No. It is very easy to see steps and to ignore them. You do not have to follow them. Saccades are used voluntarily—at least in adults.

HALLETT: There could be variations in different people's data, then, of the sort observed by Rashbass.

STEINMAN: Yes, I think that Rashbass' instruction to track may not have been explicit enough. Alternatively, Rashbass' subjects may not have been able to see small target steps for one reason or another. I do not think that this was the case and suspect that the difference in our results was due to instructional or motivational factors.

CORNSWEET: There is another possible explanation of Rashbass' results. If a target steps to the right, stays there a second or so, and then returns, a subject will usually follow it, but if it repeats that pattern a few times, many subjects, and maybe all of them, stop responding. They just keep looking at the original location of the target.

STEINMAN: But I do not see how this explains the difference between Rashbass' and Wyman's results because unpredictable target steps were used in both experiments.

CORNSWEET: Even if the time of occurrence and the size of the step are unpredictable, the subject will fail to respond if the target always returns to its original position at the end of the step. I have been a subject in this situation, and, although I am not really aware of it during the experiment, it is as if I just keep looking at the place where the target used to be because I know it will be coming back there sooner or later. Sometimes the brain that is hooked up to the eyes messes up our neat system models.

YOUNG: Did you say how long you waited for this corrective miniature saccade?

STEINMAN: A short time. Average latencies ranged from 400 to 200 msec as steps ranged from 3.5 to 28.4 min arc (Wyman & Steinman, 1973b). Rashbass reproduced a record to show his "dead zone" in which no saccade was observed in about 800 msec. We waited half as long and got consistent saccadic tracking of very tiny steps.

YOUNG: I was looking up some old records we had taken on the probability of a corrective saccade as a function of target step size and latency. For our longest allowable interval, 750 msec, the probability of a corrective saccade decreased from over .9 for large steps (50 min arc) down to .4 for the smallest steps we used (5 min arc).

STEINMAN: Rashbass reported "no responding with quarter- to half-degree" steps after a wait of 800 or so msec. No quantitative treatment of the results is presented in his paper, however, which makes it difficult to know precisely what he found.

YOUNG: We found a probability of a corrective saccade which decreases monotonically with step sizes below about $\frac{1}{2}°$. For the shortest allowable interval (250 msec) and smallest target step (5 min arc), the probability of a corrective saccade was down to less that .2 (Young, 1971).

STEINMAN: In our experiment both the experienced subject and the inexperienced subject tracked on 98–99% of the trials. The latency depended on the step size, but even 3.4-min steps were tracked in 400 msec.

YOUNG: In our experiments, in which subjects were not specifically instructed to attempt corrective saccades, we did not get those high probabilities.

STEINMAN: I do not think this issue can be resolved by counting up experiments for or against dead zones. Let me explain by saying something that may seem outrageous to some of you. I am not an engineer and had no commitment to a saccadic dead zone (which seems to be useful in modeling certain kinds of servosystems) when I ran in the tracking experiments. In fact, I had quite the opposite expectation based on my work on fixation of stationary targets. I also knew, however, that I could perform as though the oculomotor system does have a saccadic dead zone by deliberately ignoring fixation errors. I could have used this strategy in the tracking experiment and obtained data that supported the dead-zone notion quite easily, or I could have run naive subjects and seen what they would do. However, I do not think that this strategy is useful in developing models of the oculomotor machinery. The dead-zone notion implies that the oculomotor system *cannot* do something. If it can be shown that the oculomotor system can, in fact, do it, models that use the notion must be prepared to put the dead zone in a decision process box and not somewhere deep down in the oculomotor machinery. This, of course, may leave you (as it does me) with the feeling that it may be hard to use the model to make predictions about performance without telling the subject precisely what you want him to do.

Afterthoughts[5] YOUNG: I think that you misinterpret the system's ideas. The "dead zone" is a system function—not sensory or motor. If the system, subject to instructions and needs for extracting visual information, is *indifferent* to the target location on the fovea, then there is a functional dead zone. The fact that under different instructions (e.g., "move your eyes to fixate") there are smaller saccades indicates that the functional dead zone seen in normal tracking is not based on any hard sensor or motor resolution limit.

STEINMAN: It is my impression that Rashbass interpreted his results as a hard-wired limit and not simply a performance characteristic of his subjects. It is this interpretation that I have been discussing. Wyman and Steinman (1973a) have discussed this as well as other interpretations of the dead zone in some detail elsewhere.

SENDERS: I find myself frustrated by the fact that although the expressed subject of the session was the phenomenon of the apparently clear and stable visual world, we have heard only about its stability and nothing about its clarity. To me the world, whether it be the external visual world of things, people, landscapes, or the world of the printed page, appears subjectively to be all there, all clear and not subject to the degraded image quality which we know must exist for objects seen far from the point of regard. The experiments on reading show that what is *seen* is only a very small part of what there is. That is to say, as will be described later, one can alter drastically the form and the content of

[5] Conferees were invited to submit additional thoughts after the conference. Some of these follow.

words only a few degrees removed from the point of regard without interfering in any way with the reading process. I imagine that under these conditions the printed page looks whole and stable. When I look at a page, I think I see all the words on it and when I look at the world I have the illusion that even those parts of it in my periphery are clear. It is only when I artificially constrain my eye to stop moving that this clarity fades and the true fuzzy quality of visual space becomes apparent. The clarity in both cases is in the head. Presumably, the saccades and fixations of normal vision, that we make when we are not constrained in the laboratory, are designed to fill in this picture and make it whole and thus preserve the illusion. Perhaps at some future meeting we'll know more about this question.

II.6

References

Alpern, M. Movements of the eyes. In H. Davson (Ed.), *The eye.* Vol. 3. New York: Academic Press, 1969.

Beeler, G. W., Jr. Visual threshold changes resulting from spontaneous saccadic eye movements. *Vision Research,* 1967, 7, 769–775.

Boyce, P. R. The effect of change of target field luminance and colour on fixation eye movements. *Optica Acta,* 1967, **14**, 213–217.

Bridgeman, B. Metacontrast and lateral inhibition. *Psychological Review,* 1971, **78**, 528–539.

Brooks, B. A., & Fuchs, A. F. Influence of stimulus parameters on visual sensitivity during saccadic eye movement. In preparation.

C., J. Living without a balancing mechanism. *The New England Journal of Medicine,* 1952, **246**, 458–460.

Chase, R., & Kalil, R. E. Suppression of visual evoked responses to flashes and pattern shifts during voluntary saccades. *Vision Research,* 1972, **12**, 215–220.

Cleland, B., Dubin, M., & Levick, W. Sustained and transient neurones in the cat's retina and lateral geniculate nucleus. *Journal of Physiology,* 1971, **217**, 473–496.

Cornsweet, T. N. Determination of the stimuli for involuntary drifts and saccadic eye movements. *Journal of the Optical Society of America,* 1956, **46**, 987–993.

Davidson, M. L., Fox, M. J. & Dick, A. O. Effect of eye movements on backward masking and perceived location. *Perception and Psychophysics,* 1973, **14**, 110–116.

Davidson, M. L., & Whiteside, J. A. Human brightness perception near sharp contours. *Journal of the Optical Society of America,* 1971, **61**, 536–538.

Ditchburn, R. W. Eye-movements in relation to retinal action. *Optica Acta,* 1955, **I**, 171–176.

Ditchburn, R. W., & Foley-Fisher, J. A. Assembled data in eye movements. *Optica Acta,* 1967, **14**, 113–118.

Dodge, R. Visual perception during eye movement. *Psychological Review,* 1900, **7**, 454–465.

Dodge, R. The illusion of clear vision during eye movement. *Psychological Bulletin,* 1905, **2**, 193–199.

Duffy, F. H., & Lombroso, C. T. Electrophysiological evidence for visual suppression prior to the onset of a voluntary saccadic eye movement. *Nature* (London), 1968, **218**, 1074–1075.

Enroth-Cugell, C., & Robson, J. G. The contrast sensitivity of retinal ganglion cells of the cat. *Journal of Physiology*, 1966, **187**, 517–552.

Fender, D. H., & Nye, P. W. The effects of retinal image motion in simple pattern recognition task. *Kybernetik*, 1962, **1**, 192–199.

Findlay, J. M. The magnitude of translational head movements. *Optica Acta*, 1969, **16**, 65–68.

Fukada, Y. Receptive field organization of cat optic nerve fibers with special reference to conduction velocity. *Vision Research*, 1971, **11**, 209–226.

Gerrits, H. J. M., & Vendrik, A. J. H. The influence of stimulus movements on perception in parafoveal stabilized vision. *Vision Research*, 1974, **14**, 175–180.

Gouras, P. Antidromic responses of orthodromically identified ganglion cells in monkey retina. *Journal of Physiology*, 1969, **204**, 407–419.

Gross, E. G., Vaughan, H. G., & Valenstein, E. Inhibition of visual evoked responses to pattern stimuli during voluntary eye movements. *Electroencephalography and Clinical Neurophysiology*, 1967, **22**, 204–209.

Haddad, G. M., & Steinman, R. M. The smallest voluntary saccade: Implications for fixation. *Vision Research*, 1973, **13**, 1075–1086.

Haddad, G. M., & Winterson, B. J. Effect of flicker on oculomotor performance. In P. Bach y Rita & G. Lennerstrand (Eds.), *Basic mechanisms of ocular motility and their clinical implications*. London: Pergamon, 1975.

Hallett, P. E. Rod increment thresholds on steady and flashed backgrounds. *Journal of Physiology*, 1969, **202**, 355–377.

Holt, E. B. Eye-movement and central anaesthesia. I. The problem of anaesthesia during eye-movement. *Psychological Monographs*, 1903, **4**, 3–46.

Hubel, D. H., & Wiesel, T. N. Receptive fields and functional architecture of monkey striate cortex. *Journal of Physiology* 1968, **195**, 215–243.

Jones, A. (Ed.). *The Jerusalem Bible*. New York: Doubleday, 1966. Genesis 2:5–10.

Kaufman, L., & Richards, W. Spontaneous fixation tendencies for visual forms. *Perception and Psychophysics*, 1969, **5**, 85–88.

Keesey, U. Tulunay. Effects of eye movements on visual acuity. *Journal of the Optical Society of America*, 1960, **50**, 769–774.

Keesey, U. Tulunay, & Riggs, L. Visibility of Mach bands with imposed motions of the retinal image. *Journal of the Optical Society of America*, 1962, **52**, 719–720.

Krauskopf, J., Graf, V., & Gaarder, K. Lack of inhibition during involuntary saccades. *American Journal of Psychology*, 1966, **79**, 73–78.

Latour, P. L. Visual threshold during eye movements. *Vision Research*, 1962, **2**, 261–262.

Latour, P. L. *Cortical control of eye movements*. Unpublished doctoral thesis, Institute for Perception RVO-TNO, Soesterberg, The Netherlands, 1966.

Lederberg, V. Color recognition during voluntary saccades. *Journal of the Optical Society of America*, 1970, **60**, 835–842.

MacKay, D. M. Elevation of visual threshold by displacement of retinal image. *Nature* (London), 1970, **225**, 90–92.

Marquis' *Who's Who in America* (37th ed., Vol. 1). Chicago: Marquis, 1972. p. 992.

Matin, E. Saccadic suppression: A review and an analysis. *Psychological Bulletin*, 1974, **81** 899–917.

Matin, E. The two-transient (masking) paradigm. *Psychological Review*, 1975, **82**, 451–461.

Matin, E., Clymer, A., & Matin, L. Metacontrast and saccadic expression. *Science*, 1972, **178**, 179–182.

Matin, E., Matin, L., Pola, J., & Kowal, K. The intermittent light illusion and constancy of visual direction during voluntary saccades. Paper presented at the meeting of the Psychonomic Society, St. Louis, 1969.

Matin, L. Eye movements and perceived visual direction. In D. Jameson & L. Hurvich (Eds.), *Handbook of sensory physiology* (Vol. 7, Pt. 4: *Visual Psychophysics*). New York: Academic Press, 1972.

Matin, L., & Matin, E. Visual perception of direction and voluntary saccadic eye movements. *Bibliotheca Ophthalmologica,* 1972, **82**, 358–368. (Also printed as a chapter in J. Dichgans & E. Buzzi (Eds.), *Cerebral control of eye movements and motion perception.* Basel: Karger, 1972.)

Michael, J. A., & Stark, L. Electrophysiological correlates of saccadic suppression. *Experimental Neurology,* 1967, **17**, 233–246.

Mitrani, L., Mateeff, St., & Yakimoff, N. Smearing of the retinal image during voluntary saccadic eye movements. *Vision Research,* 1970, **10**, 405–409. (a)

Mitrani, L., Mateeff, St., & Yakimoff, N. Temporal and spatial characteristics of visual suppression during voluntary saccadic eye movement. *Vision Research,* 1970, **10**, 417–422. (b)

Mitrani, L., Mateeff, St., & Yakimoff, N. Is saccadic suppression really saccadic? *Vision Research,* 1971, **11**, 1157–1161.

Mitrani, L., Yakimoff, N., & Mateeff, St. Dependence of visual suppression on the angular size of voluntary saccadic eye movements. *Vision Research,* 1970, **10**, 411–415.

Murphy, B. J., Haddad, G. M., & Steinman, R. M. Simple forms and fluctuations from the line of sight. *Perception and Psychophysics,* 1974, **16**, 557–563.

Murphy, B., & Kowler, E. To pursue or not to pursue. . . Paper presented at the Association for Research on Vision and Ophthalmology, Sarasota, Florida, May 1974.

Murphy, B. J., Kowler, E., & Steinman, R. M. Slow oculomotor control in the presence of moving backgrounds. *Vision Research,* 1975, **15**, 1263–1268.

Nachmias, J. Two-dimensional motion of the retinal image during monocular fixation. *Journal of the Optical Society of America,* 1959, **49**, 901–908.

Novak, S. The effect of electrocutaneous digital stimulation on the detection of single and double flashes of light. *Psychological Monographs,* 1965, **79**, 1–19 (Whole No. 608).

Polyak, S. L. *The retina.* Chicago: University of Chicago Press, 1941.

Puckett, J. deW., & Steinman, R. M. Tracking eye movements with and without saccadic correction. *Vision Research,* 1969, **9**, 695–703.

Rashbass, C. The relationship between saccadic and smooth tracking eye movements. *Journal of Physiology,* 1961, **159**, 326–338.

Ratliff, F. The role of physiological nystagmus in visual acuity. *Journal of Experimental Psychology,* 1952, **43**, 163–172.

Rattle, J. D. Effect of target size on monocular fixation. *Optica Acta,* 1969, **16**, 183–192.

Richards, W. Visual suppression during passive eye movement. *Journal of the Optical Society of America,* 1968, **58**, 1559.

Richards, W. Saccadic suppression. *Journal of the Optical Society of America,* 1969, **59**, 617–623.

Riggs, L. A., & Johnstone, J. R. Saccadic suppression and retinal image displacement. In preparation.

Riggs, L. A., Merton, P. A., & Morton, H. B. Suppression of visual phosphenes during saccadic eye movements. *Vision Research,* 1974, **14**, 997–1011.

Riggs, L. A., & Ratliff, F. Visual acuity and the normal tremor of the eye. *Science,* 1951, **114**, 17–18.

Riggs, L. A., Ratliff, F., Cornsweet, J. C., & Cornsweet, T. N. The disappearance of steadily fixated visual test objects. *Journal of the Optical Society of America,* 1953, **43**, 495–501.

Riggs, L. A., & Tulunay, U. Visual effects of varying the extent of compensation for eye movements. *Journal of the Optical Society of America,* 1959, **49**, 741–745.

Robinson, D. A. The mechanics of human smooth pursuit eye movement. *Journal of Physiology,* 1965, **180**, 569–591.

Schiller, P. Von Die Rauhigkeit als intermodale Erscheinung. *Zeitschrift für Psychologie,* 1932, **127**, 265.

Skavenski, A. A. Inflow as a source of extraretinal eye position information. *Vision Research,* 1972, **12**, 221–229.

Skavenski, A. A., & Steinman, R. M. Control of eye position in the dark. *Vision Research,* 1970, **10**, 193–203.

Starr, A., Angel, R., & Yeates, H. Visual suppression during smooth following and saccadic eye movements. *Vision Research,* 1969, **9**, 195–197.

Steinman, R. M. Effect of target size, luminance, and color on monocular fixation. *Journal of the Optical Society of America,* 1965, **55**, 1158–1165.

Steinman, R. M. Oculomotor effects. In P. Bach-y-Rita & G. Lennerstrand (Eds.), *Basic mechanisms of ocular motility and their clinical implications.* London: Pergamon, 1975.

Steinman, R. M., & Cunitz, R. J. Fixation of targets near the absolute foveal threshold. *Vision Research,* 1968, **8**, 277–286.

Steinman, R. M., Haddad, G. M., Skavenski, A. A., & Wyman, D. Miniature eye movement. *Science,* 1973, **181**, 810–819.

Steinman, R. M., Skavenski, A. A., & Sansbury, R. V. Voluntary control of smooth pursuit velocity. *Vision Research,* 1969, **9**, 1167–1171.

Timberlake, G. T., Wyman, D., Skavenski, A. A., & Steinman, R. M. The oculomotor error signal in the fovea. *Vision Research,* 1972, **12**, 1059–1064.

Uttal, W. R. On the physiological basis of masking with dotted visual noise. *Perception and Psychophysics,* 1970, **7**, 321–327.

Volkmann, F. C. Vision during voluntary saccadic eye movements. *Journal of the Optical Society of America,* 1962, **52**, 571–578.

Volkmann, F. C., Schick, A. M. L., & Riggs, L. A. Time course of visual inhibition during voluntary saccades. *Journal of the Optical Society of America,* 1968, **58**, 562–569.

Weisstein, N. Metacontrast. In D. Jameson & L. M. Hurvich (Eds.), *Handbook of sensory physiology,* Vol. VII, pt 4: *Visual psychophysics.* New York: Academic Press, 1972.

Winterson, B. J., Steinman, R. M., Skavenski. A. A., Hansen, R., & Robinson, D. A. The minivor–Mother Nature's image stabilization technique. *Proceedings of the IEEE International Conference on Cybernetics and Society,* San Francisco, 1975.

Woodworth, R. S. Vision and localization during eye movements. *Psychological Bulletin,* 1906, **3**, 68–70.

Woodworth, R. S. *Experimental psychology.* New York: Holt, 1938.

Wyman, D., & Steinman, R. M. Small step tracking: Implications for the oculomotor "dead zone". *Vision Research,* 1973, **13**, 2165–2172. (a)

Wyman, D., & Steinman, R. M. Latency characteristics of small saccades. *Vision Research,* 1973, **13**, 2173–2175. (b)

Yarbus, A. L. *Eye movements and vision.* New York: Plenum Press, 1967.

Young, L. R. Pursuit eye tracking movements. In P. Bach-y-rita & C. Collins (Eds.), *Control of eye movements.* New York: Academic Press, 1971, 429–443.

Zuber, B. L., & Stark, L. Saccadic suppression: Elevation of visual threshold associated with saccadic eye movements. *Experimental Neurology,* 1966, **16**, 65–79.

Zuber, B. L., Stark, L., and Lorber, M. Saccadic suppression of the pupillary light reflex. *Experimental Neurology,* 1966, **14**, 351–370.

Part III

MEASUREMENT AND RECORDING OF EYE MOVEMENTS

The purpose of this session was to bring the participants up to date on important and interesting developments in recording and measurement techniques. There are many ways to measure the movements of the eyes. These all differ with respect to cost, stability, accuracy, precision, bandwidth, and ease of use. It is the hope of the editors that this discussion of methodology will make some of these problems clear and assist researchers in making intelligent choices of method and apparatus.

This session was chaired by Prof. Laurence R. Young of the Massachusetts Institute of Technology.

III.1

Physical Characteristics of the Eye Used in Eye-Movement Measurement[1]

Laurence R. Young

Massachusetts Institute of Technology

The great variety of techniques employed for eye-movement measurement illustrates the inadequacy of any one method for all applications. A number of new methods have been brought forth in recent years, permitting improvements in convenience, accuracy of assessing point of regard, and freedom of head movement. Before delving into the papers on techniques for measurement of certain properties of eye movements, a light overview of the relevant physical characteristics of the eye is in order. For references and greater detail, the reader is referred to the full report (Young & Sheena, 1975a) from which this summary is excerpted.

1. The retina. The eye has no proprioceptive feedback in terms of conscious position sense. It does, however, contain the retina which moves with the eye and makes possible the subjective assessment of eye movement. Among the earliest quantitative techniques for determining the velocity of the eye during pursuit and saccadic eye movements was the use of afterimages. A small light, flashed periodically, will leave a trace of afterimages, the density of which indicates fixation duration and the spacing of which indicates the velocity of eye movements. Afterimages separated by as little as 15 arc min can be resolved, and the technique is usable over the entire range of eye movements. Its chief drawbacks are, of course, the subjective nature of the measurement and the fact that it can be used only for a brief interval, after which the subject must report

[1] This summary is taken from an extensive report, Survey of Eye Movement Recording Methods by L. R. Young and D. Sheena, July 1974, prepared for the Conference on Eye Movement Research and Technology, Task Force on Essential Skills, National Institute of Education. See also: Young and Sheena (1975a, 1975b).

on the number and placement of his afterimages. It is of practical use currently only for the measurement of ocular torsion where it provides a convenient and relatively accurate measurement and for which there are no readily available automatic methods which are economical, simple to apply, and easily analyzed.

The fovea contains thousands of light-absorbing radially oriented crystals which selectively absorb linearly polarized light. Rotating polarized blue light has been used to form a "spinning propeller" afterimage on the subject's fovea allowing him to identify his own fixation points.

2. Corneoretinal potential. A potential difference of up to 1 mV between the cornea and the retina (cornea positive) normally exists in the eye, and is used as the basis of the most widely applied clinical eye movement technique—electrooculography. The precise basis of this potential difference, once attributable to the electrical activity of the retina itself, is now in question once again. This potential has important variations diurnally and also with the level of light adaptation, decreasing following steady periods in the dark. For stable electrooculographic measurements, especially in the dark, the subject should be permitted to adapt to the ambient illumination level to be used in the experiment for at least 30 min prior to the experiment.

The negative electrical pole lies approximately at the optic disk, 15° displaced from the macula. Since the electric field is not aligned with the optic axis, any torsional rotation of the eye introduces a potential change which can be mistaken for horizontal or vertical eye movement. This very geometry, however, makes electrooculography a possible, though difficult, method for measuring ocular torsion.

3. Electrical impedance. The impedance measured between electrodes placed at the outer canthi of the two eyes varies with eye position. The variation in this resistive component is associated either with the nonhomogeneous or anisotropic nature of electrical characteristics of the tissues in the globe or with the nonspherical characteristics of the globe so that the resistivity of the path between the two electrodes changes with position.

4. The corneal bulge. The cornea, attached to the sclera at the front of the eye and centered close to the optic axis, has a smaller radius of curvature than the eye itself. This forms the basis for a number of important methods of eye-movement measurement. In the early days of research on eye movements, attachments were made directly to the cornea by a plaster-of-paris ring and mechanical linkages to recording pens. The bulge of the retina can be felt through the eyelid of the closed eye, and pressure transducers placed over the eyelid can detect these changes. In more recent times, the cornea has acted as a mechanical post, to center tight-fitting scleral contact lenses to which other measurement devices are attached. It should be noted that the cornea itself slips slightly with respect to the sclera when forces are applied to the cornea, and probably slips slightly during the eye acceleration phase of saccadic eye movements. Contact lenses applied to the cornea itself are not an adequate base for the accurate measurement of eye position, and large contact lenses conforming to the sclera as well as the cornea are necessary for systems in which stability of better than a few minutes of arc is desired. The nominal curvature of the cornea for an adult human is approximately 8 mm radius for an eye of 13.3 mm radius. Once a contact lens is fitted, its position can be measured by any of a number of methods, including optical levers and magnetic search coils.

5. *Corneal reflections.* The front surface of the cornea, although not a perfect optical surface, approximates a spherical section over its central 25°. As with a convex mirror, reflections of a bright object from this surface form a virtual image behind the surface which can be imaged and photographed or recorded. The position of the image commonly seen as the highlight in the eye, the corneal reflection, is a function of eye position. Rotation of the eye about its center produces a relative translation as well as rotation of the cornea, forming the basis for the important class of eye-movement instruments known as corneal reflection systems.

6. *Reflections from other optical curvatures in the eye—purkinje images.* Although the brightest reflections of incident light come from the front surface of the cornea, light is also reflected from each surface of the eye at which there is a change in refractive index. Reflections come also from the back surface of the cornea, the front surface of the lens, and the rear surface of the lens. These four are referred to as the Purkinje Images. After the bright front-surface reflection, the next most visible Purkinje image is the fourth, coming from the posterior surface of the lens. Measurements of the relative displacement between the first and fourth images, representing, as they do, point-focused images from planes of different depths in the eye, represent one technique for actively measuring the orientation of the eye in space independent of it relation to head position.

7. *The limbus.* The iris of the eye is normally visible and clearly distinguishable from the sclera, and is the basis for the normal visual assessment of the angle of gaze. The position of the iris-scleral boundary (the limbus) may be measured with respect to the head. The ratio between dark iris and bright sclera observed on the left and right side of the eye may be measured either directly with photosensors or indirectly on an image of the eye. This ratio is directly related to the horizontal position of the eye. The best wavelength for making the distinction between iris and sclera depends to some extent on the iris color; however, white light is normally reasonably effective.

8. *The pupil.* The pupil is easily distinguished from the surrounding iris by its difference in reflectance. The pupil can be made to appear much darker than the iris under most lighting conditions when the majority of light does not come in

directly along the axis of measurement, and consequently is not reflected out. On the other hand, the pupil can be made to appear very bright (as is often seen in amateur full-face flash photography) when most of the light enters along the optic axis and is reflected back from the retina. In either case the pupil can be separated from the surrounding iris optically. This can be especially sharpened with the use of infrared light which will be nearly entirely absorbed once entering the eye, consequently make the pupil much darker than the surrounding iris. The pupil normally varies between 2 and 8 mm in diameter in adult humans. Although it is actually slightly elliptical in shape, it can be approximated closely by tracing the best-fitting circle to the pupil circumference with an image-dissector technique. The center of the pupil is also easily located electrooptically or on film for hand analysis.

The pupil appears elliptical when viewed other than along the optic axis, with the minor axis shortening in the axis of eye rotation. The pupil eccentricity could serve as a basis for eye-angle measurement.

9. Other optical and nonoptical landmarks. In addition to the iris and the pupil, other optical landmarks can be traced. Scleral blood vessels or folds of the iris can be identified by hand or traced with optical tracing techniques. (These are of practical application only in the measurement of ocular counterrolling.) The retinal vessels, which can also be imaged and tracked, provide one of the most accurate techniques for determining the place on the retina where a given target is imaged, and consequently the exact fixation point of the eye. The retinal vessels, approximately .2 mm in diameter, radiate from the optic disk.

Some artificial landmarks have also been placed on the eye, and their positions recorded. A globule of mercury, chalk, and egg membrane have been used for optical tracking. A small piece of metal imbedded in the sclera has been used for magnetic tracking of eye position.

III.2

The Purkinje-Image Method
of Recording Eye Position

Tom N. Cornsweet

Baylor College of Medicine

If you want to know where somebody is looking, with an accuracy of no better than about $1/2°$, then almost any old eye tracker will do. If you want better than $1/2°$ or so, you have to tolerate a quantum jump in difficulty. Let me explain very briefly what that is all about.

Suppose somebody looks at a spot on a screen 10 m away. Then suppose his eye rotates in its socket just enough so that the outer edge of the iris moves .1 mm. That will change the position on the screen that is imaged on the fovea. In other words, the subject is now looking at a different place on the screen; he's made what is usually called an eye movement. In fact, that is roughly a $1/2°$ eye movement. The subject, after the eye movement, will be looking at a spot on the screen that's about 100 mm from where he was originally looking.

On the other hand, suppose he translates his eyeball sideways by .1 mm, say by moving his head. The point on the edge of his iris will undergo exactly the same movement as it did for the $1/2°$ rotation, but the subject will now be looking at a point only .1 mm from his original fixation point. So, if someone is looking at a scene 10 m away and you look at the front of his eye and see that it moves .1 mm, you don't know whether he is now looking .1 mm from where he used to be or 100 mm from where he used to be or anywhere between those two. In fact, he might be looking at a point 200 mm away, having made an angular rotation one way and a translation the other way.

If it were possible to eliminate translation of the eye altogether, most of the techniques that were described here could be made to be very accurate. In fact, of course, you can't keep the eyeball from translating. You can do a pretty good job of holding the head steady with a good bite bar and head constraints, but even when you do that, the eyeball can still translate in its socket. After all, the eye is sitting in a bag of fat in a hole in your head, and there are six big muscles pulling on the sides of it.

It seems to be virtually impossible to hold the translation of the eye to less than about .05 mm; in other words, even if you try your best, you still get translation that corresponds to an eye movement of about $1/4°$. (The image formed by reflection from the cornea moves only about half as far as the edge of the iris per unit of eye rotation. Therefore, corneal-reflection recording techniques are worse. Half a tenth of a millimeter of translation is indistinguishable from a half degree rotation.)

Therefore, when you are doing work that requires very accurate tracking, for example when you want to stabilize an image accurately enough to make it disappear or when you want to see fixational eye movements, you have to do something to avoid artifacts caused by translation. The classic Riggs technique involves placing a plane mirror on a contact lens. If collimated light is incident on a plane mirror, and the reflected light is imaged by a lens, the motion of the reflected image is unaffected by translation of the mirror. Therefore, the technique has no translational artifact in it (as long as the subject is looking at a target that is not too close to his eye).

It is true that tracking the motion of retinal blood vessels, not scleral ones, is uncontaminated by translation (Cornsweet, 1958), but apparently nobody has developed a usable system for doing that yet.

The *double Purkinje* eye tracker uses a different principle for avoiding translation artifacts. It solves the problem in the following way: if you shine light onto an eye, about 2.5% of it is reflected from the front surface of the cornea. This convex mirror forms what is usually referred to as a virtual image behind the cornea: the first Purkinje image.

There is another, very much dimmer, image reflected from the back surface of the cornea: the second Purkinje image. The second is virtually coincident with the first and much dimmer, so it is very hard to see at all.

Then there is another dim image, 100- or 200-fold less intense than the corneal reflection, that comes off the front surface of the lens: the third Purkinje image. When you change your accommodation, this front surface of the lens is the one that changes its curvature strongly, so the third Purkinje image changes radically with accommodation. In fact, it is sometimes used to measure accommodation.

Last, there is the light reflected from the back surface of the lens: the fourth Purkinje image. The concave lens surface forms a real image in the eyeball. This image is affected only very slightly by accommodation. The fourth Purkinje image turns out to be in almost exactly the same plane as the first, it is about three-quarters as big, and it is inverted.

When the eye rotates, the first and fourth Purkinje images both move, but they move through different distances, whereas if the eye translates, they move through the same distance. Therefore, if the two images are tracked, changes in the distance between them provide an accurate measure of rotation of the eye independent of translation.

In order to put together a practical system for recording eye position using the first and fourth Purkinje images, we had to assemble a complex collection of optical and electronic equipment. The equipment is described in detail in Cornsweet and Crane (1973), but briefly it works as follows. The eye of the subject is illuminated with flickering infrared light. This light is reflected as if it emanated from two small spots, the first and fourth Purkinje images. The optics are arranged so that the first and fourth images do not overlap for any eye position within a 20° field. This means that we can deal with them independently. Light from both images is reflected from a servo-controlled mirror and the first image is then reimaged on a quadrant photodetector. Whenever the image moves off the center of the photodetector, the output of its associated circuitry causes the mirror to rotate in such a way as to return the image to the center of the quadrant photodetector. The signal used to drive the mirror is thus proportional to both the translation and rotation of the eye.

Light from the fourth Purkinje image is reflected from the same mirror before it, in turn, is projected onto another quadrant photodetector whose position is servo-controlled so that the detector follows the image wherever it goes. It is the position of this second servo-driven quadrant photodetector that is the true output of the system. It is proportional to that component of the movement of the fourth Purkinje image that is due exclusively to rotation of the eye. The servo mechanisms are relatively fast and respond in about 5 msec to a saccade of about 5°.

The instrument can track eye movements over a square field about 20° on a side. The raw output is not completely linear with rotation because the difference between the angle and the tangent of the angle becomes significant at large angles. This means that if one wants to have high accuracy over a large field, a small non-linear correction must be applied. The overall accuracy is limited largely by the photodetector noise level and is of the order of 1 min. of arc.

More recently, H. Crane, R. Savoie, and C. Steele at Stanford Research Institute, have made some very significant modifications to the design, which I would like to mention here. These improvements help to overcome two problems inherent in the design of the tracker described by Cornsweet and Crane (1973). First, in order to stay within the mechanical range of some of the movable elements of the tracker, and in order for the images to remain in focus, the head had to be tightly constrained with a dental impression plate and forehead rest. The new version permits head movement anywhere within a cube 1 cm on a side. Second, because of the geometry of the moving mirrors, a distortion was introduced into the records which became noticeable for large tracking angles. The mirror geometry has now been changed to eliminate this distortion.

In addition, the tungsten source and motor-driven chopper wheel have been replaced by an electronically flickered light-emitting diode, and an automatic search mode has been introduced so that, should tracking be lost, for instance because of a long blink, the system automatically searches until tracking is reacquired. This search requires a maximum of 1 sec and an average of .5 sec.

DISCUSSION

YOUNG: You didn't say anything about accommodation.

CORNSWEET: The fourth Purkinje image moves only very, very slightly with strong accommodation and we set up the geometry so that even if this motion were large, it would hardly affect the tracking.

YOUNG: Were you going to talk about the application of the same principle to accommodation or is it not built into the same instrument?

CORNSWEET: No, this instrument has nothing to do with recording accommodation.

KOLERS: You were going to say something about the third image that you never got around to.

CORNSWEET: We deliberately set up the geometry so that the third Purkinje image never gets onto the photodetectors.

KOLERS: Why do you never want to use the third image?

CORNSWEET: Because it moves strongly with accommodation.

KOLERS: If your target is at a fixed distance, the accommodation isn't a problem.

CORNSWEET: If you assume that the subject's accommodation does not fluctuate, that's right. But that is not a safe assumption.

KOLERS: Even with the target at a fixed distance?

CORNSWEET: Yes.

HALL: Isn't it true that there is a sort of oscillation or scanning activity of the lens' front surface, a fine tremor, if you will, that is essentially scanning the image in focus? This might be a problem for you, too.

CORNSWEET: It is true that under most conditions there is a continuous fluctuation of accommodation, that is, a fluctuation in the bulging of the front surface of the lens, at about 2 Hz. That is not a problem because we are looking at the back surface of the lens.

FUCHS: What is the frequency response with all those servo motors?

CORNSWEET: It is flat to almost 100 Hz, so the system does a pretty good job of tracking a 20-Hz eyeball.

COOPER: What are the mechanical factors that limit the usefulness of this instrument to within 20° and 1 min. of arc?

CORNSWEET: I believe the 1 min. of arc limitation is not a mechanical factor. It is the noise level of the instrument, primarily from the photodetector surface itself. We might reduce that noise substantially by replacing the silicon detectors with two quadrant photomultiplier tubes, but that is extremely expensive.

If we did that, I am sure we'd find some other things that would limit the accuracy. I don't know what they are offhand. My guess is that fluctuations in the position of the lens in the eye will constitute the ultimate limit. We don't really know that the lens is well fixed inside the eyeball. It may be that for large saccadic movements, the lens flops around in there.

The 20° range limitation is really inherent in the design of this particular version of the instrument. If you go farther to one side, the pupil starts cutting off the view of the fourth Purkinje image, and on the other side the two images start overlapping. However, there is another version on the drawing board that, in principle, can track 360°, and eventually might get built.

III.3

Recent Developments
in High-Speed Data Processing
and Unobtrusive Monitoring of the Eyes

Robert H. Lambert

U.S. Army Human Engineering Laboratory

Since the principal measurement schemes have been explained elegantly by Dr. Young I won't bother with a discussion of geometry. I will simply mention that the system I am going to describe utilizes the corneal-reflection–pupil-center measurement technique.

There are two notable features of this system. The first is that unlike the other systems that we have talked about, there is no restraint of the subject other than that he sits normally in a relatively comfortable chair as shown in the artist's illustration of Fig. 1. The other unique feature is the on-line data-reduction capability.

Starting at the front of the system, the subject is generally not aware that his eyes are being monitored. An image of his eye is viewed through what looks like a speaker enclosure. Behind the grille covering the enclosure are concealed mirrors, as shown in the cutaway of Fig. 1, which track the head movements of the subject and maintain an image of the eye centered on the vidicon face.

The stimulus is presented on a rear-projection screen surrounded by illuminated, polarized panels as shown in Fig. 2. A small nonpolarized portion of the surround located directly above the speaker enclosure produces a clearly defined highlight that is reflected from the front surface of the cornea to the TV camera via the concealed mirrors. This system uses only visible lighting and the light that provides the illumination of the subject eye is subdued relative to the light emanating from the stimulus itself.

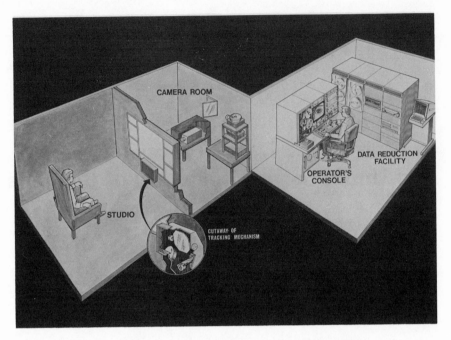

FIG. 1. Artist's illustration of the system. (After Monty, 1975.)

The projectors shown in the camera room are actually random-access slide projectors, but could be video projectors, movie projectors, etc. In this case the projectors are computer controlled as are all the events which constitute an experiment.

The system does require an operator although he is necessary only for initial acquisition of the pupil and for its reacquisition if the subject walks around the room, sneezes, rubs his eye, or whatever. The console shown in Fig. 3 contains the heart of the oculometer, namely the analog electronics that track the pupil, and detect the displacement of the pupil center from the highlight.

A video tape recording is made in real time not only of the picture of the eye, but also of the data that are collected at the rate of 60 frames per sec. As the subject is being tested, eye-movement data are recorded on the video tape and are also sent to the computer. The computer is a PDP-11/20 with a disk and two tape units. In the event that the computer is down during an experimental sequence the data can be stored on the video tape and read into the computer at a later date as the computer doesn't differentiate between a real-time data link and a recorded video link. The data, having been recorded on one of the tape units, are then summarized and read to the second tape unit in various formats. In general, what we have been interested in is fixation time, number of fixations, variability of fixation duration, and so forth. These data are computed in real time and recorded in summarized form if need be.

The next step in the data-handling process is that of statistical analysis. Any number of statistical analyses can be handled without manual manipulation of data. For example, a popular program has been the analysis of variance prepared by Butler, Kamlet, and Monty (1969). In short, every step of the process from the control of the stimulus to taking of data, through the sorting and formatting, through complete statistical analyses, can be done automatically without the operator ever seeing the data themselves.

On the right side of Fig. 3 is a graphics display terminal which, generally, is used to project eye-movement behavior in real time. It is primarily an operator aid, but it is also used at the onset of an experiment to collect calibration data. Calibration is a simple process which takes only a few seconds. One technique is

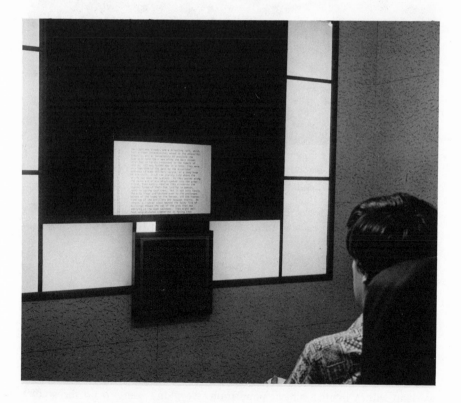

FIG. 2. A subject seated comfortably in the studio. The camera is concealed behind the speaker grille and the highlight is generated by the bright spot between the grille and the screen. (After Monty, 1975.)

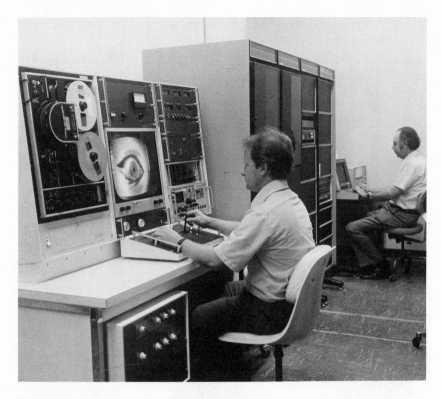

FIG. 3. The operator's console and the data-reduction facility. (After Lambert et al., 1974.)

to show the subject a set of Landolt C's, one in each corner of the screen, and to direct his attention to each in turn, under the guise of focusing the projector.[1]

DISCUSSION

KOLERS: Are your restricted to 60 frames per sec?

LAMBERT: Yes, we are restricted by the camera as we use standard TV equipment.

KOLERS: Have you studied the difference between allowing the subject to know that his eyes are being monitored and not letting him know that?

LAMBERT: We haven't studied that yet for the simple reason that we were working with a limited subject population. We didn't want to do the studies

[1] At this point Lambert showed a video film of the system in operation. The film was self explanatory and was immediately followed by discussion. For a more detailed description of the system see Lambert, Monty, and Hall (1974) and Monty (1975).

where they were aware until we were finished with the studies where they were unaware. Otherwise, we'd lose our whole naive population. Both Dr. Fisher and Dr. Hall will cover several of the studies that have been conducted to date.

ANLIKER: The Honeywell Oculometer, at least when I had access to it some years ago, has some problems about reacquiring the image after it is lost as a result of an eye blink or a rapid movement, etc. There is a dead time during which the image must be reacquired. How do you deal with that type of problem?

LAMBERT: That is the operator's function and he has to manually reacquire the image. Normally, you don't lose track during blinks. It is generally from rubbing the eye or sneezing.

ANLIKER: When the eyelid closes, what do you assume is happening during that interval?

LAMBERT: Some of the information that is recorded along with where the eye is looking has to do with how the system is performing, and one of the things to look for is highlight loss. As soon as it detects a highlight loss, the system tries to fit data between the point where the highlight was last seen and where it is next seen. That is sometimes an arbitrary thing.

ANLIKER: Can you give me some ball park figure of the amount of time it would take the operator to acquire the image from scratch?

LAMBERT: When the operator starts out he usually doesn't even have a picture of the subject. There are indicator lights on the operator's console which tell him where a subject's head would be and he first gets into that ball park. He then uses the joy stick to superimpose a circular cursor on the image of the pupil. Once that is accomplished, the operator switches out of the manual mode and the automatic tracker assumes control and tracks until the pupil is again obscured. It generally takes the operator only a couple of seconds to lock onto the pupil.

YOUNG: I might add, there is no inherent reason why the corneal-reflection–pupil-center method requires much time to acquire. The Honeywell version of it does require time, but that's not inherent in the method.

ANLIKER: There is no inherent reason except that this image is in a large field which must be narrowed down.

LAMBERT: If the head were held still, there would be no need for manual acquisition.

COOPER: Could you give us some indication of the level of accuracy of the instrument, and the angular range over which it is effective? Could you also go into a more detailed explanation about how the instrument tracks head movements and compensates for them?

LAMBERT: The uncertainty is within $2°$ over a $30°$ field. That's the worst case. You can detect eye movements of less than $1°$.

During initial acquisition, a circular cursor is positioned in such a way as to outline the image of the pupil on the TV screen. The tracking system then continuously monitors the video level at the points defined by the cursor and, if need be, repositions the cursor to overlay the area of maximum contrast gradient which occurs at the pupil/iris boundary. Similarly, the cursor is expanded or contracted to accommodate changes in pupil diameter. This is a fairly fast servo loop; it is limited only by the frame rate of the video. Since the electronic system knows the location of the pupil, only the highlight location remains to be determined to have the two points necessary to define a geometric vector which is fixed to the eye. Now, as the head moves, so will the above-mentioned cursor. There is a second, slower servo loop which compares the cursor position with the physical center of the TV picture. As the cursor moves from this position, appropriate signals are generated and fed to the motors which rotate the tracking mirrors in front of the TV camera. The mirrors are commanded in such a way as to recenter the cursor, and hence the image of the pupil. The mirror servos just described do not respond to rapid eye movements, but are sufficiently fast to track normal head movements.

NICKERSON: Is it correct that the computer doesn't distinguish between eye movements and head movements; that it is just tracking fixations and changes in fixation points?

LAMBERT: Correct. It is just looking at fixation points. It doesn't get confused terribly by head movements.

NICKERSON: It doesn't differentiate between translation and rotation?

YOUNG: Perhaps we should explain. The basic system tracks the orientation of the line of sight in space and it does not distinguish between eye movements with respect to the head and head movements with respect to the body. Is that correct?

LAMBERT: Yes, and this is really the limitation right now on the static accuracy of the system. We do not presently take that into our computation. With improved software now being developed, I think it will be much better than it is.

III.4

Ways of Recording Line of Sight

Norman H. Mackworth

Stanford University

I have a many-sided interest in ways of recording the line of sight to understand more fully the nature of cognitive processes. My interests in fact are fivefold. First, I am an *investigator* interested in learning what we can from such devices. Second, I am a *user* who likes to administer such procedures. Third, I am an *equipment designer,* and fourth, also a *constructor* since I like to build these devices myself. Last of all, I speak as an *adviser* on their use. (For instance, over the last 20 years, more than 100 separate investigators have discussed with me their points of view on lines of sight. They have asked how to convert their mental projections into appropriate hardware to give them the fixation-point measurements they need from the kind of line-of-sight changes they expect from their own particular visual situations.)

Before providing a brief glimpse of my new Digital Eye Camera, I would like, with your indulgence, to lay before you some general words of wisdom. It is well known that creative research persons often have a strong sense of humor [and of modesty, (eds.)]. Therefore, most of you may appreciate the expression of my serious convictions in this lighthearted form of five fables for our times.

1. The simpler the rig, the simpler the deed. The hard-headed expert knows when to bring in a complicated device, and when to avoid it like the plague. He knows that the research aim is to collect relevant data and nothing but the relevant data. Let us not go overboard and try to measure the height of all the waves in sight. The resulting data may obscure the tip of the iceberg you are looking for. Most people (like myself) start off with devices that are much too complex for the tasks in hand. Simpler procedures can often obviate the need for complex equipments with all their accompanying headaches. No one uses a Boeing 747 for a ten-mile journey when the trusty Datsun is available. But people sometimes do this with elaborate eye-tracking machines, and they usually end up still talking about the flight plans with the programmers when the Datsun has done the job. (The record here is 6 years spent in shaping up the equivalent of the 747, and still no maiden flight.)

2. The pause is mightier than the move. The eyes travel merely to arrive at important places on the visual scene. Cognitive researchers are usually much more interested in the pauses than they are in the jumps that get the eyes to areas where there are new pieces of information. This meeting could be said to have the wrong title. That is, *eye fixations* are far more significant for cognitive research than *eye movements*. The visual pause gives much of value, especially when we know the spatial location of the visual fixations on the stimuli comprising the visual situation: this is true whether the stimuli are pictures (Mackworth & Bruner, 1970), words (Mackworth, 1975), or symbols (Mackworth, Grandstaff, & Pribram, 1973). A good case can be made for stressing this distinction between *line-of-sight research* which studies the visual *pauses* for cognitive investigations, and *eye-movement research* which studies the visual *moves* for eye-tracking investigations. The paradoxical situation is that the highly complex cognitive processes can often be studied by relatively simple photographic recording devices. Conversely, the biologically simpler processes involved in the precise aiming of the eyes and accurate oculomotor control really do need complex electronic equipments. This distinction between line-of-sight and eye-movement research is more than just a verbal quibble. The objectives are so very different that the methodology must be at a different level of complexity.

3. To bite bar, or not to bite bar, that is the question. The decision of whether or not to bite bar often rests on the permissible positional errors in the recording method. Suppose we consider five kinds of research situations requiring different levels of percisions.

(1) *Studies of oculomotor control* demand exquisitely precise devices such as those by Cornsweet and Crane that give exact positional information. The drawback here is that they usually have to employ a bite bar to fix the head position.

(2) For most studies of *visual search* in which one has to know the position of the gaze within at least $\pm 1°$ of some spatial position in the outside world, then the unfortunate fact is that the bite bar also has to be used for reliable readings, unless enormous expenditures can be made.

A decade of experience has shown that the Mackworth (1967) Stand Eye Camera is still worthwhile in the hands of many investigators. My own most recent experience is contained in the paper entitled the "Stimulus Density Limits the Useful Field of View" given in another section of this conference.

Briefly, the bite bar system works well but the procedure is not too popular with the subjects, and is quite slow.

4. Overaccuracy is the thief of time. Most cognitive researches do not need superaccurate recording devices. Most cognitive researches involve

(3) reading,

(4) *picture processing,* or

(5) *visual choice between two or more alternatives.*

I designed the new Digital Eye Camera with *no* bite bar, merely a head rest, specifically to cover this range of requirements. I have tried it out mostly in the *reading* situation because in some ways this is the most demanding. I wished to find the limits of accuracy of this very simple device, consisting essentially of a viewing box and a recording camera. The main fact is that the Digital Eye Camera can break up a 8-in. line of large typescript into *eight* distinguishable segments for data analysis, despite the fact that no bite bar is used. I tested 22 children from Grades 2 through 6, and I found that there was another advantage of removing the bite bar: they could read aloud from the printed material. The most significant measure was fixation time while reading aloud; the reading-aloud fixation time (RAFT) was very closely related (inversely) to every other measure of cognitive ability considered in this study (Mackworth, 1975). One minute spent with the child reading aloud in this Digital Eye Camera is the fastest way to measure his reading ability in either school or clinic.

Throwing away the bite bar buys you so much time that you may well be laughing all the way to the data bank. I believe that 20 subjects per day or even more is not at all an unreasonable estimate. My experience suggests that once you have thought out the basic idea, just one month need be spent undertaking a sizable study: one week to make the stimulus materials, one week to run the subjects through the Digital Eye Camera, one week to analyze the motion picture films, and a final week to write the scientific paper.

5. Ask not the absolute accuracy of the device, but what it can do for you (especially in terms of columns and rows). I am saying that for cognitive researches such as reading, picture processing, and visual choice between items we should throw away the bite bar, and use something like the Digital Eye Camera rather than the Stand Eye Camera. This sounds as if I were in favor of sin. Here I am, calling for a lowering of accuracy standards, just to make life easier for the experimenter and his subjects. Let me hasten to explain why the resulting accuracy loss is negligible or at any rate, less than you might think. This is really, therefore, only a very small sin. The rationale behind this claim is that cognitive researches have different needs. Recording systems for this type of study have to be evaluated in a way which is quite different from the evaluative visual angle yardsticks applied to systems for oculomotor studies.

The way to judge the accuracy of a system intended to record the position of eye fixations on a stimulus scene is to ask the simple question: *How many columns and rows does the system provide in the analysis matrix?* The question has to specify the size of the page that is being subdivided in this manner and also the distance from which it is being viewed. If we consider a display 8 inches X 8 in. then we find the Digital Eye Camera to be just as accurate as the Stand Eye Camera on this columns and rows anterior. The Digital Eye Camera gives at best eight columns and eight rows; the Stand Eye Camera also gives 8 columns and 8 rows. (The display can be brought so much closer with the Digital Eye Camera that the column accuracy level is quite considerably improved. The Digital Eye Camera can have a picture 8 inches wide, 14 in. from the eyes, whereas the Stand Eye Camera can deal with this width only when the page of print or picture is much further from the eyes).

I maintain that this is a much more valid way of comparing the two systems than is the visual angle or oculomotor approach which would be as follows. The Digital Eye Camera subdivides a page subtending about $32°$ of width into eight columns which are, therefore, each $4°$ wide, giving an accuracy of $±2°$. The Stand Eye Camera subdivides a 10 inch wide page subtending about $20°$ at a distance of 28 inches into ten columns which are, therefore, each $2°$ wide, giving an accuracy of $±1°$. This second method is the classical way of expressing the precision of a system of recording, but it assumes that the important feature is the misalignment of the line of sight in terms of the number of degrees that the gaze is off target. This assumption is certainly true for oculomotor tracking and visual search studies. But I question whether it is true for cognitive studies. Here it becomes permissible to gain finer resolution (of reading matter, not degrees) by bringing the page closer to the eyes, to the normal reading distance of 14 in.

In summary, the important way to assess a recording system which is measuring the position of visual fixations on a page is to use the columns and rows criterion rather than the visual angle measure. Go ahead. Throw away your bite bars. Sin a little. (For most *cognitive* research, the Digital Eye Camera is just as precise as the Stand Eye Camera.) It is quite all right because in cognitive research you want to know simply where the subject is looking in terms of the item or region being inspected. This does *not* have to be expressed in terms of the visual angle accuracy with which the eyes are being aimed. *R*emember the columns and rows. Relax and enjoy!

The Digital Eye Camera

a. Line-of-sight recording. This new method gives the spatial coordinates of the eye fixations directly from the record in numerical form. Scales for this purpose are automatically placed on the pictures of each eye as in Fig. 1. This sample picture shows how the readings are made. The X coordinates come from the

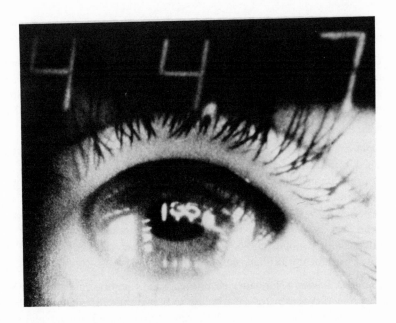

FIG. 1.   This is a direct copy of a typical recording obtained from the Digital Eye Camera. Time to the nearest tenth of a second is shown as "44.7," from the start of the test run. Every frame of the film is indexed automatically in this manner. The grid scale reflected around the pupil gives the current position of the eye. The picture shows an 8 X 8 grid, with the subject now looking directly at that area of the picture which lies at the intersection of column 3 and row 1. Number 3 can be seen vertically above the pupil center and the left-hand scale mark 1 is horizontally in line with the pupil center. A 6-min film record can be completed within 10 min from the moment the subject first enters the test room. Figure 1 illustrates the most difficult situation, because the subject had dark brown irises and was wearing her contact lenses.

horizontal scales for the columns above and below the eye. The Y coordinates come from the vertical scales for the rows at the sides of the eye. The X (columns) reading is where the vertical diameter of the pupil cuts the horizontal scales. The Y (rows) reading is where the horizontal diameter of the pupil cuts the vertical scales. The sample picture shows the eye on position 35 since the vertical pupil diameter is on column 3 and the horizontal diameter is on row 5. Many studies need only a 5 X 5 or even a 3 X 3 analysis grid rather than 8 X 8 shown here. Only the relevant numbers are shown on the eye, e.g., with the 2 X 2 display, only the reference numbers 1 and 2 appear around the eye.

b. Time marking.   Each frame of the 9 frames per sec motion picture film is also automatically time marked by a four-digit display which appears along the top of the picture. This gives time in seconds from the start of the test run, the accuracy being to the nearest tenth of a second.

c. Operation. Everything possible has been done to help the operation and administration of the testing, e.g., the camera is cartridge loaded, and can be focused throughout the test; the camera is fixed in place as it needs no aiming. The viewing box (into which the subject peers) is small enough to be taken by car between laboratory, school, and clinic.

d. Data analysis. The X-Y coordinates for eye position and the time reading are typed out from each frame of the motion picture recording. For most studies, this immediate and direct procedure is sufficient. But it is worth repeating from Mackworth (1967) that nine-tenths of the analysis time is spent in the period *after* this eyeballing of the eyeballs. Clearly, then, the occasional user who can type the X-Y readings directly onto magnetic tape for later computer analysis should do so. Many different researchers have devised computer programs for this off-line analysis.

e. Stimulus Scenes. Normally the printed text or picture comes from a 8 × 8 in. slide-projection screen to make it easy to prepare the stimulus materials. But the scale numbers for the grid analysis can also be placed around real scenes when these are viewed through the window obtained by removing the projection screen.

f. Conclusion. This Digital Eye Camera may be one answer to the recent call by Baer and Wright (1974) for "a practical high-speed, eye-movement recorder." It is undoubtedly a practical, high-speed, *eye-fixation* recorder. A simple device is all that is needed for most cognitive studies.

III.5

Pattern-Recognition Techniques for Extraction of Features of the Eye from a Conventional Television Scan

David Sheena

Whittaker Corporation/Space Sciences Division

Many of the eye-position measurement instruments involve scanning or television methods of extracting some feature of the eye such as the iris, the pupil, or the corneal reflection. These particular elements must be acquired to the exclusion of portions of eyelids, eyelashes, and the sclera. Their presence also has to be determined in the midst of nonuniform illumination and noise of various sources, as well as shading in the viewing system and coloration differences. These conditions make such an automatic acquisition generally difficult.

Two things were found very useful in making a proper and successful recognition of the feature of the eye which one is seeking. The first is the use of some characteristics peculiar to the elements in question which allow for increased certainty of recognition; the second is the use of feedback indicators to the operator to show him just what is being acquired and the quality of the measurement. This way he knows if it is necessary to make some adjustments.

These techniques will be described as they apply to an eye-movement measurement instrument. In Fig. 1, one television camera is shown viewing the subject's left eye while he is looking at a scene and the other views the scene directly. The operator has two items of visual feedback available to him. He sees the eye of the subject with various superimposed indicators and he sees the scene being viewed by the subject on another monitor with a superimposed dot or cross hairs indicating the subject's point of fixation.

Figure 2 shows, as an example, the eye-movement method employed here which utilizes the recognition and feedback techniques being described. It uses a conventional horizontal television scan across the pupil and corneal reflection. The N is the number of television lines from the beginning of the field to the

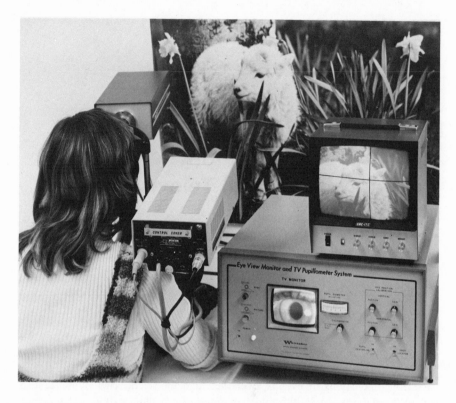

FIG. 1. Television scan type eye-movement measurement system with various operator indicators.

bottom of the pupil; n is the number of scan lines which intersect the pupil. Pupil diameter PD is therefore proportional to n. As indicated in the figure, if the head is fixed, the vertical eye position is proportional to $N - n/2$. If the time from the beginning of the scan to the first intersection with the left edge of the pupil is LE, then the horizontal eye position is proportional to $LE + PD/2$. The same technique is employed to measure the position of the center of the corneal reflection which generally falls inside the pupil. For a free-head situation, the eye's angle of gaze is proportional to the distance between the center of the pupil and the center of the corneal reflection (Merchant & Morrissette, 1974). Figure 2 also gives the relationship between these measurements and the eye angle when the viewing device is off to the side.

The matter here is not so much measurement technique but rather the implementation of the recognition and feedback schemes in the acquisition of the pupil and the corneal reflection which can be subsequently used to determine eye position in any desired manner. Figure 3 shows TV monitor pictures of the eye, viewed by the operator, as he sets up his discrimination level to detect the pupil and the corneal reflection. This is done using a simple threshold comparator. As the video level on a particular TV scan line reaches the comparator level, it switches the latter and, as an indicator to the user, places a tiny white spot at that point on the monitor in real time. This shows the operator precisely which points on the eye are being detected. These dots are combined, as may be seen in the various pictures, to form continuous white lines. A black dot corresponding to each white dot is placed at the end of the horizontal scan line, forming a vertical black bar.

As the operator turns up his discrimination level, he begins to see a little bit of the pupil as in Fig. 3a. It is clearly not sufficient, so he turns up his level until he sees a full crescent around the left edge of the pupil as in Fig. 3b. This is precisely what he wants to get. The instrument tells him that this measurement is now correct by placing a white horizontal line right through the vertical center of the pupil. This centerline tells him which segment of the eye the instrument is recognizing as the desired feature. The rule used for this recognition scheme must be a relatively simple one. Clearly, if one has a computer and can perform sophisticated analysis, all one needs is a little portion of pupil arc, and the entire pupil can be extrapolated from it. However, this simplified recognition method will require only that the pupil being detected be of some minimum diameter as a first criterion. As can be seen in Fig. 3a there is no such segment, and therefore there is no centerline. Once the minimum is reached, the centerline comes into view indicating that the segment bisected has been acquired as the pupil.

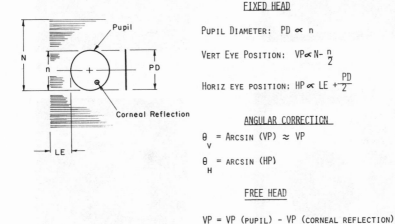

FIXED HEAD

PUPIL DIAMETER: $PD \propto n$

VERT EYE POSITION: $VP \propto N - \dfrac{n}{2}$

HORIZ EYE POSITION: $HP \propto LE + \dfrac{PD}{2}$

ANGULAR CORRECTION

$\theta_V = \text{ARCSIN } (VP) \approx VP$

$\theta_H = \text{ARCSIN } (HP)$

FREE HEAD

$VP = VP \text{ (PUPIL)} - VP \text{ (CORNEAL REFLECTION)}$

$HP = HP \text{ (PUPIL)} - HP \text{ (CORNEAL REFLECTION)}$

FIG. 2. Eye point of gaze-determination geometry.

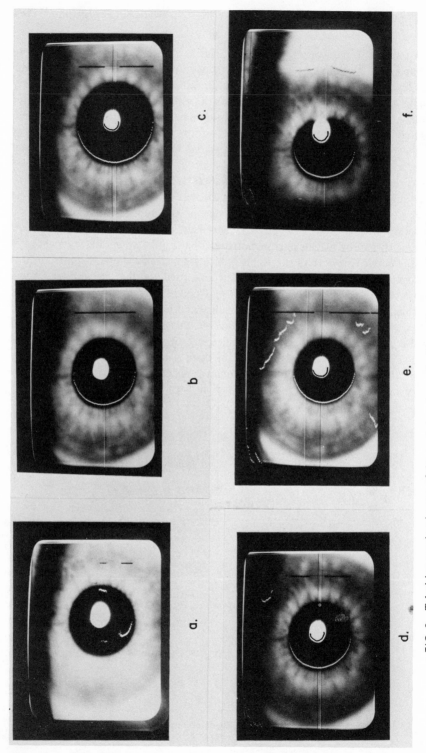

FIG. 3. Television monitor images of the eye being observed with pupil and corneal-reflection crescents and centerlines.

182

In Fig. 3c the same procedure is employed with reverse coloration of indicators to detect the corneal reflection. A black centerline goes through it with a black crescent and a white dot at the end of the line. The same rules apply to the corneal reflection detection as to the pupil detection.

If the threshold level is turned up further, or the eye moves, or lighting conditions change, the system may start detecting some elements of the iris, the eyelids, or eyelashes and superimpose more white dots as in Fig. 3d. The centerline, however, is still correctly placed because of the second criterion employed, which is that none of the additional detections are contiguous to the major segment that is found. The feedback indicators tell the operator that all is still correct. Should conditions change even further or should he have his discriminator turned up even higher, he may have even more firings as shown in Fig. 3e, so that there is detection on scan lines immediately above and/or below the pupil. This makes for one continuous vertical segment and the centerline jumps out of its correct position and immediately indicates to the operator that the setting is incorrect and so is the measurement. The same thing occurs in Fig. 3f where the discrimination for the corneal reflection has gone too far. There are additional black dots contiguous to it above and below, and the black centerline is clearly not in place.

This detection scheme operates in the vertical direction which is amenable to the conventional TV scan. It can also be applied horizontally by measuring the time from the beginning of the scan line to the detection point or white dot. The same continuity criterion can be applied in the horizontal direction. One can therefore do better than Fig. 3 shows and can, for example, accept cases such as Fig. 3e where there is clearly a horizontal discontinuity above and below the pupil to separate it from the additional firings. Any discontinuity, therefore, in the vertical or horizontal direction would be sufficient to separate the element being sought and allow the measurement of its position.

This technique works very efficiently when coupled with the various operator feedback indicators. The operator may instruct the subject to fixate on some points, and as the operator views the monitor image of the scene presented to the subject with superimposed cross hairs, he can clearly see if the cross hair position agrees with the subject's fixation point. If not, he can check the pupil monitor with crescents and centerlines. In this way there can be no doubt as to the quality of the measurement, and the operator can make any necessary adjustments.

III.6

Eye Movements: On-Line Measurement, Analysis, and Control [1]

James Anliker

NASA Ames Research Center

As an organizational basis for my remarks I shall recall some of the highlights of the ancient Greek myth concerning Perseus and the Gorgon Medusa. As you may remember, the wicked king of Seriphos, Polydectes, sent Perseus on what was presumed to be an impossible mission: he was to slay Medusa and bring back her head. The Gorgon's head with its horrible face and snaky locks symbolizes Ineffable (unutterable) Truth which cannot be grasped directly. . .

KOLERS: Especially when it is a can of worms!

ANLIKER: You have anticipated one of my points, namely, that the serpents covering the gorgon's head in place of hair symbolize the frightful complexity of Ineffable Truth. Please notice, however, that Medusa's head was covered with deadly vipers, not benign worms. Medusa, as her name implies, was "queen" of the Gorgons, i.e., the most frightening.

To continue with the myth, it was said that mortal man could not look directly at the face of Medusa without being petrified, which is to say, paralyzed or rendered impotent. Fortunately for Perseus, and possibly because of his heroic virtues, he was befriended and aided by Hermes, the messenger of the gods, and by his sister Athene, goddess of wisdom. The goddess, Medusa's sworn

[1] This work was supported in part by NASA under grant NGR-05-020-575 and by the Advanced Research Projects Agency of the Department of Defense under contract DAHC-72-C-0232 to Stanford University.

enemy, warned Perseus not to look directly at Medusa's terrible face but to observe her image reflected in his mirror-bright shield. According to the version given by Hesiod, Athene also taught Perseus how to distinguish the vulnerable Medusa from her two sister Gorgons who were immortal (possibly because one, Stheno, was too "strong" and the other, Euryale, was too "wide-leaping" to be conquered by man). From Hermes, Perseus obtained a sharp, unbreakable sword to be used in decapitating Medusa. Perseus also needed to find the three Stygian Nymphs who could lend him some equipment which was essential for his expedition: a pair of winged sandals which could magically transport the wearer to otherwise inaccessible places (and times?), a magic pouch in which he could conveniently and safely carry the awesome head of Medusa, and the helmet of invisibility which would allow Perseus to approach the Gorgons without being seen and, after seizing the trophy, to escape the fury of Medusa's sister Gorgons. The secret of where the Stygian Nymphs lived was known only to three ancient ladies, the swanlike Graeae, who shared a single marvelous eye and a single tooth. Perseus snatched the eye and the tooth from them during a moment when they were completely blind, namely, when the eye was being handed from one sister to another as they took turns using it [the first description of saccadic suppression (eds.)!]. With their most precious possessions in hand, Perseus was able to persuade these three ladies to reveal to him the location of the Nymphs in exchange for the return of their eye and tooth.

Well, as you know, Perseus succeeded in slaying Medusa and, returning to Seriphos, he petrified Polydectes and all of his courtiers by showing them the Gorgon's head.

I hope that you will not be disappointed when I confess that I cannot open my briefcase and dazzle you with the Unutterable Truth concerning eye movements, images, and memories. Instead I plan to describe for you a *P*rogrammed *E*yetrack *R*ecording *S*ystem and *E*ye-coupled *U*biquitous *S*cene generator which provides all the letters for constructing the acronym PERSEUS. Moreover, I believe that you will see, as my description of the system unfolds, that there are some thought-provoking parallels between the myth of Perseus and the electronic PERSEUS and its goals.

Rapid advances in eye tracking, digital display generation, signal classification, signal estimation and prediction, and control technology have made it increasingly tempting to apply real-time eye-tracking and computerized control techniques in the analysis of the relationships between eye movements and visually dependent performances. After discussing the problem on and off for several years, Professor David Lai of the Information Systems Laboratory, Stanford University, and I finally decided to stop talking only and to start working on the problem. Accordingly, for the past two years we have been collaborating in the design and implementation of a computer-based real-time eye-tracking system with associated digital scenic display capability. The completed system will be capable of moving and modifying the display contents so as to compensate effectively for a wide range of eye movements while keeping an accurate record of any or all data and operations of interest. We wish to obtain maximal freedom in controlling the placement (and displacement) of *scenic* images on the retina while permitting a rather wide range of eye movements.

Our ultimate objective in conducting this research and development is to gain a better understanding of visual memory for "concrete" or scenic images (as opposed to simple spots or printed text). We would hope that we might discover ways to control and enhance this type of visual memory. Whereas the recognition memory for complex, recognizable scenes is very large (Nickerson, 1965; Shepard, 1967; Standing, 1973) and of long duration (Nickerson, 1968), the ability to sustain a positive impression or image in the absence of an eliciting stimulus is, ordinarily, extremely limited and of very short duration. Therefore, any clues concerning how concrete visual images can be sustained or recalled in the absence of the original stimulus pattern would be of considerable practical value. In our opinion, a successful analysis of visualization strategies will not be accomplished without mobilizing the most powerful measurement and control techniques available. Our approach is to bring together into one coherent system the best available techniques for the real-time analysis and control of eye movements, scenic displays, and visual memory. Whereas it is a relatively straightforward task to study each of these variables separately, it is much more complex and demanding to analyze and control all three simultaneously, interactively, and in real time. Nevertheless, that is the difficult task that we have set for our electronic PERSEUS. Although the system as we envision it is not yet complete and ready to tackle its Medusa, I believe that you may be interested in hearing about some of the progress that has been achieved in the development of this programmed eye-track recording system and ubiquitous scene generator known as PERSEUS.

Eye tracking. Our plans for the development of PERSEUS call for the inclusion of an advanced eye tracker as a source of eye-position signals. The accurate two-dimensional eye tracker developed by Cornsweet and Crane (1973) has been selected for this purpose; its installation is expected before the end of the year. Meanwhile, in order to proceed with the development of the rest of PERSEUS, we have been using a simpler, less accurate, eye-movement monitor (Biometrics) as a sort of stand-in capable of generating real-time electrical signals corresponding to vertical and horizontal components of eye movements. We selected the Cornsweet–Crane eye tracker for this major front end role in PERSEUS because it is (a) sufficiently accurate (better than 5 min. of arc), (b) insensitive to translational movements of the eye, (c) convenient and non-contacting (uses reflected images from the eye), (d) noninterfering (uses infrared light), (e) capable of a nearly linear response over a sufficiently wide angle (10°

to 20°), and (f) only moderately expensive (being neither the least expensive nor the most expensive eye tracker available). Since Tom Cornsweet has already described his double Purkinje image method for eye tracking, I shall pass over this part of the system, but not without a few passing observations about some parallel relationships between this device and certain features of the Perseus myth. For example, the use of infrared light by the eye-tracker provides the electronic PERSEUS with the invisibility required for the stalking of its Medusa. The Purkinje images reflected from the eye are detected by a system which, like the magical great orb of the Graeae, "sees" images which are undetectable without instrumental assistance and which, like the gray ladies' divining tooth, interprets the meaning of these obscure images. And, of course, the great speed of electronic signal processing both here and throughout the PERSEUS system is competitive with that of the winged sandals used by the mythical Perseus and the 'mercurial' speed of the messenger of the gods.

Automatic detection of fixations and saccades. The eye tracker delivers continuous output voltages which are proportional to horizontal and vertical eye positions. It does not analyze the temporal *patterns* of these voltages into fixations and saccades. But PERSEUS to avoid disrupting visual perception, must be able to move the display only during the relatively blind period of the saccade, literally "in the twinkling of an eye". In other words, PERSEUS requires real time information concerning the moments of saccadic initiation and saccadic termination, i.e., the fixation-saccade and the saccade-fixation boundaries. One of our first programming efforts was directed, therefore, toward solving this problem of discriminating, on an automatic basis, between fixations and saccades. Various classification schemes were tried out by Arun Shah and Michael Stauffer, graduate students in Stanford's Information Systems Laboratory. I will give a brief account of one successful automatic classification scheme.

A fixation/saccade classification program has essentially two problems to solve: (a) deciding where, in the sample series, the fixational mode begins and the saccadic mode ends, and (b) deciding where the fixational mode ends and the saccadic mode begins. In this program both decisions are based on parameters which are largely empirical in nature. For determining whether a fixation is present, the program checks to find out if, of N points, M lie within a certain distance D of the mean location. The values of N, M, and D are set on the basis of Yarbus' observations (1967) and our own measurements of the duration and spatial extent of fixations. To detect the end of a fixation, the program examines the eye-position data to find out if a certain number of consecutive points falls outside of a prescribed distance from the mean. Again, the parameters are set as described above. When the fixation-saccade boundaries and the saccade-fixation boundaries have been identified, it is a relatively simple task to

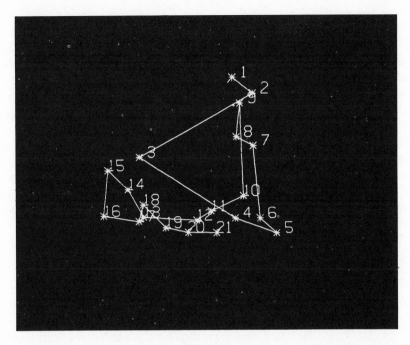

FIG. 1. Automatic scanpath analysis. Fixations are marked by stars and numbered in their order of occurrence in the scanpath. Sequential fixations are connected by straight lines; no attempt has been made to preserve the original saccadic paths.

generate some basic statistics about fixations and saccades such as durations and locations of fixations and distance, direction, velocity, etc. of saccades.

Automatic scanpath analysis. When you have developed the capacity for automatic detection of fixations and saccades, you are close to achieving automatic scanpath analysis. For his study of scanpath sequences Noton (1970) first recorded on analog tape the horizontal and vertical output voltages from his eye-tracking device while his subjects scanned projected test figures. After digitizing these data, he plotted them slowly enough to be able to detect the fixations by direct inspection and to number them by hand. This approach is not only very time consuming but also relies heavily upon subjective judgments by the scorer. However, it also avoids the problems inherent in communicating to a computer the detailed instructions it requires for the performance of a completely automatic scanpath analysis. The automatic fixation/saccade detector described above and a programmed assignment of ordinal numbers to successive fixations together generate an automatic scanpath analysis. Figure 1 shows the result of such a process. Arun Shah implemented two different fixation/saccade classification schemes which I shall describe next.

The first of these is a *position-variance method,* based on the fact that a fixation is characterized by relative immobility (low position variance) whereas a saccade is distinguished by rapid change of position (high position variance). For a sliding window of sample times, the means and variances are computed. The variance of the data inside a time window containing only fixation samples is lower than some empirically determined threshold value. When a saccade starts, the variance rises, reaches a peak, and subsides toward the fixation level again. By selecting an appropriate threshold value for the position variance, we can objectively and automatically detect the initiation and termination of a saccade. Furthermore, by fitting curves to the variance function, we can make predictions about future variance values which, along with the straight-line assumption, serve to predict the time and location of the next fixation. The position-variance method suffers somewhat from a time lag attributable to the width of the sliding window, and its calculation is burdensome.

An alternative approach that relieves some of the difficulties just mentioned, is the *velocity detection method.* In this method, the threshold is set for an empirically determined velocity level above which the eye is assumed to be in the saccadic mode and below which, in the fixational mode. This discrimination can be given added stability by specifying further that a run of N samples is required in each new mode before the system recognizes a change of state; however, it should be noted that the inclusion of this criterion entails a delay equivalent to the length of the run specified. At any rate, Fig. 2 shows that the position-variance and the velocity methods give similar results.

It is feasible to combine these two methods to obtain an even more reliable fixation/saccade discriminator under circumstances where reliability is more important than speed. The combined position-variance/velocity method could be based either quite simply upon the two threshold detector outputs (agreement, disagreement) or, more elaborately, upon the state-probability estimates derived from the magnitudes of the position-variance and the velocity measures.

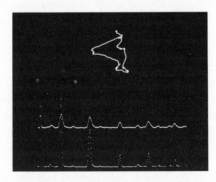

FIG. 2. A comparison of the sample mean velocity function (middle) and the position-variance function (bottom) for eye-movement data (top). Observe the close correspondence between the peaks of the two functions.

Michael Stauffer has programmed a velocity-based prediction scheme that derives from Yarbus' observation (1965) that the eye-movement velocity function during a saccade is nearly symmetrical around a peak velocity located approximately half-way to the next fixation. In other words, the saccadic velocity function rises above the fixational velocity level, accelerates to a peak velocity about half-way to the next fixation, then decelerates to land on the next fixation point. Therefore, by detecting the peak of the saccadic velocity function, measuring the elapsed time and the distance traveled between the beginning of the saccade and the peak of the velocity function, and by taking into account the saccadic direction, we can project these values forward to predict the approximate arrival time and location of the next fixation.

Figures 3a–3d illustrate such a predictive sequence. Although Yarbus (1965) reported a good fit for the velocity function using a sine wave, the velocity function is, in fact, more or less asymmetrical depending upon the magnitude of the peak velocity. Consequently, the prediction of saccadic termination time and saccadic termination distance can be improved by creating and consulting a look-up table containing the empirically determined correction factors needed to adjust for the asymmetry of the saccadic velocity function.

Fixation-conditional stimulation. In many visual experiments, although there is a requirement that the subject's eye be fixated on a specified target at the time of exposure of the test object, the actual direction of eye pointing at the moment of stimulation is seldom monitored. Instead, the experimenter relies upon his subjects to carry out his instructions (and upon statistics to clean up the mess). In fact a subject's ability to monitor his own eye movements is very limited. Yarbus (1967) reported that subjects were frequently unaware of rather sizeable saccades. Occasional studies can be found in which the experimenter, in order to insure fixation, directly observed the subject's eye position, or monitored eye position with electronic techniques, or photographed the eye for off-line classification of trials.

As a part of the development of PERSEUS, Robert Floyd and I have implemented a scheme for the real-time monitoring of fixations and the automatic control of computer-generated displays on an SEL-840 computer. The fixation-monitoring portion of this program recognizes two states, namely, ON TARGET and OFF TARGET. The experimenter may specify the following parameters of fixation: (a) the location of the fixational target center, (b) the acceptable range or radius of ON TARGET values, and (c) the duration of continuous within-range eye pointing that is required before an ON TARGET state is recognized. Whenever the eye moves outside the ON TARGET radius, the fixation monitor switches to the OFF TARGET state. The stimulus-controlling portion of the program can then require that the ON TARGET conditions be met as a prerequisite (additional conditions may be required) for the display of a stimulus object. If the eye moves OFF TARGET before the prescribed stimulus exposure has been completed, the display is instantly blanked. It is a relatively simple

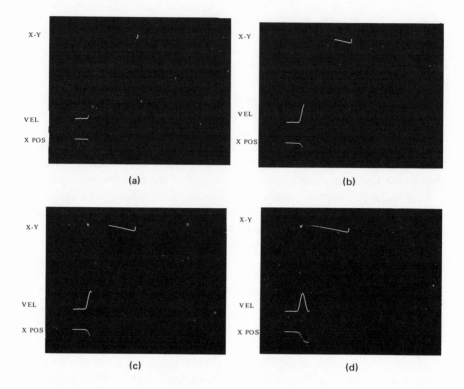

FIG. 3a. Prediction of the saccadic target. Eye position (X, Y) is near beginning of saccade. Note the increase in velocity (VEL).

FIG. 3b. Prediction of saccadic target. Velocity function approaches peak.

FIG. 3c. Prediction of saccadic target. Velocity has just passed its peak and a prediction is made as to the location of the next fixation (star).

FIG. 3d. Prediction of saccadic target. Shows saccade terminating at the predicted fixation location.

matter for the computer to keep an account of the complete and incomplete stimulus exposures. Such a fixation-conditional stimulus controller is extremely useful both from the standpoint of (a) preventing the leakage of stimulus information to the subject through other than the experimentally specified retinal routes and (b) eliminating response data associated with incomplete stimulus presentations. It can speed up experimentation by allowing trials to proceed as soon as fixational requirements are met and simultaneously eliminate a serious source of experimental error, namely, the fallible experimenter —monitor. An interesting application of this fixation—conditional stimulus controller is found in the study of eye pointing as an operant response. I am currently studying reinforcement of eye pointing responses to visible and invisible targets in an attempt to determine to what extent eye pointing can be divorced from visual contents.

I will proceed with the description of a recent version of the program. The new version is more general and provides for real-time monitoring and recording of sequences of free-scanning fixations or scanpaths. The development of this program is a large step toward the implementation of biocybernetic schemes for the prediction and control of eye pointing behavior. and the generation of eye position–conditional displays. This scheme has been programmed on an SEL-840 computer and utilizes the associated Evans and Sutherland line-drawing system. Two 21-inch CRT's are exercised simultaneously: one CRT is used as a monitor for the display of various analyses and experimental parameters that may be of interest to the experimenter; the other CRT is used to display stimulus patterns for viewing by the subject at a distance that allows $1.66°$ of visual angle per inch of display surface. The subject's head is fixed and his eye position is monitored. I shall skip over the rather extensive calibration procedure. Following the calibration (which is repeated at intervals), the subject may be asked to inspect a displayed test pattern. During his visual scanning the program creates time-varying amplitude histograms using the digitized horizontal and vertical voltages received from the eye tracker. The entries in the separate horizontal and vertical amplitude histograms (see Figs. 4a and 4b) are accumulated in accordance with a

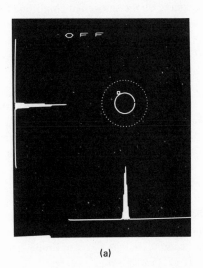

(a)

FIG. 4a.   Real-time fixation–conditional controller. Amplitude histograms for horizontal and vertical eye positions are located at bottom and left side, respectively. Fixation circle is smaller solid circle. The dotted circle designates the spatial limit. Small square indicates location of instantaneous eye position; notice that small square is *outside* the solid circle, so monitor scope displays OFF.

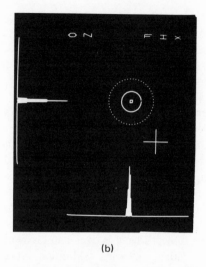

(b)

FIG. 4b.   Real-time fixation–conditional controller. Similar to Fig. 4a except instantaneous eye position (small square) is *inside* the solid circle; therefore display shows ON. FIX indicates that program is in scanpath mode. All fixations are designated by cross marks.

sliding window of time (the width of the window is specified in milliseconds by the experimenter). The peaks of the smoothed amplitude histograms are treated as the best estimates of horizontal and vertical eye positions within the time window. The eye position (X, Y) is made the center of a circle (solid circumference) the radius of which is controllable by the experimenter (or the program), enabling him to tighten or relax the fixational requirements imposed upon the subject's eye pointing. By setting an amplitude threshold detector to monitor the peak of the amplitude histogram we have a basis for defining the initiation of a fixation. A second circle (dotted circumference), sharing the same center as the fixational or target circle previously described, has an independently variable radius which must be equal to, or greater than, the target (or fixational) circle's radius. This dotted circle, displayed on the monitor CRT, is used by the experimenter to set spatial limits for the fixational mode. That is, when the instantaneous eye position (designated in the figures by a small square) exits through the boundary defined by the dotted circle, it is assumed that the eye is making a saccadic movement (i.e., the fixation has terminated). It is also assumed that the data accumulated in the amplitude histograms is no longer relevant; consequently these distributions are reset to zero and the monitor circles vanish until a new fixation is established. An important feature of this program is that, in addition to ON TARGET and OFF TARGET state detection, it provides for the storage of scanpaths of up to 100 fixations. In the scanpath monitoring mode, the program displays numbered cross marks on the monitor CRT in locations corresponding to the various fixations in a scanpath. This real-time monitoring and storage of scanpath locations makes possible the recreation at a subsequent time of the scenes located at the various fixation points. One of the questions we hope to answer through the use of this program is whether guiding the subject through his earlier scanpath has a favorable effect upon image recognition. We are considering the hypothesis that one characteristic of superior concrete imagery is an uncommon consistency in the retracing of scanpaths during the reviewing of familiar scenes. In other words, one possible difference between excellent concrete visual memory and poor concrete visual memory could be that the former remembers both *what* was seen and *where* it was located whereas the latter has more difficulty with *where* than with *what* (or vice versa). The ability to recall *where* environmental information is located is obviously helpful in finding or recognizing patterns located there. What effect extraordinary powers of location might have is not clear. A tantalizing clue that seems to point in the direction of benefits associated with superior powers of location is found in the ability of some eidetic individuals to experience emergent perceptions based on the integration of two scenes presented separately (Leask, Haber, & Haber, 1969; Stromeyer & Psotka, 1970). There is, of course, in musical skills a clear-cut distinction between the ability to recognize a musical pattern that is heard and the ability to summon the same pattern by means of executing from memory the operations required to produce this pattern of sounds from a musical instrument. Using this analogy, it seems possible that the visual perception of familiar material might depend—especially in difficult perceptual tasks—upon the skilled execution of a complex sequence of eye movements, predominantly under the guidance of memory rather than being serially elicited by the stimuli encountered at each successive fixation point. To return to the musical analogy, the memories that guide the pianist's fingers not only accurately predict the physical properties of the keyboard mechanics and the notes of the composition, but also predict the auditory feedback that will result from the patterned motor output to the keyboard. Although the training process may be very time consuming and tedious—as in programming and debugging a complex computer operation—the concert performance is rapid, smooth, and can be so automatic that the performer himself experiences a strong sense of detachment from the performance similar to that of a Zen master who says of his extraordinary skill, "it happens." It seems likely that the development of complex motor skills associated with superior powers in memorizing concrete images (scenery) will be far more difficult to analyze than the eye movements associated with the reading of texts and technical diagrams.

In line with the previously mentioned study of fixation—conditional reinforcement, this real-time scanpath analyzer can be used to study scanpath-conditional reinforcement. The response I am trying to obtain from subjects is a sort of eye-movement slalom or the successive fixation of a course or sequence or targets (visible or invisible) within progressively narrowing time limits. The basic question being asked is essentially the same as before, namely, to what extent can eye-movement patterns be divorced from, or integrated with, visual contents?

Digital scene generation   So far I have said very little about the scenic stimulus materials except to indicate that they are derived from a digital data base. While a digital source for images is highly desirable from many points of view, it is seldom utilized to any very large extent. The reason for this is not far to seek. There are many, many problems that attend the building of a digital data base and there are many more problems in trying to make a digital display compete with an analog display. The poorest photographer can set a standard that is difficult to match in a digital system. Nevertheless, the advantages offered by computerized speed and flexibility have lured us in the digital direction. With the able assistance of Kenneth Jacker, Alan Huang, and Lynn Strickland, I have been developing a flexible program for the creation, storage, and display of digitized patterns. This program, called SEER, currently accepts data from a grafpen (ultimately it will employ an automatic scanner on the input), digitizes, catalogues, and stores segmented patterns in disk memory. It provides for the equalization of sample densities along contours as well as the modulation of sample density so that a display of the tracing at a constant sampling rate appears to "slow down" on sharp curves and to "speed up" on straighter segments, allowing close tracking by a subject's eye of the moving spot on a display CRT. The SEER program can draw at very high speed on a CRT that can either hold the tracing in its storage mode or rely upon rapid refreshment from the computer. With these arrangements it is possible to obtain precise eye-movement tracings of stimulus patterns by asking the subject to track (pursue) a moving spot which traces the contours of the figure. This can be done in two different ways: (1) the entire figure may be drawn rapidly onto the storage CRT so that it is present while the subject tracks a slowly moving spot around the contours of the displayed figure; or (2) the subject may be allowed to see only the spot that he is currently tracking. If you happen to be using an eye monitor that is significantly nonlinear, you may find it useful to have the subject make a nonlinear tracing (i.e., by collecting the eye positions corresponding to the stimulus contours as measured through the nonlinear eye tracker). It is convenient to superimpose scanpath data upon such a tracing because both share the same nonlinearities. If the goal is simply to detect which features the eye is fixating, this approach is far easier than attempting to linearize the nonlinear data; however, we are also incorporating linearization algorithms in the design of PERSEUS.

The final, most difficult step for the electronic PERSEUS to accomplish consists of controlling the display of scenic patterns of light so that images falling upon the retina are confined (though not completely stabilized) to specified locations on the retina regardless of the subject's eye movements. The problem with this is that scenes, in contrast with single spots, are much more affected by perspective—especially when projected upon a relatively flat display surface. Although we have not been able as yet to exploit it (because of the extensive programming effort I have been describing), we are exceptionally fortunate in having access to a quite remarkable display system (Wempe & Palmer, 1970; Chase, 1972; Palmer & Cronn, 1973) developed by the Man-Machine Integration Branch of the NASA Ames Research Center. This advanced computer graphics system, utilizing the same SEL-840 computer and Evans and Sutherland line-drawing system mentioned previously, can be programmed to display to a pilot a view in dynamic perspective of the night scene of an airport landing area. Figure 5, a photograph of one frame of the simulated out-the-window night scene at the airport of San Jose, California, gives some idea of the exceptional realism that can be achieved by using some 1200 points of light. This all-digital approach to scenic simulation not only eliminates the camera optics and electromechanical servomechanisms of TV-model systems of simulation but also opens the way to the virtually unlimited sequencing of data-base contents and perspectives thereof. In other words, not being limited by the structure and inertia of physical models or of actual events, it is possible to generate either unnaturally "realistic" scenes or, conversely, to generate utterly fantastic "events" or sequences of events which would not be possible in the physical world. Furthermore, these images emerging from the digital data base (where, say, a particular "airport" is stored as a three-dimensional matrix of points) can be selected, modified as to content, modified as to perspective,

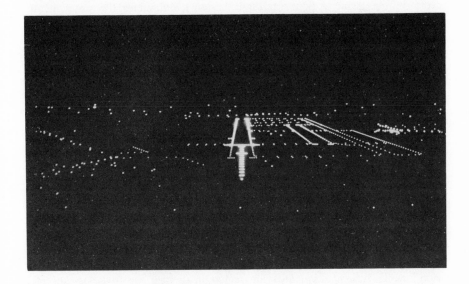

FIG. 5. Digital simulation of the night scene of the landing area of the airport at San Jose, California. This frame is composed of 1200 points of light.

offset, and so forth, at a rate of 30 "frames" per sec, where each frame consists of a picture utilizing 1200 to 2000 points and/or lines connecting points. It should be evident that such an advanced system, which is already able to modify its output in accordance with input information concerning aircraft position and attitude, is admirably suited to respond equally well to inputs about eye position with a minimal amount of reprogramming.

The domain of Medusa. Before closing I would like to make a few observations on the nature of memory for concrete or scenic images (as distinguished from abstract or verbal images). Recent research on the perception of visual chimeric images by patients with sectioned interhemispheric connections (Levy, Trevarthen, & Sperry, 1972) indicates that the minor hemisphere, sometimes known as "silent" hemisphere, is distinctly more adept than the major hemisphere in dealing with concrete images. On the other hand, the major hemisphere (as has long been known) excels in the processing of abstract or verbal materials. It seems reasonable to assume that, on a continuum ranging from the smallest part or detail to the largest whole that can be screened on the retina, the parts would be easier to transcribe into verbal behavior than the whole (the "unutterable All"). Thus, I cannot resist making the suggestion that the domain of the silent Medusa (Ineffable Truth) lies in that verbally dark, but experientially bright, region of concrete images.

If Levy, Trevarthen and Sperry (1972) are correct in their analysis, it seems likely that Medusa still reigns over the minor hemisphere while her articulate adversary, the divine Athene (cultural Wisdom), dominates the major hemisphere. The hatred of Athene for Medusa might be explained by the observation that they were, at an earlier (preverbal) age, twin sisters (balanced hemispheres). But Athene, ambitious for immortality, worked her way up to divine status by developing her latent powers of abstraction to the extent of being able to defy Time (in the sense that cultural products survive the death of the individual whereas inarticulate personal experience cannot). Consequently, the talkative parvenu (Athene) is perpetually trying to dissociate herself from her ancient sisterhood with Medusa (silent, sensuous Truth). Much in the manner that (male? eds) mathematicians attempt to exalt their paramour as "queen of the sciences" (a phrase used by the mathematician Gauss) and deny her humble origins, Hesiod tries to persuade us that Athene sprang straight from the brow of Zeus, fully armed, with a mighty shout.

The Perseus myth suggests that Ineffable Truth, which leaves man speechless, can only be approached *indirectly.* Therefore, if I may be permitted to continue this line of thought, I am strongly inclined to suggest that Medusa is identified more with the periphery (or perhaps the whole nonfoveal retina) or "indirect vision" while Athene dominates the region in or near the fovea or "direct" vision. In other words, that which is singled our for foveal fixation will tend to be closer to the possibility of verbal accounting than are the vast polymorphous contents of the periphery (and the largely intuitive regions located just beyond the retinal limits). Peering into my own crystal ball, I predict that the most interesting use for the electronic PERSEUS will be found in the analysis of peripheral visual functions—especially as they relate to the perception and memorization of concrete or scenic images. The foveal precinct is, after all, a very small portion of the retina, a part that is heavily dependent upon the periphery for orientation and for guidance toward worthwhile visual targets. One cannot fit a very large scene upon the fovea during one fixation and yet there is little evidence that the eye attempts to systematically process the scene by a series of foveal aliquots. While it seems to be true that some features require more foveal attention than other features, it seems to me that we have largely forgotten the fact that fixations also serve to *center* the entire scene of interest upon the retina so as to include simultaneously peripheral objects on opposite edges of the retina just as a photographer may have as his goal the fitting of all present into his group picture rather than excluding all but one. Stated in more general terms, some visual problems are solved by obtaining a larger field of view while sacrificing details (or resolution) whereas other visual problems require an opposite compromise. There appears to be a trade-off between memory and eccentricity of image placement on the retina. Thus memory or familiarity with visual objects permits their recognition at more eccentric locations than is possible for less familiar objects. In this way, memory acts to relax the data-processing load in the more central regions of the retina. A consequence of developing familiarity, therefore, would be to reduce dependence upon foveal contact and to encourage the giving of attention to the larger, extrafoveal panorama.

In summary, I have tried to give you an outline of the plans for, and the progress in, the development of a Programmed Eye-track Recording System and Eye-coupled Ubiquitous Scene-generator, otherwise known by the acronym PERSEUS. I have attempted to give some indications why a comprehensive electronic system intended for the analysis of the visualization of concrete scenes must provide real-time counterparts for the eye movements, images, and memories of its flesh-and-blood partner in this complex biocybernetic interaction. The myth of Perseus and the Gorgon Medusa was introduced to appeal to the imagination in dealing with an abstruse area of vision that is not, at least at present, translatable into satisfactory objective terms.

III.7

References

Baer, D. M., & Wright, J. C. Developmental Psychology. In M. R. Rosenzweig & L. W. Porter (Eds.), *Annual review of psychology* (Vol. 25). Palo Alto: Annual Reviews, 1974.

Butler, D. H., Kamlet, A. S., & Monty, R. A. A multi-purpose analysis of variance FORTRAN IV computer program. *Psychonomic Monograph Supplements,* 1969, **2,** 301–319 (Whole No. 32).

Chase, W. D. Performance with computer generated and TV-model visual displays for visual simulation of the landing approach. Paper presented at the International Society for Information Display, San Francisco, 1972.

Cornsweet, T. N. A new technique for the measurement of small eye movements. *Journal of the Optical Society of America,* 1958, **48,** 808–811.

Cornsweet, T. N., & Crane, H. D. Accurate two-dimensional eye tracker using first and fourth Purkinje images. *Journal of the Optical Society of America,* 1973, **63,** 921–928.

Lambert, R. H., Monty, R. A., and Hall, R. J. High speed data processing and unobtrusive monitoring of eye movements. *Behavior Research Methods and Instrumentation,* 1974, **6,** 525–530.

Leask, J., Haber, R. N., & Haber, R. B. Eidetic imagery in children: II. Longitudinal and experimental results. *Psychonomic Monograph Supplements,* 1969, 3, 25–48.

Levy, J., Trevarthen, C., & Sperry, R. W. Perception of bilateral chimeric figures following hemispheric deconnexion. *Brain,* 1972, **95,** 61–78.

Mackworth, N. H. A stand camera for line-of-sight recording. *Perception & Psychophysics,* 1967, **2,** 119–127.

Mackworth, N. H. The line-of-sight approach to children's reading and comprehension. In S. F. Wanat, H. Singer, & M. Kling (Eds.), *Extracting meaning from written language.* Newark: International Reading Association, 1975.

Mackworth, N. H., & Bruner, J. S. How adults and children search and recognize pictures. *Human Development,* 1970, **13,** 149–177.

Mackworth, N. H., Grandstaff, N. W., & Pribram, K. H. Orientation to pictorial novelty by speech-disordered children. *Neuropsychologia,* 1973, **11,** 443–450.

Merchant, J., & Morrissette, R. Remote measurement of eye direction allowing subject motion over one cubic foot of space. *IEEE Transactions on Biomedical Engineering,* 1974, **BME-21,** 309–317.

Monty, R. A. An advanced eye-movement measuring and recording system featuring unobtrusive monitoring and automatic data processing. *American Psychologist,* 1975, **30,** 331–335.

Nickerson, R. S. Short-term memory for complex meaningful visual configurations, a demonstration of capacity. *Canadian Journal of Psychology,* 1965, **19,** 155–160.

Nickerson, R. S. A note on long-term recognition memory for pictorial material. *Psychonomic Science,* 1968, **11,** 58.

Noton, D. Scanpaths in eye movements during pattern perception. Doctoral Dissertation (Part 4), University of California, Berkeley, 1970.

Palmer, E. A., & Cronn, F. W. Touchdown performance with a computer graphics night visual attachment. *Proceedings of the AIAA Visual and Motion Simulation Conference,* Paper No. 73-927, Palo Alto, Calif., 1973.

Shepard, R. N. Recognition memory for words, sentences, and pictures. *Journal of Verbal Learning and Verbal Behavior,* 1967, **6,** 156–163.

Standing, L. Learning 10,000 pictures. *Quarterly Journal of Experimental Psychology,* 1973, **25,** 207–222.

Stromeyer, C. F., & Psotka, J. The detailed texture of eidetic images. *Nature,* 1970, **225,** 346–349.

Wempe, T., & Palmer, E. A. Pilot performance with a simulated pictorial landing display including different conditions of resolution and update rate. *Proceedings of the Sixth Annual Conference on Manual Control,* Wright-Patterson Air Force Base, Ohio, 1970.

Yarbus, A. L. The motion of the eye in the process of changing the points of fixation. *Biofizika,* 1965, **1,** 76–78.

Yarbus, A. L. *Eye movements and vision.* New York: Plenum Press, 1967.

Young, L. R., & Sheena, D. Survey of eye movement recording methods. *Behavior Research Methods and Instrumentation,* 1975, **7,** 397–429. (a)

Young, L. R. and Sheena, D. Eye movement measurement techniques. *American Psychologist,* 1975, **30,** 315–330. (b)

Part IV

THE RELATION OF EYE MOVEMENTS TO THE PERCEPTION OF MOTION, POSITION, AND TIMING OF VISUAL STIMULI

Session IV is concerned with matters relating to the effect of eye movements on the perception of the location, the movement, and the timing of visual stimuli. Problems arise basically from the fact that even though identical patterns of stimulus change on our sense organs may be produced either by movements of things in the environment or by movements of the body, we normally do not confuse the two. That is to say, the world appears to remain stable and to present a constant picture independent of the voluntary and the involuntary eye movements which lead to changes in retinal stimulation. However, there are differences between two different kinds of "involuntary" eye movements: those which are made by the organism, perhaps at some less-than-conscious level, which yield a stable world, and those which are made by external forces applied to the eyes in which the world appears to move in a way strongly related to the movement of the eye. Such a difference immediately suggests the very strong influence on visual space perception of signals derived from the oculomotor control system. Whether these are "outflow" or "inflow" or both is still not completely settled.

However, this stability is not universally true. Both pursuit movements and saccades significantly alter the perceived position, movement, and timing of stimuli which are in fact stationary or moving in other directions from those perceived. In a sense it may be difficult for the visual system to do two things at the same time. That is to say, when the eye is engaged in pursuit tracking of one stimulus, another stimulus moving in the visual field may suffer distortions of position and direction of movement. These problems regarding visual direction have been studied by a number of investigators, several of whom have employed brief flashes in close temporal proximity to the eye movement. Although some of the important issues are clarified by the work described below, it is also clear that much remains to be done.

This session was chaired by Dr. Leonard Matin of Columbia University.

IV.1

Saccades and Extraretinal Signal for Visual Direction [1]

Leonard Matin

Columbia University

I am going to tell you about the influence of the extraretinal signal on reports of visual direction. There are, however, three other items that must concern us: (1) It is possible for the presence of other visual stimuli (visual context) to influence the report of visual direction for any particular stimulus being judged. (2) Visual stimuli presented as flashes for any particular duration persist in perception for a considerable time beyond the actual duration of the visual stimulus. (3) Eye movements result in smears and masking. I will be showing you that visual context, visual persistence, and smears and masking all control the perception of visual direction. But in order to study the extraretinal signal a situation must be employed that allows its influence to be separated from influences from these other sources.

When I originally began working on how the perception of a stable world is maintained when we make saccadic eye movements, it was possible to entertain as a working hypothesis the simple view that the controlling mechanism was essentially a cancellation mechanism, that even though the stimulus at the retina was shifted when we moved our eyes, there was another process which maintained stability by knowing exactly how far the eye moved, feeding this information back or forward, and doing the algebra appropriate to maintaining stability. Now the cancellation model doesn't fit anything that we have found, and in Figs. 3 and 4 I will indicate the sloppiness of the visual perception of

[1] This work was supported by grants from the National Eye Institute, National Institutes of Health (EY 00375) and the National Science Foundations (NSF GB 5947 and NSF BM S73-01463 A01).

direction when visual context, smears, and masking play no role, leaving the extraretinal signal as the most substantial controlling influence.

A Digression—Perceived Stability and Involuntary Fixation Eye Movements

For a variety of reasons it is useful to first digress and look at a case where the eye movements are not saccadic. In this case the following sequence was presented: 400 msec following extinction of a fixation target two vertical lines were sequentially flashed (2 msec each) for vernier judgment by the subject (Fig. 1). For the data in Fig. 2 the same pair of lines was presented on every trial: the horizontal offset of the lines was 21" of visual angle and the time between their presentations was 100 msec. In the actual experiment this stimulus was randomly alternated on different trials with others containing different spatial and temporal separations.

Since the subject was attempting to hold his eye steady in a position determined by the previous fixation target, any eye movements that took place

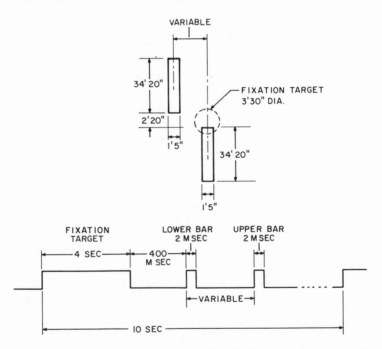

FIG. 1. Experimental paradigm employed in dealing with influence of involuntary fixation eye movements on visual direction. (a) Spatial array consisting of fixation target and two bars. (b) Temporal sequence of stimuli on a trial. Subject reported on vernier offset of the two bars. For data in Fig. 2 the variable offset was fixed at 21". (Matin, Matin, & Pola, 1968).

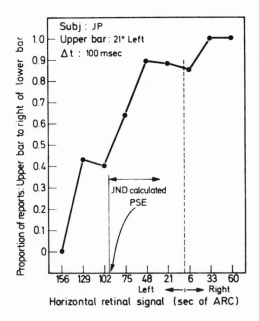

FIG. 2. The ordinate displays the proportion of trials on which subject JP reported that the upper vertical bar (Fig. 1) appeared to the right of the lower vertical bar. On each trial the upper bar was flashed 100 msec after the lower one and was located 21″ to the left of the lower one. The abscissa is the horizontal offset between the retinal loci of the two flashed bars; trial-to-trial variation in this retinal distance is wholly due to trial-to-trial variation in the eye movement between presentation of the two bars. (Matin, Matin, & Pola, 1968).

between presentation of the two lines were totally involuntary. If the subject knew where his eyes were going, presumably he would take this information into account and carry out the appropriate cancellation leaving the same accurate perception on every trial. But instead, as is normally the case in psychophysical experiments, on some trials the subject reported that the upper line lay to the left and on other trials to the right of the lower line although on all trials the upper line was exactly 21″ to the right of the lower line. Clearly, if a cancellation mechanism was at work it was not working with perfect reliability. Since the eye movements were monitored by a contact lens technique (Matin, 1964; Matin & Pearce, 1964) it was possible to calculate the total offset in the stimulus at the retina produced by the combination of 21″ offset of the two target lines and the involuntary eye movements that took place in the 100 msec between their presentation. Variation in this quantity (the horizontal retinal signal) among trials—wholly produced by the involuntary eye movements (abscissa in Fig. 2)—produced a substantial part of the variability in psychophysical response, generating the regular psychophysical function in Fig. 2. Although we do not show the other data here (see Matin, 1972) the response variability increased from about .5' at zero interstimulus interval to reach about 6' at an interval of 800 msec. The fact that some variability in response remains after the influence of variation in magnitude of the eye movement on the retinal signal has been removed, and the existence of change in this response variability with interstimulus interval, suggest another process at work—failure of memory in the interstimulus interval for the location of the first flashed line (Matin, Pearce, Matin, & Kibler, 1966; Matin, 1972)—a process for which Kinchla has developed a quantitative model (Kinchla & Allen, 1969).

It is now important to note that the failure of cancellation shown by the imperfectly reliable response in Fig. 2 does not mean that the cancellation mechanism is not operative at all. However, further analysis has not yielded any clear connection of this failure to a "canceling extraretinal signal" (Matin et al., 1966; Matin, 1972).

Nevertheless, since the eye movements we have dealt with so far are involuntary, the failure—or lack of participation—of a canceling extraretinal signal probably isn't too surprising to many of you, particularly if you believe that the extraretinal signal is guided by "outflowing" or "efferent" neural signals. If efferent signals are the sole direct source of information regarding the occurrence of eye movements (besides information coming in via visual stimulation), then it is not too surprising that a subject does not know that his eyes have moved if he was attempting to hold them steady (however, see Matin, 1972).

We now return to the saccadic case.

The Extraretinal Signal for Saccades Does Not Cancel

The results of an experiment that was actually done four years ago probably give the simplest and clearest indication of why I have concluded that the extraretinal signal related to saccades is sloppy. On each trial the subject first fixated one point in an otherwise dark room. Shortly after it was extinguished, a second point was flashed $2°11'$ to the right of the first point. When the subject saw the flashed point he turned his eye to it. Since the first flash was over before the saccade began, the saccade was carried out in darkness. However, when his eye reached a particular point midway into the saccade, two vertical lines were simultaneously flashed on the central fovea for 1 msec, again in a vernier configuration. These were the same two lines that were employed in the involuntary case described above and their presentation was triggered by a pulse from the eye position monitor. The horizontal physical offset of the two lines was randomly varied among trials and the subject was required to report whether the upper line appeared to the left or right of the lower line.

The important point about this experiment was that there were two main conditions and two control conditions. In each of the two main conditions the two lines differed in illuminance by two log units: in one condition the upper line was 2 log units brighter than the lower line; in the second the lower line was 2 log units brighter than the upper line. In each of the two control conditions the two lines were equally bright: in one control condition they were both set at the lower brightness employed in the two main conditions; in the other control condition they were both set at the higher brightness employed in the two main conditions.

There was no substantial difference in the response distributions among the four conditions. In addition the center of not one of the distributions deviated by as much as a minute from veridicality.

This result may not seem terribly puzzling if you believe that a "canceling extraretinal signal" is operative, for a truly effective signal would not be fooled by the difference of 4 log units of illuminance across the two main conditions in spite of the fact that such differences in stimulus intensity produce substantial differences in latency to the onset of the visual response to flashed stimuli (of the order of 30 msec for the present stimuli). A truly effective signal would correct for such differences in latency of response to stimulation from different parts of the visual field (most of which difference is produced in the retina) and generate a stable and accurate percept anyway. However, such a remarkable extraretinal signal would also have to have independent information regarding the true physical times of stimulation by the two lines if it were to correct for different times at which the responses to the two lines come out of the retina, and would thus have to come from a locus in front of the photoreceptors or at least no more proximal than the photoreceptors.

Such an unreasonable conclusion is only arrived at, however, if we believe: (1) that a canceling extraretinal signal shifts the relation between stimulated retinal locus and visually perceived direction at a rate that parallels the eye movement itself, and (2) that the process occurs in the service of maintaining stability of visual direction. For it is the combination of these two requirements that generates the need to compensate for intensity differences. A process that shifts the relation between retinal locus and visual direction in parallel with the eye movement but does not correct for latency/intensity differences would yield a special class of distortions which, in the present experiment, would have required a vernier offset of several degrees of visual angle between the two lines in order to yield an appearance of colinearity; such a prediction is a far cry from the nonsystematic, under-one-minute variation we actually obtained.

The conclusion we thus arrive at is that it is not true that a canceling extraretinal signal shifts the relation of stimulated retinal locus and perceived visual direction at a rate that parallels the actual saccadic eye movement. This conclusion is confirmed in another set of experiments (Matin & Pearce, 1965; Matin, Matin, & Pearce, 1969; Matin, Matin, & Pola, 1970; Matin & Matin, 1972; Matin, 1972). In these experiments (Fig. 3) we measured the time course by which the extraretinal signal shifted the relation between retinal locus and visual direction. This time course is shown in Fig. 4. While a time course that parallels

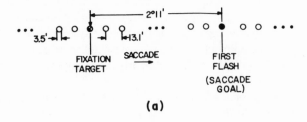

(a)

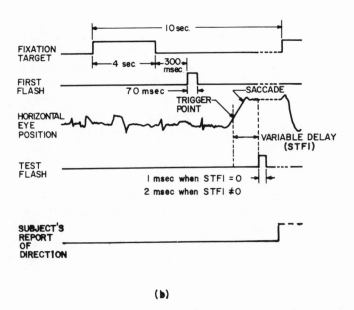

(b)

FIG. 3. Experimental paradigm employed in mapping the time course of the extraretinal signal for voluntary saccades. (a) Spatial array of targets. Any target in the array could be employed as a test flash. (b) Temporal sequence of stimulation, eye movements, and report of direction on each trial. Following extinction of the fixation target the subject attempted to hold his eye at the position of fixation until he saw the first flash, at which time he turned his eye to look at it. Since the saccade began after the first flash was extinguished, it was carried out in darkness. On each trial, either before, during, or after the saccade a test flash was presented to the subject from a randomly preselected member of the horizontal array (STFI represents saccade-test flash interval). Following test-flash presentation the subject reported whether the test flash appeared to the left or to the right of the previously extinguished fixation target.

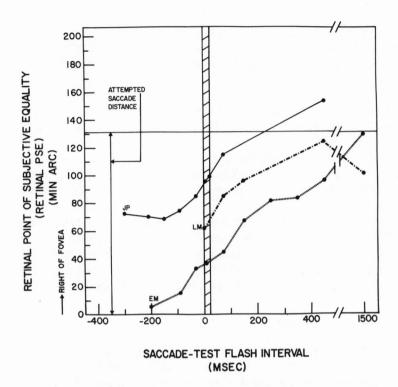

SACCADE-TEST FLASH INTERVAL
(MSEC)

FIG. 4. Variation of the point of subjective equality (PSE) of the fixation target as measured by the test flash (see Fig. 3). The PSE measures the "magnitude" of the extraretinal signal. The PSE is a distance at the retina, and is calculated from knowledge of the eye position (contact-lens technique) and target position. It is the retinal distance between the image of the fixation target and that test flash which is reported to lie to the left and to the right of the fixation target equally often; hence the PSE is the location of the test flash that we take to be the one that appears in the same visual direction as the fixation target had before the saccade. The cross-hatched bar represents the period of the saccade. If the extraretinal signal were not operative at all the data would follow a horizontal straight line at zero on the ordinate. If the inferred extraretinal signal were appropriate to maintain stability of visual direction alone it would begin to climb from zero at the beginning of the saccade and complete its climb to 131' at the moment that the saccade terminated.

the saccade would be wholly included within the cross-hatched vertical bar and extend from zero at zero time (the left edge of the bar) to 131' at roughly 25 msec (the right edge of the bar), the actual time course is very much slower and more extended in time; it begins before the saccade, changes only slightly during the saccade, and continues to change for a considerable period after the saccade. The eye and extraretinal signal are out of correspondance for a long time. Clearly such an extraretinal signal is not sufficient to explain the considerable stability of visual direction we normally experience when we carry out saccades. (See the legends to Figs. 3 and 4 for the means by which these measurements were obtained.) It could conceivably be effective, however, after the saccade is all over.

YOUNG: What was the size of the saccade?

L. MATIN: In this case it was $2°11'$. We have similar information for $5°$ and $8°$ saccades.

ANLIKER: How bright was the flash?

L. MATIN: The order of 4.5 millilamberts.

ANLIKER: And how is it presented to the eye? Is it presented through a diffusion screen?

L. MATIN: The lamps are glow discharge lamps. They each have a diffusing plastic and mask in front of them providing a circular target $3.5'$ in diameter. The test flash was either 1 or 2 msec long (depending on the experiment) with rise and decay times of about $20-30\,\mu$sec. The eye did not travel very far during the test flash, and the test flash itself appeared as a small point.

A Primitive Visual Context

The paradigm employed in the experiments of Figs. 3 and 4 was designed to isolate the influence of the extraretinal signal from—among other things—influences of visual context and masking. At this point I want to show you the substantial influence of what would seem to be a very minor sort of visual context (data from Matin, Matin, Pola, & Kowal, 1969). The data shown by open circles connected with dashed lines in Fig. 5 (memory condition) are data for one subject from an experiment exactly like the one described in Figs. 3 and 4. In this figure the ordinate represents location of the Point of Subjective Equality (PSE) at the stimulus array. The data to the left of the vertical midline are for flashes presented when the eye reached different positions in the saccade; the data to the right are for flashes presented at different times after the saccade. Although the data are displayed in a different way than in Fig. 4, the results are very similar.

The data shown by solid circles and connected by solid lines in Fig. 5 (continuous condition), however, are for a condition in which the fixation target was never extinguished. This continuously present fixation target *is* the reduced context. It leads to data that is totally different than for the case in which the fixation target is removed before the saccade. For example, in the continuous condition a close approximation to stability is arrived at quite soon after the saccade. But it is important to note that this result is not simply a consequence of the operation of an extraretinal signal; it includes influences derived from a number of things happening to the visual stimulus arising from the fixation

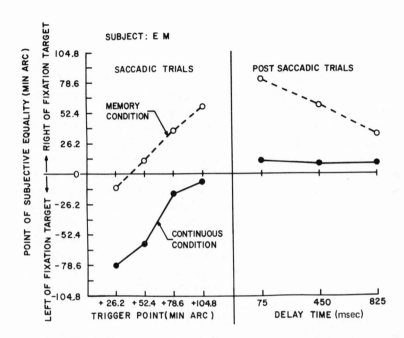

FIG. 5. Influence of a primitive visual context on the time course of the extraretinal signal related to voluntary saccades. The experimental procedures employed in obtaining the data for the "memory" condition were essentially the same as those employed in the experiments of Figs. 3 and 4. The procedures employed for the "continuous" condition were also identical, with the sole exception that a target identical to the fixation target was located .5° above the fixation target itself and was never extinguished. This target provides a rudimentary form of context.

The abscissa for saccadic trials is the distance of the eye from the start of the saccade at the moment when a test flash is presented. The abscissa for postsaccadic trials is the time after completion of the saccade. The ordinate for all data is the location at the target array of the test flash that appeared in the same direction as the fixation target. Zero on the ordinate is the location of the fixation target itself. Distances above 0 are locations in the direction of the saccade.

Although scaled on a different ordinate than those in Fig. 4, the data for the "memory" condition show essentially the same time course as those in Fig. 4 for this subject; the PSE does not begin to return to the fixation target itself until some time after the completion of the saccade. However, for the continuous condition this is not so. The PSE does return to near the fixation target very shortly after the saccade is over. (Matin, Matin, Pola, & Kowal, 1969).

target. Thus, for example, the image of the fixation target sweeps across the retina during the saccade, but is not seen as such—a fact that we deal with shortly.

Visual Persistence

I have mentioned visual persistence several times. I now want to indicate what I mean by persistence in a context outside of our concern with stability of visual direction, and then return to show its potency for influencing visual direction. By visual persistence I mean the duration for which a stimulus continues to remain in perception after it has been physically extinguished. The data on persistence in Fig. 6 (from Bowen, Pola, & Matin, 1974) show that a 1-msec stimulus persists for approximately 300 msec following its termination, a value that decreases with increasing stimulus duration or stimulus luminance. These values were obtained by use of simultaneity judgments between offset of the test stimulus and onset of a probe stimulus. New methods for measuring the total duration of the visual percept for brief stimuli yield similarly long values—for example 270 msec for a 30-msec flash (Matin & Bowen, unpublished manuscript). Thus, although we have employed brief flashes in part as a way of delimiting the time when the stimulus was acting, the long-persisting percept is something to be concerned about when our interest is in mapping the time course of the extraretinal signal.

An influence of such long-enduring persistence of visual stimuli in experiments concerned with establishing the time course of the extraretinal signal is shown by the next experiment (Fig. 7). Here we carried out essentially the same

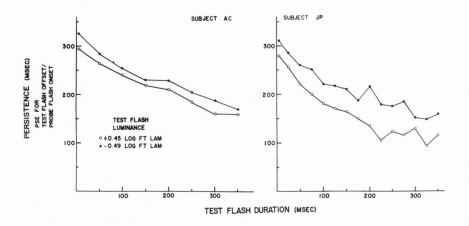

FIG. 6. Visual persistence as a function of test-flash duration at two luminance levels for each of two subjects (Bowen, Pola, & Matin, 1974.)

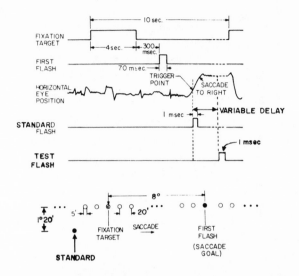

FIG. 7. Stimulus paradigm used to evaluate some effects of visual persistence on visual direction in the presence of saccades. The subject reported the location of the randomly located test flash relative to the location of the standard flash. The standard flash had a fixed location—it was set at that horizontal distance from the fixation target for which it appeared in the same visual direction as the fixation target as determined by the method in Figs. 3 and 4 (Matin, Pola, & Matin, 1972).

kind of experiment as we described in Figs. 3 and 4—that is, the subject had to report on the relative visual direction of the two stimuli presented at different times and with the eye pointed toward different positions. However, in this experiment the first of the two stimuli on each trial was a brief flash ("standard") presented from the same target location to the eye when it was at the same point early in the saccade. The test flash which followed was presented at different time intervals and locations on different trials. The subject reported whether the test flash appeared to the left or to the right of the standard flash. Thus instead of comparing visual directions of the fixation target and test flash as in Figs. 3 and 4, the subject compared the visual directions of two brief flashes. The standard flash had, on the basis of previous work like the experiment in Figs. 3 and 4, been set at a point that appeared in the same visual direction as the fixation target. Thus, among other purposes this experiment provided us with a means of testing for transitivity of the visual direction judgments: Since we had previous information on the PSE between fixation target and test flash, and also the PSE between fixation target and the standard flash, we could also predict the PSE between test flash and standard flash if the judgments were transitive.

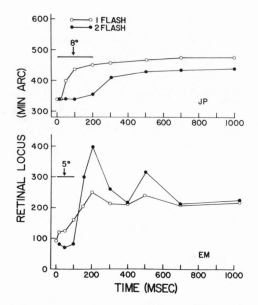

FIG. 8. Experiment employing paradigm shown in Fig. 7 (solid points) and data from experiment employing paradigm in Fig. 3 (open points). Subject JP executed an 8° saccade, subject EM executed a 5° saccade (Matin, Pola, & Matin, 1972).

The results are in Fig. 8. Two sets of data are shown for each subject. One set (open circles) is essentially a repeat of the experiment and results shown in Fig. 4—measurement of temporal variation of the extraretinal signal from visual direction judgments between a flash and previously viewed fixation target. The second set (solid data points) are the measurements obtained from judgments of the relation between two flashes. Among other differences on which we do not comment here, these two sets of data differ in an important way: the PSE for the two-flash data does not begin to change until a temporal interval of about 100–200 msec intervenes between the two flashes; after this interval the two-flash PSE changes and begins to look somewhat like the one-flash data. This interval is a period during which the PSE for the flash against the fixation target undergoes a substantial change, however. Since the standard flash in the two-flash data was set at the PSE for the fixation target, transitivity between the two experiments would require that the data be superimposed. Clearly this is not the case.

The main question presented to us by the difference between the two sets of data in Fig. 8 is: Why does the PSE in the two-flash data remain essentially constant during the first 100 to 200 msec or so after the standard flash? The result is concordant with the result on vernier targets presented during saccades, but is much stronger. It also helps us in dealing with those data: clearly if essentially no change occurs in the PSE for 100 to 200 msec after a flash then a 30-msec or so latency difference introduced by intensity differences between the two lines would not influence the appearance of relative offset.

The main message we derive from these results is: when saccades occur, a substantial duration must intervene between two flashes before the PSE measuring their relative visual directions can reflect something more than their relative offset at the retina. This duration is in the same neighborhood as the values we find for visual persistence that are obtained for the same visual stimuli. This suggests—but does not prove—that before a shift of relative visual direction between two visual stimuli can occur as a result of mediation by an extraretinal signal, the visual persistence of the first flash must have dissipated, perhaps moving the visual image into something like a memory bank for long-term storage (Matin, 1972).

I will now discuss the prepotent mechanism by which visual persistence may normally be reduced in the presence of saccades: saccadic suppression.

Saccadic Suppression

In Fig. 9 I show the results of an experiment (Matin, Clymer, & Matin, 1972) which demonstrates that metacontrast is the most potent means by which saccadic suppression is produced: on each trial the subject viewed the row of dots (upper right of Fig. 9), fixating the leftmost one. He saccaded to the rightmost dot. At the moment that the eye reached the point marked "trigger" the vertical slit underneath the saccadic target was illuminated. The duration of the flash was varied between 1 msec and 300 msec (abscissa, Fig. 9). What the subject saw was a smear whose length increased with flash duration up to 20–40 msec (depending on slit illumination) and decreased for longer flash durations. (Apparent flash length was measured by a length-matching technique which involved flashing the comparison line for 2 msec when the eye was steady). While the increase in apparent length with flash duration is simply related to the length of the streak at the retina, the decrease in apparent length with longer durations involves no corresponding decrease in the length of the streak at the retina. For stimuli whose durations are sufficiently long so as to continue into the postsaccadic period, the retinal streak is as long as the streak for the stimulus that terminates with the termination of the saccade. However, for such long-duration stimuli a substantial portion of the streak is not seen at all, and in fact for a sufficiently long-duration stimulus the appearance is as narrow as the appearance of the slit during a 1-msec presentation or as narrow as a continuously illuminated slit viewed with a steadily fixating eye.

The fact that the streak appears shorter when more stimulus energy piles up at the end of the streak on the retina in the postsaccadic period implies that this additional energy serves the function of suppressing perception of the smeared retinal image produced by the saccade—an effect which under other conditions would be labeled "metacontrast." Since each visual stimulus in our environment normally produces a streak at the retina when we saccade and then comes to approximate rest at a particular retinal locus, each stimulus carries its own inhibitor when we move our eyes. Dim stimuli do not act as self inhibitors as

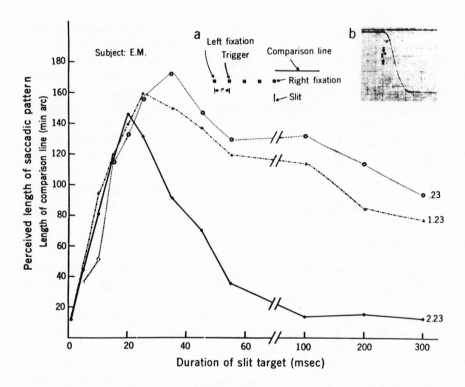

FIG. 9. Perceived length of the "smear" shown as a function of the duration of presentation of the slit. Numbers to the right are slit luminance in mlamberts. Inset a shows the stimuli as they appeared to the subject when all fields were illuminated, the eye was still, and the comparison line was at full length. Light and dark in the inset are reversed relative to the actual view, and the figure is only approximately to scale. Only the two extreme small fixation squares were present throughout trials; the other three were used only for calibration purposes. Inset b is a recording of the variation of eye position during a 4° saccade; the vertical lines are 10-msec time markers (Matin, Clymer, & Matin, 1972).

well as bright ones (Fig. 9). This finding reminds one of the observation that in very dim illumination entire visual fields may appear to jump when we turn our eyes, an observation that may be due to the fact that there isn't enough saccadic suppression to do a good job.

Relations between the Extraretinal Signal, Visual Persistence, and Saccadic Suppression

We now return to the seminal question of this discussion regarding why the world continues to look stationary when we change our direction of gaze by means of saccades.

The original measurements from which we inferred the time course of the extraretinal signal (Fig. 4) yielded a signal that appeared too slow to function as a simple canceling signal. However, if the conclusions regarding the influence of visual persistence are accurate we must question whether the failures in stability of visual direction obtained in Fig. 4 are wholly due to the slowness of the extraretinal signal itself or whether the long-enduring visual persistence of the test flash which we employ to measure the extraretinal signal is involved in such a way as to yield an appearance of such slowness. We ask this because our experimental situation differs from normal viewing in two related ways that could conceivably obscure the normal operation of a cancellation mechanism: (1) in normal viewing the retinal stimulus during saccades is not perceived as such; (2) in normal viewing the occurrence of flashes is not contingent on the occurrence of a saccade nor are objects visually available to us only as flashes.

We deal with the first difference by noting that our finding of an extraretinal signal that is too slow to function effectively in a simple cancellation mechanism (Fig. 4) does not provide any difficulties regarding the smeared retinal image for continuously present stimuli during the saccade. Since the smeared image of the continuously present stimulus that is generated during the saccade is not seen (Figure 9), whether a cancellation mechanism provides stabilization of visual direction or not for the stimulus *during* the saccade is—to a first order— unimportant for perception, although it is of considerable theoretical importance (Matin, Matin, & Pearce, 1969).

However, the utilization of a test flash against a dark background provides a stimulus that persists for a duration considerably beyond the flash itself. The perception of visual direction of such a flash presented at one moment might then be determined by the value of extraretinal signal during the entire subsequent 300 msec corresponding to the duration of perception of the flash itself. Such an "average weighting function" applied to the test flash might yield a slowly changing PSE as we have found (Fig. 4), but instead of being due to a slowly changing extraretinal signal, this would be due to the large segment of overlap in durations during which the extraretinal signal acts on test flashes presented at different moments. The actual prediction from such a hypothesis, however, is a PSE that reaches a value close to the asymptotic PSE much before the saccade, and gradually moves to reach the asymptote itself at the completion of the saccade—a result quite different from Fig. 4. Hence we must conclude that however flashes might provide abnormal stimulation, the abnormality does not lead to peculiar results simply by virtue of removing the stimulus conditions by which saccadic suppression can act to reduce the persistence of stimulation during the saccade. This conclusion lends considerably more credence to the interpretation of Fig. 4 as showing the time course of the extraretinal signal itself. Other aspects of the above, which I do not have time to analyze here, provide additional support for this conclusion.

IV.2

Eye Movements, Efference, and Visual Perception

Harold A. Sedgwick
Leon Festinger
New School for Social Research

We are currently investigating a class of visual illusions, or misperceptions, which arise during visual tracking and which we think may serve as useful tools in analyzing the functioning of the smooth-pursuit eye-movement control system and its relation to the visual perception system. We will describe the phenomena we have been looking at, explain our reasoning, and discuss briefly some of the preliminary results we have obtained.

Let me begin by giving an example. If, in a darkened room, an observer visually tracks a spot of light moving back and forth horizontally with a moderate, sinusoidally varying velocity, then the perceived extent of motion of the spot is much less than its true extent of motion. A spot moving through 4° of visual angle, for instance, may be perceived as moving only 1° or 2°. If a second spot of light, moving in phase with the first but at some angle to the horizontal, is included in the display, then the perceived direction of this second spot is much closer to the direction of relative motion between the two spots than to the true direction of motion of the second spot alone. If, for instance, the second spot is moving vertically, as shown in Fig. 1a, then its perceived direction of motion may be tilted nearly 45° away from the vertical, as shown in Fig. 1b.

This double phenomenon—the systematic misperception of extent of a tracked spot and of direction of other spots moving nonparallel to the first—is quite robust and is easily obtained in darkness under conditions which permit the eyes to follow the tracked spot well. Three such conditions are sinusoidal motion, which allows for the gradual deceleration and acceleration of the eyes each time the spot reverses direction, frequencies of back-and-forth motion of no more

221

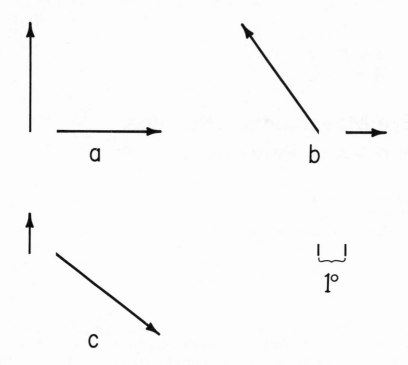

FIG. 1. Example of misperception of direction and extent of motion. Arrows represent direction and extent of one half cycle of motion of spots moving sinusoidally at .5 Hz in a darkened room: (a) physical motion of spots; (b) approximate perception when tracking horizontally moving spot; (c) approximate perception when tracking vertically moving spot.

than about 1 Hz, and velocities of no more than about 15° of visual angle per second.

Both aspects of this phenomenon can be accounted for, at least qualitatively, by saying that the perceptual system radically underregisters the velocity of smooth-pursuit eye movements. The reasoning underlying this explanation is that in the reduced visual environment of a few spots moving in a darkened room the perception of motion must depend principally upon the combination of two forms of information. The first is information concerning motion of the spot relative to the eye, which is equivalent to motion across the retina, and the second is information concerning the movements of the eyes, head, and body. In the situation we are considering, the eyes do the tracking while the head remains still so that this second form of information is reduced to information concerning eye movements. If we assume for the moment that motion across the retina is adequately registered by the perceptual system, then the accuracy of perceived motion will depend directly on the accuracy with which eye movements are registered by the perceptual system. If smooth-pursuit movements are accurately registered, then perceived motion should be accurate. If, at the other extreme, pursuit movements are not registered at all by the perceptual system, then perceived motion during smooth pursuit should be the same as motion relative to the eye. In this case, if the eyes could track a moving spot with perfect accuracy, which of course they never can, then the spot would not be perceived to move at all since it would not be moving relative to the eyes.

It is easy to see how both aspects of the phenomenon I have described would follow from the inadequate registration of smooth-pursuit velocity. The underestimation of the extent traveled by the tracked spot would arise directly from an underregistration of the extent traveled by the eyes in their pursuit movement. The underregistration of smooth-pursuit velocity as the eye tracked a horizontally moving spot would also entail the misperception of the horizontal component of motion of the second, untracked spot and so would lead to a misperception of its direction of motion. In a case such as that shown in Fig. 1a, the vertically moving spot has a retinal component of horizontal motion equal to and in the opposite direction of the horizontal tracking motion of the eye. The underregistration of eye movement would thus make the perceived path of motion of the spot approach 45°. We have informally looked at many such configurations of spot motion, and all of them have conformed qualitatively to this interpretation.

Several other observations also suggest that this perceptual phenomenon arises from a failure to adequately register the tracking movements of the eyes. If a third, stationary spot is added to the display in some position where it does not interfere with tracking, it has little or no effect on the misperception—either of the extent of motion of the first spot or of the direction of motion of the second spot. If the observer now stops tracking the first spot, however, and fixes his eyes on this third, stationary spot, then the motion of the spots is immediately seen veridically. This shows that the original misperception is not due simply to the relative physical motion of the three spots since the physical configuration of motion remains the same whether the observer is tracking the first spot or fixating the third. This observation also supports our assumption that the perceptual system receives rather accurate information about motions relative to the eyes under these conditions. A similar argument can be made with the two-spot display if in looking at it the observer switches from tracking one spot to tracking the other; here, too, the perception changes dramatically. In the case where the second spot is moving vertically, the result of tracking this spot is that its direction of motion is now seen veridically, while the first spot now appears to be moving along a path sloping downward at an angle of almost 45° from the horizontal, as shown in Fig. 1c.

What I have said so far has been only qualitative, as was our first series of observations, and indicates only that there is considerable underregistration by the perceptual system of information concerning pursuit eye movements. A more precise assessment of the nature and extent of such information requires simultaneous quantitative measures of the visual display, the observer's eye movements, and his perception as he watches the display. Without the eye-movement information it is impossible to tell how much of the perceived extent of motion of a tracked spot is due to the registration of information about eye movements and how much is due to the slippage of the spot across the retina that arises from tracking error. If we know, however, what the optical stimulus at the eye of the observer is and how his eye moves in response to it, we can then calculate the relative angular motion between the spots and the eye—that is, the motion of the spots on the retina. From this information we can directly estimate what perception would correspond to the perceptual system having no information concerning pursuit movements of the eyes.[1] If the actual perceptions of the observer deviate from this estimated perception, this is evidence that the perceptual system does have some information about the smooth-pursuit movements, and these deviations can be used as the basis of quantitative inferences about the nature and extent of that information.

For the preliminary results that I shall describe now, our display of moving spots was created by multiplexing the analog signal from a waveform generator and was presented on an oscilloscope with a fast-decay phosphor screen so that the moving spots left no perceptible trace behind them. The observer viewed the display with his head position held constant by a bite bar at a fixed distance from the screen. To measure the observer's eye movements we used the double Purkinje image eye-tracker designed by Cornsweet and Crane (1973). This method gave us a continuous eye-position measure, to within a few minutes of arc, which we sampled and printed out on paper tape every 35 msec. We measured the observer's perceptions by the method of adjustment, using an additional spot which moved along with the horizontally moving, tracked spot. On trials on which we wished to measure the observer's perception of the extent of movement of the tracked spot, the additional spot was always directly beneath the tracked spot but at a variable vertical distance from it. The observer indicated his perception of extent by adjusting the vertical offset of the additional spot from the tracked spot until the vertical distance between the two spots looked equal to the horizontal extent through which they were perceived to be moving back and forth. For trials on which we wished to measure the observer's perception of the slope of the path of the second spot, the additional spot was always 1° below the tracked spot but at a variable horizontal offset from it. The observer indicated his perception of slope by adjusting the horizon-

---

[1] Because visual tracking always involves a mixture of saccadic and smooth-pursuit eye movements, it is also necessary for us to have a way of dealing with saccades when we encounter them in our analysis. It seems most reasonable to us, and is most consistent with our results, to assume that saccades are superimposed on the on-going smooth-pursuit movement and that the perceptual system has accurate information concerning the saccadic component of eye movements.

tal offset of the additional spot from the tracked spot until the line defined by these two spots looked parallel to the path of the second spot. This method of adjustment proved to be fairly easy for our observers after a little practice at the somewhat unnatural task of tracking one spot while paying attention to another. To control for possible constant errors, such as the well-known tendency to overestimate vertical relative to horizontal extent, that might enter our observers' perceptual measures, we adjusted the observers' settings in accordance with comparable settings which they made while fixating a stationary spot. In obtaining quantitative data from which to estimate the velocities of smooth-pursuit movement registered by the perceptual system, our own observations, combined with some pilot work we had done, had led us to concentrate initially on obtaining estimates based on slope judgments and on extent judgments for several different frequencies of spot motion. On each trial, which lasted 32 sec, the observer made either an extent judgment or a slope judgment. Four frequencies of spot motion—.125, .25, .5, and 1.00 Hz—were used. The basic angular extent of motion of the tracked spot was 4°, so the average velocities of spot motion were 1°, 2°, 4°, and 8°/sec. Because the spot motion was sinusoidal, the actual velocity varied from zero to about $1^1/2$ times the average velocity.

For each frequency the observer made two judgments of slope at each of eight different angles chosen so that the retinal slopes, with perfect tracking, would cluster in 5° steps between 60° and 75° and between 105° and 120°. The variation in angle was primarily to prevent the development of habitual responses, since pilot-work measurements on widely different slopes yielded little difference in estimates of the registered eye velocity. The observer also made four judgments of the 4° extent at each frequency. For these extent judgments no vertically moving spot was present since pilot work had also shown no discernible effect of the vertically moving spot on extent judgments. Two judgments of another extent, which was 2° for 1.0 Hz and 6° for the lower frequencies, were also included to help prevent habitual responses from developing.

So far we have gathered and analyzed data from two naive observers. Table 1 shows our estimates, based on the discrepancies between the perceptual measures of slope and of extent and the corresponding retinal motions, of the average velocities that the perceptual system is attributing to the eye at each of the four frequencies. Three features of this data may be noted. First, the average velocity of pursuit movement registered by the perceptual system is quite low, and in several cases it is not appreciably different from zero. Second, the perception of extent of motion of the tracked spot gives a higher estimate of registered eye velocity than does the perception of slope of the untracked spot. This result is at present still a puzzle to us. It may be due in part to the different response measures which we used for extent and slope, since the extent measure required the perceptual system to integrate velocity information received over an entire half cycle and may consequently have led to the use of somewhat

TABLE 1
Estimates of the Average Velocity of
Smooth-Pursuit Eye Movement
Registered by the Perceptual System

	Frequency (in Hz)			
	.125	.25	.50	1.00
Average spot velocity (in °/sec)	1.00	2.00	4.00	8.00
Estimate based on slope (in °/sec)	.17	.29	.14	−.02
Estimate based on extent (in °/sec)	.68	1.00	1.52	1.15

different, and perhaps higher-order, information than the slope measure, where the direction of spot motion was perceived continuously. Third, it seems clear that as the frequency, and consequently the average velocity, of spot motion increases the average registered velocity of the eye does not increase proportionally. The proportion of registered to actual eye velocity is lower at high frequencies of motion. The registered eye velocity is so small and changes so little with changes in frequency that we cannot yet say with confidence whether it does increase somewhat as spot frequency and velocity increase or whether it remains essentially constant or even decreases. We are currently installing an on-line computer system for display, data gathering, and analysis, which should substantially increase the quantity and accuracy of the data we have to work with and may make it possible for us to resolve this question. The new system will also make it easier for us to obtain the additional data necessary to distinguish between the effects of frequency and those of velocity.

What does seem clear from our results so far is that although the human perceptual system has some information about smooth-pursuit movements of the eyes this information is very poor, often reflecting only a small fraction of the true movement. What does this signify? Our present belief is that whatever information the perceptual system has about eye movements comes from monitoring the efferent commands to the eyes rather than from any proprioceptive information coming back from the extraocular muscles. This belief is based on studies such as that of Brindley and Merton (1960) which shows that passive movements of the eye are not consciously registered and, more recently, that of Skavenski and his colleagues (Skavenski, Haddad, and Steinman, 1972) which shows that the perception of direction is not affected by inflow information. Further support for this belief comes from the easily made observation that afterimages viewed in the dark appear stationary when the eye is passively moved, but are seen to move when they trigger an active movement of the eye.

If the perceptual system is in some sense monitoring the commands coming from the efferent system, then the information which the perceptual system obtains should tell us something about the content of the efferent commands at the level at which they are monitored. Thus, our experiment may give us some access to the internal operation of the efferent system. One way of interpreting our present results is to say that the initial central command to the eyes to execute a smooth-pursuit movement is rather crude, and that it is only at a level peripheral to that at which the command is monitored by the perceptual system that it is elaborated and made precise. A good deal more work needs to be done, however, before we can be sure of this interpretation or can describe it in detail.

DISCUSSION

RIGGS: It seems to me that another variable of importance might be latency. As one spot is being tracked, the other spot that is being observed would be going away from the fovea as it is moving in one direction, and then going back toward the fovea as it is moving the other way. Since latency varies a great deal with eccentricity, one might anticipate that there would be a sort of hysteresis effect so that the arc of apparent motion going one way would not be a straight line, but a curve that represents the slowing of the information coming in as the spot gets farther and farther from the fovea. Then as the spot comes back the other way, the arc would be brought down in the other direction.

SEDGWICK: We have not noticed any curvature in the path of apparent motion during our informal observations. Could you estimate what the magnitude of such an effect might be?

RIGGS: An estimate could be arrived at from measurements of latency as a function of eccentricity. There are some old data of Sweet (1953) on that point that could be used. I think these considerations would not apply for the very slow spot motions that you described, but inasmuch as the spot in your 8°/sec condition actually goes even faster than that in the middle of its excursion, I think that an effect might be found there.

YOUNG: I think I was very happy to hear of your results because they support the perceptual feedback hypothesis and the Yasui work that I related earlier in that they say that the cancellation of the perceived motion for true eye movement is only a partial cancellation. On the other hand, I am not sure that I understood the experiment correctly. You are saying that for sinusoidal motion of the horizontal and vertical spots, you perceived the vertical spot as moving in a tilted straight line and that this perceived slope varied with the frequency of the spot?

SEDGWICK: Roughly, yes. The vertically moving spot is seen as moving along a straight path but tilted as much as 45° away from the vertical. When we use this perceptual measure along with our calculation of retinal motion to estimate the average velocity attributed to the eye by the perceptual system, this velocity does seem to be somewhat greater, in proportion to the true velocity, at very low frequencies of spot motion.

YOUNG: Then I do not understand your results. I would assume that one would not see a straight line, but rather see a curved line. If the illusion that we are discussing is associated with eye velocity, then, since the pursuit eye velocity is varying sinusoidally and, therefore, the inadequacy of the cancellation could also be varying sinusoidally, I would expect the slope to have a sinusoidal variation as well. This would give the perception of an S-shaped curve.

SEDGWICK: What you are suggesting is certainly correct in that if the proportion of information concerning smooth-pursuit eye movements that was available to the perceptual system varied inversely with eye velocity, then we might expect the perceived slope to vary approximately sinusoidally, giving an S-shaped curve, when the eyes were attempting to track a sinusoidal motion. That we do not see this sinusoidal variation, but rather see the vertically moving spot as moving along a tilted but straight path indicates that we cannot adequately describe our results by saying that the available information varies inversely with velocity. Several points may help to clarify this. First, although there is broad agreement between the results of the two subjects we have run so far in showing that the perceptual system utilizes little information about the velocity of the eyes during pursuit movements, there are sufficient differences in detail between these first two subjects to make very tentative any conclusions that may be suggested about how this effect varies with frequency. It is not at all clear that the registered velocity is a continually changing function of frequency. Second, in our experiments so far, angular extent has been held constant so that average velocity varied with frequency. It seems clear that in dealing with the perceptual system, which integrates information over time, one cannot directly make inferences from how the system behaves at different frequencies, where frequency here describes the over-all pattern of velocity over time, to how the system would behave at different instantaneous velocities.

STEINMAN:: Do you see the illusion when the motion of the spots follows a triangular rather than a sinusoidal waveform and when the amplitude of motion is small, say $1°$ or $3/4°$?

SEDGWICK: I do not recall having looked at just the configuration you are describing, but I would expect that the perception would be quite different, and closer to veridical. My reason for saying this is that although the eye can track a linear motion very well, it cannot handle the virtually instantaneous change in velocity that occurs at each end of the spot's path. Thus, each time the spot reverses direction there is a period of up to several hundred msec during which the eye must slow down and change directions. As the eye slows down, all the spots in the display are moving relative to the retina at close to their real angular velocities and directions, and the perceptual system is thus getting fairly good retinal information about their motion. The effect of this information will persist in the perceptual system for some time so that even after the eye has caught up and resumed good tracking, the motion of the spots that was picked up while the eye was stationary may continue to be seen for some time, perhaps a few hundred msec.

KINCHLA: A somewhat different emphasis is possible, I think, than you are putting on your analysis, although I do not think it is the whole story by any stretch of the imagination. The correlated movement of points across the visual field has always been a very strong cue for the points being on the same object. Gestalt psychologists talk about phenomena like that, and pattern recognition utilizes that sort of a cue to indicate that two points are on one object. Now, I suspect that it would be relatively straightforward to analyze the kind of movement that you are generating as the two-dimensional projection on the subject's retina of an appropriate movement in three-dimensional space in front of the subject of two points of light on a rigid object, say a straight rod, for example. This relates to higher mental processes, to which you alluded a little.

SEDGWICK: You are suggesting, I think, that our results might be explained by the sort of analysis that Johansson (1950) has used extensively in his investigations. In fact, the kind of configurations that we are looking at are very similar to some of the ones that he has used, and my first attempt at understanding our phenomena was to look for an explanation in terms of the perceptual analysis of motion configurations. Such an explanation would say that the visual system has completely veridical information about how the spots are moving, but is organizing that information in a way different from what we might expect. Rather than perceiving the second spot in Fig. 1a as moving vertically, as it really is, the system might perceptually factor this motion into two components—a horizontal component of motion common to both spots and a motion along a 45° path which was the residual motion of the second spot relative to the tracked spot. None of us has been able to perceive the configuration in this way, however. A common horizontal motion of the tracked spot and the second spot is not perceived when the display is viewed in a completely darkened room. The sloping path of the second spot does not appear to translate horizontally along with the tracked spot and, more conclusively I think, the horizontal extent of motion of the tracked spot is greatly underestimated. If there is enough light in the room so that the edges of the screen or of some other frame are visible, then what is perceived is closer to what Johansson describes. Thus, while it is clear that some analysis of motions can be carried out perceptually and that common motion can be, as you suggest, very salient information for the perceptual system, I do not think that this is the primary explanation of our observations.

SENDERS: I have two questions. First, your Fig. 1a shows the two spots starting at the fovea and then diverging at 90°. Does the illusion occur with any other configuration of the initial starting point? For example, could we put the second spot at the end position of the first?

SEDGWICK: We have looked informally at quite a number of other configurations such as the one you describe and have been unable so far to find any appreciable difference in the basic illusion. Our conclusion at present would be that configuration does not play a critical role in the effects we have been observing.

SENDERS: My second question is, what happens if you begin to shift the phase of the vertical sinusoidal motion relative to the phase of the horizontal or tracked motion? Does the illusion then break down with some amount of phase shift?

SEDGWICK: No, the illusory perception does not break down. It alters in about the way that we would expect, given the geometry of the situation and the hypothesis that not much eye movement information is being registered by the perceptual system. What happens is that as the second spot is shifted more and more out of phase with the tracked spot, it begins to move elliptically on the retina. At 90° out of phase it generates something close to a circle.

SENDERS: So you *do* perceive the figure you would expect as a result of the phase shift?

SEDGWICK: Yes, if I move the second spot back and forth horizontally and the tracked spot back and forth vertically, 90° out of phase with the second spot, I see the second moving in approximately a circular path.

IV.3

Extraretinal Influences on the Primate Visual System

Robert H. Wurtz

National Institute of Mental Health

The perceptual changes accompanying eye movements in man have been considered extensively in this symposium. What I would like to consider now is several possible physiological correlates of these perceptual changes. In this brief presentation, I decided to concentrate on work in the monkey since most of the work relating visual behavior to single-cell activity has been done in this cooperative primate. I also decided to limit consideration to recent work on the striate area of cerebral cortex and the superior colliculus in the midbrain.

The striate cortex is the primary receiving area for retinal input to the cerebral cortex; it probably receives all the fibers from the lateral geniculate body of the thalamus (Wilson & Cragg, 1967) which in turn receives a direct input from the retina. Cells in this cortical area appear to have the properties necessary for a precise analysis of stimulus qualities including shape, orientation, and direction of movement (Hubel & Wiesel, 1968; see Brooks & Jung, 1973, for further references). The superior colliculus receives fibers directly from the retina and also a projection descending from striate cortex (Wilson & Toyne, 1970). Most cells here respond to stimuli of any shape or orientation moving in any direction and located over comparatively large areas of the visual field (Cynader & Berman, 1972; Goldberg & Wurtz, 1972a; Schiller & Koerner, 1971; see Sprague, Berlucchi, & Rizzolatti, 1973, for further references). Both structures have a clear retinotopic organization and can be regarded as early way stations for visual processing in the central nervous system. I think there is sufficient physiological evidence at these points in the nervous system to comment on three general questions: (1) Is there any shift from a retinal specific visual map to a spatial specific map? (2) Is there input accompanying saccadic eye movements which modify the response of cells to visual stimuli? (3) Is there any modification of cell response dependent upon the monkey's use or response to the receptive field stimulus? To indulge in a little disclosure, the answers to the questiona are essentially, no, maybe, and yes, in that order.

In order to answer these questions, we trained monkeys on a visual fixation task and recorded the activity of single cells (using the methods of Evarts, 1968) while the monkeys performed this task. As shown schematically in Fig. 1, the monkey learned to depress a bar in order to turn on a spot of light (labeled fixation light) which remained on for random periods of several seconds' duration. The light then dimmed briefly and if the monkey released the bar during the dim period, he received a drop of water or fruit juice. In that way we required the monkey to hold his eyes steady for a few seconds. During these fixations, we introduced a second stimulus (labeled the receptive field stimulus in Fig. 1) and used this stimulus to study the relation of a cell's response to such stimulus characteristics as position, shape, and movement. Moving this fixation point produced tracking eye movements; turning it off in one place and turning it on someplace else elicited saccades from one point to another. Eye movements were recorded using electrooculograms (EOG); the microeye movements occurring during fixation were neither recorded nor controlled in our experiments but must certainly have contributed to the visual stimulation falling on the retina.

The answer to the first question, on retinotopic versus spatial localization, falls out almost automatically from receptive-field mapping experiments. While the monkey looked at the fixation point the area of the visual field where the stimulus modulated the activity of the cell (the visual receptive field of the cell) was determined as illustrated in Fig. 1. From this experiment, however, we did not know whether the cell discharge related to the visual stimuli at that particular point in space or to that particular part of the retina which happened at the moment to be directed toward that point in space. These two variables were easily separated in our task simply by moving the fixation point. If the cell was in fact related to a point on the retina, a new fixation point, say 20° to the

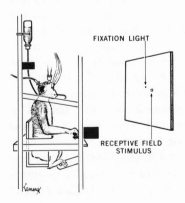

FIG. 1. Drawing of an experimental arrangement for recording single-cell activity in response to visual stimulation. Monkey's head is held steady via implanted bolts in the skull. Eye movements are recorded with implanted EOG electrodes and single cells by the hydraulically driven microelectrode. (After Wurtz 1969a.)

left, would move the retinotopic map $20°$ to the left and consequently the position of the receptive field would move $20°$ to the left. For cells in both the striate cortex and the superficial layers of the superior colliculus, as the fixation point moved, the receptive field moved correspondingly; these cells were responding only to stimulation of one point on the retina. Our visual perception is clearly not tied to such a fixed retinotopic organization and presumably at some point in visual processing, cells will also be more closely related to a position in space rather than to a position on the retina.

The second general question concerns the influence of the oculomotor system on activity of cells in visual areas. The simplest type of question is whether the discharge of cells is modulated by the occurrence of eye movements in the absence of any visual input, that is, when the monkey makes eye movements in total darkness. In the extrafoveal area of striate cortex no clear relationship between eye movements and cell discharge was observed (Wurtz, 1969b). Buttner and Fuchs (1973) have recently done similar experiments on the lateral geniculate nucleus, and they also concluded that cells did not discharge in close association with eye movements. In net, in the awake monkey, cells in the geniculostriate system do not seem to be influenced by eye movements in the absence of light.

The more psychologically relevant question, however, is whether the response of cells to light might be modified during an eye movement. To study this question, I compared the response of cells in the striate cortex to a stimulus moved across the receptive field by a saccadic eye movement with the response of the cells to a stimulus moved equally fast across the receptive field while the eye was stationary (Wurtz, 1969c). Figure 2 illustrates the response of a striate cortex cell during such an experiment. Cell discharges are indicated by dots as are the beginning and end of each line. Successive lines represent successive fixation trials. In Fig. 2A a slit of light was swept across the receptive field of the cell and across an adjacent photocell which started the line in each case. The stimulus velocity is indicated in the left margin. (The shift in latency is largely a matter of how fast the stimulus reached the photocell and the receptive field, respectively.) The cell continued to discharge in response to the stimulus even with velocities up to $900°/sec$. This high velocity was chosen since, according to Fuchs (1967a), the peak velocity in the middle of a $20°$-long saccade is in the neighborhood of $900°/sec$. By placing the same stimulus in the middle of the trajectory of a horizontal saccadic eye movement that was $20°$ long, I then determined the response of the cell when the retina swept across the receptive field at about $900°/sec$; the results of this experiment are shown in Fig. 2B. This cell responded during the rapid eye movement in ways quite similar to its response when the stimulus was moved rapidly in front of the stationary eye. All cells responded in a very similar way during rapid eye movement across a stationary stimulus and to rapid stimulus movement across a stationary eye (Wurtz, 1969c). Under these experimental conditions I did not see any evidence

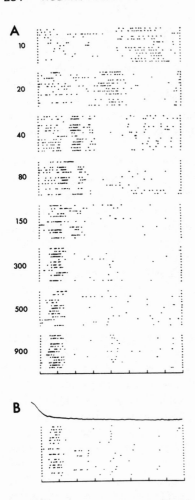

FIG. 2. Excitatory response of a striate cortex cell to increasingly higher speeds of stimulus movement (indicated in degrees per second in left margin) in A or to a rapid eye movement across the stationary stimulus in B. Eye-movement trace showing saccadic eye movement is shown above unit responses in B. In this and all succeeding figures, time between successive points on the time line at the bottom of the figure is 50 msec. (After Wurtz, 1969c.)

in the extrafoveal areas of the striate cortex for an oculomotor input accompanying saccadic eye movements.

In spite of this lack of oculomotor input, I want to emphasize that most cells in the striate cortex responded very differently to the fast stimulus movements accompanying eye movements than they did to slower stimulus movement. Only about one-quarter of the cells in striate cortex continued to respond at all to high velocities of stimulus movement, and about half of the cells stopped responding to stimulus velocities over 200–300°/sec. The remaining quarter of the cells behaved in a very interesting fashion: instead of increasing their discharge rates or just dropping out, they had an excitatory response to a slowly moving stimulus but then showed a suppression of the background rate during rapid stimulus movement (Fig. 3A). Rapid eye movement (Fig. 3B) produced the same type of suppression. However, if the eye swept across either a dark field or a uniformly illuminated area of the screen, no suppression was evident (as is illustrated for a different cell in Fig. 4B). Introduction of a patterned background again produced the suppression of discharge associated with eye movement (Fig. 4, C and D).

This suppression is not an indication of oculomotor input but rather is a visual concomitant of eye movements made over a patterned background. Since these experiments were performed, MacKay (1970) has shown that saccadic suppression under certain conditions can be largely accounted for by a suppression effect of a moving background, since threshold for detection of a briefly presented stimulus was raised whether the eye moved across the textured background or the textured background was jerked in front of the stationary eye. Those cells that showed a suppression of discharge at higher-stimulus velocities provide an excellent physiological correlate of the psychophysical observations of MacKay and might provide at least a partial explanation of saccadic suppression. This possibility is made more plausible by the demonstra-

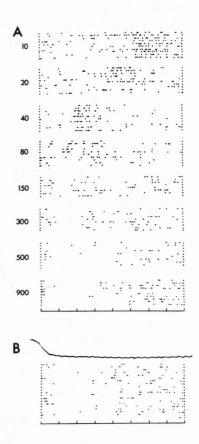

FIG. 3. Conversion of an excitatory response of a striate-cortex cell to a suppression response, with increasing speed of stimulus movement (A) and suppression of response with a rapid eye movement across a stationary stimulus (B). (After Wurtz 1969c.)

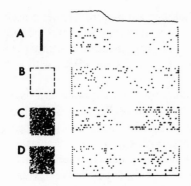

FIG. 4. Suppression of discharge of a striate-cortex neuron during eye movements across a slit of light .5° by 6.0° (A) or textured backgrounds (C and D). No such suppression occurs with eye movement over a homogeneous background (B). (After Wurtz 1969b.)

tion of saccadic suppression in monkeys by Mohler & Cechner (personal communication). More recent experiments in cats have also suggested that rapid stimulus movements, such as must occur during eye movements, selectively alter the discharge of certain groups of cells (Noda & Adey, 1974; Singer & Bedworth, 1974).

In the other branch of the visual system, the superior colliculus, M. E. Goldberg and I have also investigated the effect of eye movements on visual processing. In order to explain these experiments, I must first indicate that the superior colliculus can be divided into at least two subgroups of cells. Figure 5

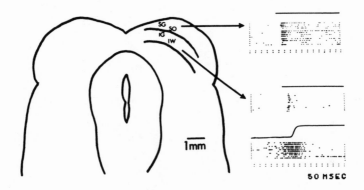

FIG. 5. Drawing of a coronal section through the superior colliculus of a monkey. An example of the response of a typical cell in the superficial gray (SG) or stratum opticum (SO) layers is shown in the upper right. Response of a cell in the intermediate gray (IG) or intermediate white (IW) layers is shown to a visual stimulus in the middle on the right and with an eye movement in the lower right. Horizontal lines above the cell displays indicate onset of the visual stimulus; EOG trace indicates time of the saccade. (Cell responses on the right after Goldberg & Wurtz, 1972a, and Wurtz & Goldberg, 1972a.)

shows a drawing of a coronal section through the colliculus and a sample of the type of responses found in cells lying in superficial and intermediate layers. Cells in the superficial layers (stratum opticum and superficial gray) discharged following the onset of a stimulus but did not have such an excitatory response before eye movements made in the dark (Goldberg & Wurtz, 1972a). The cells in the intermediate layers sometimes gave a little burst of cell discharge at the onset of a visual stimulus but always gave a vigorous burst preceding an eye movement made toward one area of the visual field, generally the same area in which the visual stimulus was effective (Wurtz & Goldberg, 1971, 1972a; Schiller & Koerner, 1971). Since I want to concentrate on oculomotor influences on visual processing, I will consider only the superficial-layer cells that are directly concerned with visual processing. I mention these cells discharging before eye movement to emphasize that these cells lie within 1 mm of the visually activated cells in the upper layers and may influence the activity of these upper-layer cells.

For cells in the superficial layers we first determined whether there was any modulation of cell discharge during eye movements made in the dark as I had done in the striate cortex. An example of a cell recorded in the superficial layers that showed such modulation is shown in Fig. 6 (Goldberg & Wurtz, 1972a). The arrow above the figure indicates the occurrence of a spontaneous saccadic eye movement made in total darkness; all eye movements were spontaneous, larger than 5°, and made predominantly in the direction indicated by the arrows on the left. The suppression of background activity started a little before and lasted a little after the eye movement. We did this experiment on 28 cells in the superficial layers and saw this modulation of discharge in roughly half of them. We are just starting the next experiment, asking whether this kind of input modifies the response of the cell to visual stimulation occurring during eye movement.

In net, the answer to the second question on extraretinal input is strikingly different for these two visual areas. For the striate cortex, there is no clear

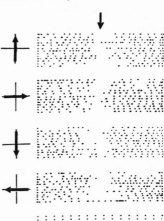

FIG. 6. Inhibition of discharge of a superior colliculus cell during rapid eye movements made in the dark. (After Goldberg & Wurtz, 1972a.)

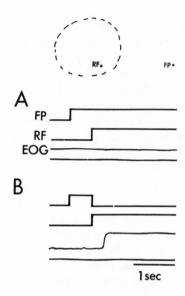

FIG. 7. Series of steps used in experiments requiring the monkey to saccade to the receptive field stimulus. See text for explanation.

modulation of activity during eye movement, although there is an effect of textured background which in turn may relate to the perceptual phenomenon of saccadic suppression. For the cells with visual responses in the superficial layers of the superior colliculus, there clearly is such modulation of cellular activity during eye movement, but we have not yet determined the functional significance, if any, of this modulation.

The third and final question concerns the possibility that the response of cells to visual stimulation might show a modification depending on the response the monkey makes to the visual stimulus. In the experiments described so far the monkey was simply required to fixate a spot of light while we used a *different* stimulus (the receptive field stimulus) to activate the cell under study. The monkey's reward was in no way contingent upon changes in the receptive field stimulus; by the time we began recording from cells the monkey had seen the stimulus thousands of times in the course of our training procedures. We now wanted to see if there were any modifications in the activity of cells when we forced the monkey to use the receptive field stimulus by requiring him to use the effective stimulus, driving a cell as the target for a saccadic eye movement (Goldberg & Wurtz, 1972b).

The paradigm for this experiment is shown schematically in Fig. 7. The experiment was done in two steps. The first step was just a mapping of the excitatory area of the receptive field of a cell in the superficial layers of the colliculus; with a small spot of light we determined the area of the visual field where a spot of light activated the cell (outlined by dashed lines in Fig. 7). We then picked a point (RF in Fig. 7) and determined the response of the cell with repeated stimulus presentations. The sequence of fixation and stimulus onset during this first phase of the experiment is shown in Fig. 7A. Then we changed the paradigm (Fig. 7B). Now when the receptive field stimulus came on, the fixation point went off. The monkey had previously learned to make a saccade to the receptive field stimulus under this condition since the receptive field stimulus might dim, and if he released the bar during this dimming, he obtained the reward. We saw that the monkey made a saccade from the EOG records. The significant time interval in this experiment was between the onset of the stimulus and the start of the eye movement. This was because during most of this time the signal that it was time to saccade to the receptive field stimulus had been given, but the monkey had not yet saccaded and thereby moved the receptive field stimulus off the receptive field of the cell. During this saccade phase of the experiment the stimulus had the same physical properties as in the original no-saccade condition but the stimulus now had a different significance to the monkey, namely, it was now the target for a saccadic eye movement.

Figure 8 shows an example of the results of one of these experiments. In the no-saccade control period (A) the monkey was simply fixating, and the cell responded after the stimulus onset (indicated by the horizontal line at the top of the figure) as in previous experiments. At B in Fig. 8, without any interruption in the sequence of trials, the other paradigm began and the monkey made saccades to the receptive field stimulus after one or two trials. The response of the cell to the same stimulus was now enhanced. This response enhancement has been observed in about half the cells studied in the monkey superior colliculus. During eye movements made without any visual stimulus present (in the dark) there was no such excitatory response related to the saccade. We are seeing the effect of the saccade on the cell's response to the visual stimulus rather than a discharge related to the eye movement alone. After reverting to the original no-saccade condition (Fig. 8C), the monkey stopped making saccades to the stimulus and the enhanced response gradually faded to its original level.

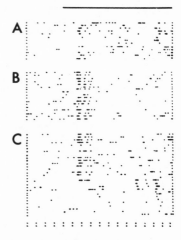

FIG. 8. Response of a superior colliculus neuron to visual stimulus (onset indicated by horizontal bar) when the monkey was fixating (A), making saccades to the stimulus (B), and again fixating (C). (After Goldberg & Wurtz, 1972b.)

Note that if we started the experiment at C in Fig. 8, we would probably regard the cell's response decrement with repeated stimulation as similar to the decrement or habituation seen under similar conditions in behavioral experiments. Fig. 9C shows an even more dramatic example of such a decrement in cell discharge, but Fig. 9, B and D, show no decrement with repetition since the monkey was using the stimulus. These experiments suggest that similar decrements of cell responses seen in acute experiments may frequently be related to decreased use of the stimulus by the animal rather than stimulus repetition alone. In our experiments, where the monkey uses the stimulus, no decrement occurs; where he does not, decrement or habituation is apparent.

I have implied that the enhancement of response is specifically related to the eye movement. But obviously there are other events such as changes in pupil size or level of arousal occurring in association with eye movement. We next determined whether the enhancement occurred in association with any eye movement (Goldberg & Wurtz, 1972b). In this experiment, in addition to the receptive field stimulus, a control stimulus far outside the receptive field was added (see drawing in Fig. 10), and in both the no-saccade and the saccade

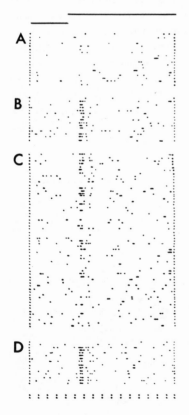

FIG. 9. Habituationlike response of a superior colliculus cell when the monkey ceases to saccade to the receptive field stimulus. In A and C the monkey was looking only at the fixation point, while in B and D he was making saccades to the visual stimulus. (After Goldberg & Wurtz, 1972b.)

.FP

FIG. 10. Control experiment for nonselective factors affecting response enhancement of superior colliculus neurons. In A the monkey was fixating, in B he was making saccades to the control stimulus (CON), and in C he was making saccades to the receptive-field stimulus (RF). Trials in B and C were not consecutive but were placed in one group or the other according to which eye movement (to CON or RF) the monkey made. (After Goldberg & Wurtz, 1972b.)

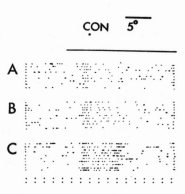

conditions both of these stimuli came on. We first determined how the cell responded when the monkey made no saccade to either stimulus (Fig. 10A) and then how the cell responded when the monkey made saccades from the fixation point to the control stimulus (Fig. 10B) or to the receptive field stimulus (Fig. 10C). For the cell shown in Fig. 10 and for all the cells studied in the superior colliculus, the response to the visual receptive field stimulus was always much more pronounced when the saccade was to that stimulus than when the saccade was to a control stimulus distant from the receptive field area. There were frequently cases where there was a slight stimulus enhancement effect with saccades to the control stimulus (as in Fig. 10B) which might be related to some sort of general arousal or other effect associated with an eye movement. This selective relation of enhancement to one area of the visual field led us to suggest that these cells might be a correlate of selective attention (Goldberg & Wurtz, 1972b; Wurtz & Goldberg, 1972b). Subsequent experiments in which a hand-movement rather than an eye-movement response was made to the visual stimulus indicated that the enhancement occurred only with the eye movement. Since the enhancement is response related, the term *attention* must be applied with caution if it is appropriate at all (Wurtz & Mohler, 1974; Mohler & Wurtz, in preparation).

The effect of this enhancement in the colliculus is that cells relating to one part of the field respond more vigorously during a series of trials when the monkey is using the stimulus in that field. Obviously the experiments that we have done represent a laboratory simplification of what normally must be a more complex task; we present one or two stimuli while a monkey in his normal environment has to select significant stimuli from a welter of visual stimuli in order to make a saccadic eye movement to them. These superior colliculus cells may be involved in that selection process.

As I noted earlier, one of the primary inputs to the superior colliculus is from the striate cortex, and it is possible that the selective enhancement seen in the superior colliculus simply reflects a similar enhancement in the striate cortex. Mohler and I (Wurtz & Mohler, 1974; Wurtz & Mohler, in preparation) have done a similar experiment on striate cortex cells. We did not find any such selective enhancement in striate cortex, and after ablation of striate cortex the enhancement effect was still found in collicular neurons. Therefore, the selective effect is not generated in striate cortex and is simply passed on to the superior colliculus. We have seen enhanced responses associated with saccades made in any direction and therefore not at all selective to one part of the visual field. This general enhancement effect may be related to a nonselective change in arousal and is possibly related to the changes seen in striate cortex and lateral geniculate neurons following stimulation of the mesencephalic reticular formation (Doty, Wilson, & Bartlett, 1973; Bartlett & Doty, 1974). So the answer to the third question is that we do see a change in the cell's response when the monkey responds to the stimulus driving the cell, but we see it in the superior colliculus, not in the striate cortex.

In conclusion it is worth noting the consistent differences in extraretinal influences found in the primary cortical visual area, the striate cortex, and a primary midbrain area, the superior colliculus. The striate cortex emerges as an analyzer par excellence for many characteristics of a visual stimulus. But no clear selective extraretinal influence on the activity of these cortical cells has yet been observed either during an eye movement or in the selective use of the visual stimulus by the monkey. In contrast, the superior colliculus cells must convey rather ambiguous information about the type of visual stimulus impinging on the retina or, for that matter, where on the retina the stimulus is located. But colliculus cells do show modulation of activity during eye movements and do show selective changes related to use of the visual stimuli by the monkey. The midbrain, not the primary receiving area of cerebral cortex, appears to be more involved in the integration of extraretinal inputs with visual processing. Presumably cortical processing beyond the striate cortex incorporates more extraretinal input, particularly since one of the major projections of the superior colliculus is upward to this cortical area via the posterior thalamus.

DISCUSSION

SKAVENSKI: What are the inputs to the colliculus besides that from the striate cortex? It seems that the striate cortex is rather unintelligent as far as the stimulus goes and there must be some other place telling the colliculus what is significant, etc.

WURTZ: The problem is not in finding possible inputs to the colliculus but in finding which ones contribute to the enhancement effect we see. While not as well studied as striate cortex, most areas of cerebral cortex have some projection to some layers of the superior colliculus; projections also arise from other areas of the brainstem. Therefore selection among the inputs would have to be on other than purely anatomical grounds; inferotemporal cortex seems like a reasonable candidate. Frontal cortex, at least the frontal eye-field area, we have ruled out experimentally (Mohler, Goldberg, & Wurtz, 1973).

CARPENTER: Humans can learn to fixate a certain point and yet attend to some other place. Can you teach your monkeys to do this and then have a look at the fields they are selectively attending to but are not going to fixate?

WURTZ: Yes, we have done the experiment much as you describe it (Wurtz & Mohler, 1974; Mohler & Wurtz, in preparation). We first trained the monkey to fixate the small fixation point and rewarded him for releasing a bar when the spot dimmed; the response of the superior colliculus cell to a stimulus was determined during the fixation period. Then we modified the experiment so that on half of the fixations the receptive-field stimulus dimmed rather than the fixation point, and if the monkey released the bar during this dim time he received the reward. The monkey did not make eye movements to the visual stimulus both because the fixation point was small and required fixation to detect the dimming and because eye movements larger than $2°$ automatically terminated the trial. We found that cells did not show the enhancement when the monkey responded to the stimulus by moving his hand rather than his eye. If on the same cell both saccade-response and hand-response experiments were done, the enhancement was clearly present with eye movements, very marginally present with hand movements. Because of this dependence of enhancement on the type of response made to the stimulus, I think we need to be very careful in talking about this enhanced response as being related to selective attention. It might be related to a selective process specifically preceding eye movements, or related to selecting visual targets for an eye movement.

I should say also that the experiment has a flaw in the design in that in one case we ask the monkey to localize the stimulus by making a saccade to it and in the other case just to respond to the stimulus but not to localize it. So it might be that if the monkey were required to reach to the stimulus, the special requirement in processing this information might lead to different effects on these cells. But it would be a much more complicated experiment and we haven't done it.

HALLETT: There seem to be some differences between the monkey and the cat. Mandl (1974) at McGill University describes receptive fields in the colliculus of the cat which are tuned to respond to certain velocities, and there is evidence of antagonistic surrounds so that the neurons function as if they are tuned to certain velocities. Would you care to comment about the possibility of this arrangement in the primate?

WURTZ: Yes, obliquely. The cat's visual system is quite a bit different from that of the monkey, both anatomically and physiologically. This is particularly true of the superior colliculus. The salient features of the superficial cells in the cat's colliculus is that they show directional selectivity. Cells respond with movement of a visual stimulus in one direction but not in the other. In the monkey we find only 10% of cells that show this type of directional selectivity; the rest respond to all directions of stimulus movement. Unfortunately, I do not have data that are adequate to say that the monkey does or does not have the velocity tuning you referred to in the cat. But in light of the differences between cat and monkey in the response of cells to movement I certainly would not assume that cat and monkey are the same.

FUCHS: There seems to be a difference in your stimulus conditions when you are mapping receptive fields and when the receptive field is the target for the saccades. When you are mapping receptive fields the original fixation point remains on, and when the monkey saccades to the receptive field, the fixation point goes off. If the central fixation point were inhibiting visual responses in the periphery of the receptive field of the cell under study, then when it goes off in the saccade condition the release from inhibition in the periphery itself might give you an apparent increase in the saccade condition.

WURTZ: This is a critical point and it is particularly critical because of an experiment in the cat (Rizzolatti, Carmarda, Grupp, & Pisa, 1973) where it has been shown that the response to a visual spot at one part of the visual field is altered if a line is moved in a very different part of the visual field.

In our case this question is also answered by the control experiments illustrated in Fig. 10. Here we have a stimulus in the receptive field and another stimulus which is far from the excitatory area of the receptive field. In this control experiment we are turning off the fixation point both when the monkey saccades to the receptive-field stimulus and when he saccades to the control stimulus; the visual stimulation is exactly the same when the monkey uses the control stimulus as when he uses the receptive-field stimulus. If it were the off of the fixation spot that were releasing a surround inhibition, I would expect to see its effect in both cases. But since the clearly enhanced response is observed only with saccades to the receptive-field stimulus, the spot in the periphery must not be an important factor for the colliculus cells. For striate cortex cells, we do see an enhancement in both cases and here a release of peripheral inhibition cannot be excluded.

IV.4

Voluntary Saccades, Eye Position, and Perceived Visual Direction[1]

Jordan Pola

The Johns Hopkins University[2]

When a person makes a voluntary saccade, the location of visually perceived objects remains undisturbed even though the image of these objects on the retina is displaced. In order to account for this discrepancy between what occurs in perception and on the retina, a number of theories have been proposed (Helmholtz, 1962; James, 1950; Sherrington, 1918; von Holst, 1954) which in general suggest that the brain, via an extraretinal signal, assigns a visual direction (local sign) to each retinal locus. During a saccade, according to this viewpoint, the extraretinal signal changes causing a shift in the relation of visual direction to retinal locus. It is implied that the shift has the same direction, time–course, and magnitude as retinal image displacement and thus "cancels" or "nulls" the displacement in perception.

Several experiments conducted by L. Matin and his co-workers (Matin, Matin, & Pearce, 1969; Matin, Matin, & Pola, 1970; Matin, Matin, & Pola, in preparation) have demonstrated the existence of a shift in visual direction and revealed some of its important characteristics. In Matin's experiments, subjects reported on the visual direction of a brief flash presented at various times before, during, or following a voluntary saccade. The direction of the flash was judged relative to the location of a fixation target viewed and extinguished before the saccade. Using this procedure it was possible each time to find a point on the retina at which the flash stimulation was perceived to come from the same direction as

[1] This research was supported by Fellowship 1-F01-MH-49678-01 from the National Institute of Mental Health, Grant R01-5-EY0037E from the National Institutes of Health, and Grant NSF GB-5947 from the National Science Foundation.

[2] Now at the State University of New York College of Optometry, New York, N.Y.

the previously viewed fixation target. Thus it was possible to determine the manner in which the visual direction of the fixation target was related as a function of time to retinal locus. The results of the experiments showed that the visual direction shifted away from the fovea in a direction compensatory for the saccade. However, in contrast to the above theories, neither the time–course nor the magnitude of the shift corresponded to those of the eye movement. Instead, the shift began before the saccade and continued for several hundred milliseconds after, and it reached a magnitude which, depending on the subject, was either somewhat larger or smaller than that of the saccade.

These differences between the characteristics of the shift in visual direction and those of the saccade suggested that a component of the shift was time dependent. The results, however, did not show the extent of this dependence. Moreover, they did not indicate whether the shift was also related, both during the course of the saccade and afterwards, to the position of the eye (although a small but significant eye position effect was uncovered at one time delay after the saccade). One would expect that if the shift were essentially time dependent, then its magnitude would not change with variations in saccade size when, for example, a person on successive trials tried to look at a given location. But if the shift were coupled to eye position, then its magnitude would vary according to the amplitude of the saccade.

With the above considerations in mind I performed an experiment to see whether the shift was related to eye position, time, or perhaps both. But the amplitude of a saccade toward a given location does not always appreciably change from trial to trial. Thus a major problem in the experiment was to obtain a range of saccade amplitudes wide enough to enable finding out whether there was in fact an eye position effect, and furthermore, to determine the general quantitative features of such an effect. This problem was solved by using two different types of experimental sessions. In one type of session (the 8° non-adjustment or 8na session) visual direction was measured for a saccade of normal amplitude when the subject attempted to look at a target 8° removed from his original point of fixation. In the other type (the 8° adjustment or 8a session) visual direction was determined for a saccade of reduced size when the subject tried to look at the 8° peripheral target (a form of preconditioning was used for the reduction—see below).

Each of the two types of sessions was divided into *two* parts: the *first* part consisted of a training procedure to establish the desired oculomotor behavior, and the *second* part involved a psychophysical procedure to measure the shift in visual direction. In both parts the subject was in complete darkness except for experimental stimuli (to eliminate the possible influence of visual context on perception), and the horizontal eye position was continuously recorded using a contact-lens–optical-lever technique. The *first* part of each 8a session was used to reduce saccadic amplitude (Fig. 1a). On each trial (there were 100 training trials in each session) the subject attempted to make a saccade to a target 8° to

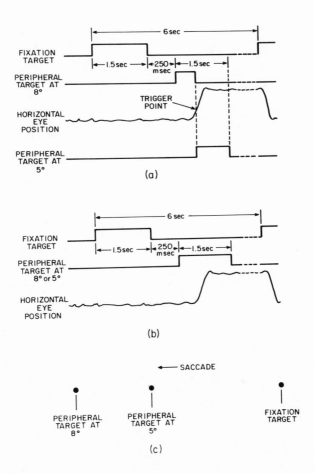

FIG. 1. (a) Temporal sequence of stimuli and eye movement on each trial in the first part of each 8° adjustment (8a) session. (b) Temporal sequence on each trial in the first part of both the 8° nonadjustment (8na) and 5° nonadjustment (5na) sessions. (c) Spatial array of fixation target and peripheral targets used in the first part of the different sessions.

the left of his original fixation position. However, at the onset of the saccade (i.e., when the eye crossed a preset trigger point 1° from the fixation position) the 8° target was switched off, and another target, 5° to the left of the fixation position, was switched on. By repetition of this sequence of events on successive trials it was possible (even though the subject consistently tried to look at the 8° target) to reduce the amplitude of the saccade from 8° to about 5°.

In the *second* part of each 8a session, the shift in visual direction was determined psychophysically during and after a saccade toward the 8° location. At the beginning of each trial (Fig. 2a) the subject viewed a fixation target

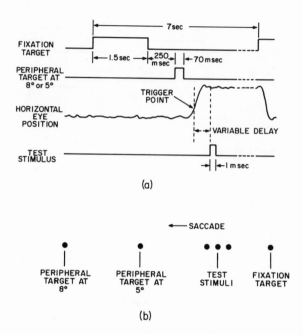

FIG. 2. (a) Temporal sequence of stimuli and eye movement on each trial in the second part of each of the three types of experimental sessions. (b) Spatial array of the fixation target, peripheral target, and test stimuli in the second part of the sessions. In the 8na and 8a sessions the peripheral target was located 8° from the fixation target, and in the 5na session it was 5° from the fixation target.

presented for 1.5 sec. This was followed, after a brief dark interval, by the presentation of the 8° peripheral target for 70 msec. Upon seeing this target, the subject made a saccade in an attempt to look at it. Either during or following the saccade (i.e., 15, 25, 50, or 200 msec from the time the eye crossed the 1° trigger point) a 1-msec test flash occurred, and the subject reported (using a hand switch) whether the flash appeared to be to the right or left of the previously viewed fixation target.

By randomly varying the test-flash location from trial to trial (the psychophysical method of constant stimuli), it was possible to determine at each time delay the physical location at which the flash appeared to be in the same direction as the fixation target (i.e., the location at which the flash appeared to be to the left of the fixation target 50% of the time and to the right 50% of the time). This location is called the target point of subjective equality (target PSE). Since eye position was recorded, it was also possible to find a point on the retina corresponding to each target PSE, that is, a retinal locus associated with the visual direction of the fixation target (called the retinal PSE).

The first part of each 8na session (Fig. 1b) was the same as the first part of each 8a session except that the peripheral target remained at 8° throughout and following the saccade. The second part of each 8na session (Fig. 2a) was identical with that of each 8a session.

Besides the above two types of sessions the experiment involved a third type, the 5na session, to determine whether visual direction was influenced by the location toward which a saccade was made. Each 5na session was the same as each 8na session except that in both the first and second parts (Figs. 1b and 2a) the peripheral target was located 5° from the fixation target.

Some general features of the subject's oculomotor behavior and psychophysical data in the second part of each type of session are shown in Figs. 3 and 4. (The data of only one of the two subjects used in the experiment are given here.) Values of mean horizontal eye position are presented in Fig. 3 (in the upper portion of the figure) at each time delay from the onset of the saccade (i.e., the trigger point). According to this figure, the training procedure in the

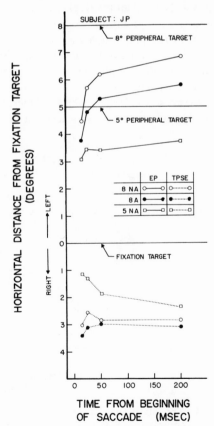

FIG. 3. Mean horizontal displacement of the eye from the fixation position (EP) plotted against time from the beginning of the saccade. Associated with each mean eye position is the location of the test flash which appeared to be in the same direction as the fixation target, the target point of subjective equality (TPSE).

first part of each type of experimental session had a clear influence on the subject's oculomotor behavior in the second part. That is, the magnitude of the subject's mean eye position was smaller at each time delay in the 8a than in the 8na condition.

If the test flash that appeared at the location of the fixation target were actually at that location, then all the target PSE's would lie along the straight line representing the fixation target. Obviously such constancy of visual direction did not occur in any of the conditions; instead, all the target PSE's were located noticeably to the right of the fixation target.

Figure 4 presents retinal PSE's plotted against time from the beginning of the saccade. In each condition the retinal PSE shifted monotonically away from the fovea in a compensatory direction (leftward on the retina) as time from the onset of the saccade increased. A substantial shift occurred early in the saccade (15 msec) suggesting that it began prior to the eye movement. Notably, at each time delay both during and following the saccade the magnitude of the retinal PSE was larger than the displacement of the eye (see Fig. 3). These results, then, are similar to those found by Matin, Matin, and Pearce (1969), Matin, Matin, and Pola (1970), and Matin, Matin, and Pola (in preparation).

A striking feature of the data in Fig. 4 is that at each time delay the amount of retinal PSE shift in the 8a condition was less than in the 8na condition. But similar differences also occurred in the values of mean eye position (Fig. 3). These two sets of results taken together, then, suggest that the magnitude of the shift was related to the displacement of the eye from the fixation position. In

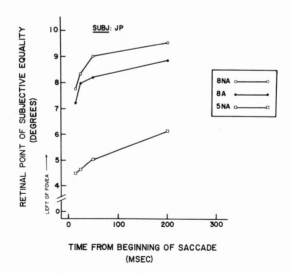

FIG. 4. The retinal locus at which the test flash appeared to be in the direction of the fixation target (retinal PSE) plotted as a function of time from the beginning of the saccade. The fovea is designated by ordinate zero.

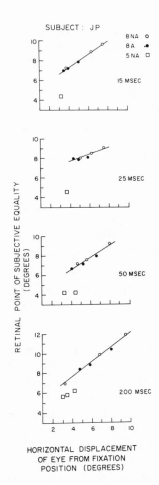

FIG. 5. The retinal PSE is shown in relation to the horizontal position of the eye. Each of the small graphs shows data at one of the time delays from the onset of the saccade. The 8na data are represented by open circles (○), 8a data by filled circles (●), and 5na data by open squares (□). At each time a linear function was fitted to the 8na and 8a data using the method of least squares.

order to find the quantitative features of such an effect, the total data at each time delay in each of the three conditions were divided into subgroups (Pola, 1973). For each subgroup both a retinal PSE and the eye position at which the retinal PSE occurred were calculated. These retinal values are plotted against corresponding eye positions in Fig. 5. The data points at each time delay (i.e., in each small graph) indicate that when the subject attempted to look at the $8°$ peripheral target, in either the 8na or 8a sessions, the value of the retinal PSE increased as a linear function of displacement of the eye from the fixation position. Moreover, both the 8na and 8a PSE's at a given time increased according to essentially the same linear function.

Another outstanding aspect of the results in Fig. 5 is that the slope of the linear relation changed over time. The slope was relatively large at the beginning and end of the saccade (.67 and .75, respectively). At about the middle (25 msec) of the eye movement, however, the slope dropped to a noticeably lower value (.40). Visual direction thus was not only related to eye position but was also time dependent.

A third influence on visual direction is suggested by the 5na data in Fig. 5. In the 5na sessions, as stated, the subject made saccades of normal length to a 5° peripheral target. The figure shows that at a given eye position at each time, the 5na retinal PSE fell significantly closer to the fovea than did either the 8na or 8a PSE's. Thus, while the size of a saccade was often the same to the 8° target as to the 5° target, the magnitude of the shift in such instances was different. This result suggests that the shift was influenced by the distance of the peripheral target from the fixation point. In other words, the "attempt" to look at a given location apparently had an effect on perception.

In summary, the present findings indicate that the shift in visual direction for a saccade was related to three parameters: (1) the position of the eye during and following the saccade; (2) time from the onset of the saccade; and (3) the "attempt" to look at a specific location. Perhaps the most important finding was the relation of the shift in visual direction to eye position. This result unequivocally shows that the oculomotor system has a significant influence on stability of visual space. The data do not reveal, however, some important characteristics of this influence. For example, either an "outflow" or "inflow" signal could underlie the linear relation. An "outflow" signal such as "efference copy" could obviously cause the position effect since it would be derived from neural activity which drives the eye globe from one position to another. But an "inflow" signal could do the same since the neural response of stretch receptors in the extraocular muscle would be related to the stretch of the muscle and thus to the position of the eye. Inflow theory has generally been rejected in favor of outflow theory (Helmholtz, 1962; von Holst, 1954; Skavenski, Haddad, & Steinman, 1972) on the basis of the observation that passive rotation of the eye does not cause any clear shift in visual direction. Nevertheless, the present results together with previous findings (Matin, Matin, and Pola; 1970) suggest that more than one type of signal may be involved with the shift. As mentioned, a substantial shift seems to occur prior to the onset of a saccade. This might be due to an outflow signal. But the eye position effect, both during and after the saccade, could be the result of an inflow signal whose influence is dependent on the "attempt" to make a saccade (Matin, 1972; Pola, 1973). If this sort of inflow signal exists, then passive rotation of the eye would yield little or no shift in visual direction.

An interesting aspect of the present data was the finding that although mean saccadic amplitude was less in the 8a than in the 8na session, no corresponding change occurred in how visual direction was quantitatively related to eye position. In other words, while substantial plasticity was found in saccadic behavior, no plasticity was evident in visual perception. This result has some interesting ramifications. It is possible, for example, that the saccade-reduction procedure in the present experiment is related to the various forms of visuomotor adaptation which occur using inverting, reversing, and displacing prisms (Harris, 1965). Both the saccade-reduction procedure and the visuomotor adaptation involve a change in the relation of motor behavior to some aspect of visual space perception. In view of this similarity the present findings provide support for a theory that the visuomotor adaptation consists of a modification of motor "programs" but not of visual perception.

DISCUSSION

STEINMAN: Do you have an opinion about what would happen perceptually if you asked a subject to make a saccade to a location halfway to an $8°$ peripheral target, leaving the target at $8°$ during and after the saccade, instead of reducing the length of his saccade via the parametric adjustment training? Would the subject's shift in visual direction be like your 8a data or similar to the 5na data?

POLA: In the $8°$ adjustment procedure, a subject always "attempts" to look at an $8°$ target, whereas when a subject looks at a point halfway to an $8°$ target he is, I believe, simply attempting to look at a $4°$ location. I would thus predict, since my data suggest that attempt can influence perception, that the shift in visual direction for a saccade halfway to an $8°$ target would be similar to the results in the 5na condition.

KINCHLA: I want to comment on some problems that might arise when one uses the PSE as a psychophysical measure. In most psychophysical procedures this measure is extremely susceptible to a number of influences. For example, if you told your subject that he was too often reporting that the test stimulus was "to the right," his PSE would be dramatically affected.

The type of data you have presented is, in a sense, a correlation between the conditions and the retinal PSE in that the subject could distinguish one condition from another. For the same reason, there is also a correlation between the PSE and the time delays. In other words, it is possible that the subject shifted his judgmental standard according to the experimental situation. The orderliness of your data is very impressive and you have shown some very interesting effects. However, it is a question about whether your findings can be attributed purely to an extraretinal effect or to the influence of instructions.

POLA: It seems to me that the only way in which the precise eye-position effect in the 8na and 8a conditions could have been produced by instruction would have been for the experimenter to tell the subject on each trial both the location of the test flash, which was randomly varied, and the position of his eye at the time of the flash. The subject would then have had to make a quick computation on the difference between his eye position and the flash location (to obtain a retinal PSE), and based on this, give his response. Needless to say this sequence of events did not occur. In fact, there was essentially no communication between the subject and experimenter during the psychophysical procedure. The only reasonable account of the effect, then, is that the subject indeed did have a sense of eye position, and this sense was the same in the 8na and 8a conditions.

E. MATIN: I would like to reply briefly to Dr. Kinchla's remarks. I think that the kind of effects that you are talking about are, of course, common in all psychophysical experiments, and it is our job to conscientiously be aware of them and fight against them, so to speak.

I can assure you that we were conscientious in the sense that we tried to reassure the subject that he didn't have to produce a response distribution of 50% "right" and 50% "left." Even if we weren't, the effects in these experiments were so enormous that they could not be the result of the kind of response biases that you are talking about unless, for example, the experimenter hypnotized the subject.

IV.5

Saccades to Flashes[1]

Peter E. Hallett

University of Toronto

Lightstone and I collected data on saccades, and the timing aspects of these have been reported (Lightstone, 1973; Hallett & Lightstone, 1973). More recently I have studied the sizes of the saccades (Hallett and Lightstone, 1976a, b) and it is this aspect that I wish to report here.

My interest in eye movements arises from studies in night vision where photons are scarce and it is difficult to believe that the visual system wastes much light (e.g., Hallett, 1971). Lightstone and I were, therefore, particularly interested to know whether there is useful visual inflow during saccades from retina to oculomotor pathways and whether the oculomotor output is based on possibly wasteful intermittent sampling of visual input. The notions of suppression, mislocation, and sampling have been contributed to and modified by a number of workers (e.g., recent reviews by MacKay, 1973, and Robinson, 1973), but the present experiments represent a rather different approach.

Most experiments in the literature are made with continually lit targets, which are stepped according to the experimenter's clocks (not according to the ongoing cycle of oculomotor neural events) and the experimental conditions are generally such that subjects' perceptions and instructions are of some importance. We (1) synchronize the target step to the very beginning of a *triggering saccade* (which should correspond to the beginning of the final motorneuron burst plus a few msec, given the findings of Robinson and Keller, 1972), (2) blank out the stimulus for a reaction time soon after stepping the target, (3) assess the use of visual information from the timing and amplitude of the fixation reflex alone, and (4) automatically randomize the target patterns from trial to trial. The net result is that the subjects' perceptions, in the ordinary

[1] This work was supported by the Medical Research Council of Canada and the Defence Research Board of Canada, grants MRC MT 4092 and DRB 9310 122.

meaning of the word, are rather poor. They typically fail to notice the blanking and are uncertain about the number of target steps, etc., although eye movements are as usual.

To summarize the results which follow, for the present conditions (dark-adapted subjects and single targets): (1) visual inflow during a primary saccade can initiate a corrective or new primary saccade, and seems to be necessary to prevent strange responses; (2) retinal position is not the stimulus that determines saccade amplitude, but rather the retinal position of the cue is corrected for any subsequent saccadic movement that happens to intervene between the cue and the saccade that it eventually elicits. Thus in our experiments saccades are typically toward the physical position of objects. These points can be supported

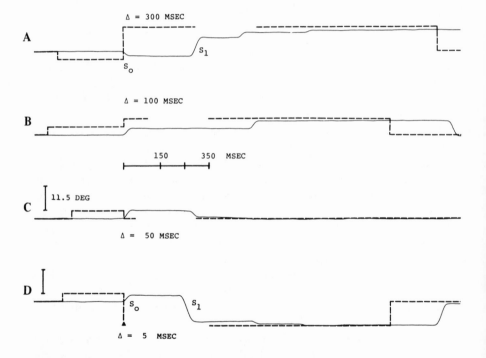

FIG. 1. (A) Saccade S_1 can be followed by a corrective saccade toward the unlit target, provided that the target is not blanked out before the start of S_1. (B) There is the tendency for cues in the direction of the triggering saccade S_0 ("uncrossed cues") to be missed on occasions. (C, D) Short cues (Δ = 1–50 msec), which are "intrasaccadic", typically elicit S_1 saccades toward the position of the unlit target, allowance being made for the size and direction of the triggering saccade S_0.

These trials are selected from an experiment in which randomization from one trial to the next provides eight major varieties of position pattern and three major varieties of timing pattern (i.e., 24 major varieties, not counting mirror-image patterns or minor varieties).

by measurements, but it will suffice here to illustrate them by means of a few trials (Figs. 1 and 2).

In a fairly typical trial the otherwise dark-adapted observer fixates a nominally 8-min arc subtense blue-green, 100X foveal threshold target as soon as it is lit. The target steps randomly left or right by 3.8° to elicit the triggering saccade S_0, the beginning of which (at an eye velocity of 37°/sec when the eye has traveled about 1 target width) triggers an instantaneous target step to one of eight randomly selected positions in the range ±11.5°. After a cue period Δ the target is blanked out for 150–350 msec before final reillumination. This describes the simplest experiment (e.g., Fig. 1), but in other experiments (e.g., Fig. 2) the arrangements are more elaborate with extra cues and blanking periods. The residual noise of our near-infrared eye-monitoring device (Lightstone, 1973) has SD = 3 min arc and the linearity is to within ±5% over the range ±12°. The device is insensitive to vertical movement or change in pupil size. Eye position and timing are read from chart paper to ±10 min arc and ±4 msec.

Figures 1 and 2 show eye position and position of the *lighted* target. The interval between the traces is retinal image position relative to the fovea. Very short target exposures are illustrated with ▲, ▼. Velocity traces are not shown but are important for defining the beginnings and ends of saccades.

In the experiments a primary saccade brings the fovea only a proportion of the way to the target and the balance is corrected (in appropriate circumstances) by one or more smaller, shorter latency, corrective saccades. Saccades are, of course, somewhat variable in amplitude and timing. In Fig. 1A the Δ cue is, by chance, longer than the reaction time, so that the target is blanked out *during* primary saccade S_1, after which there is a corrective saccade toward the unlit target. For our range of eye movements, corrective saccades to unlit targets are *never* seen unless there is some visual inflow during saccade S_1. The motor package concept for the primary–corrective saccade pair (Becker & Fuchs, 1969) is based on much larger eye movements, and is an attractive notion, but clearly visual inflow during saccades is important for the present situation, if only to *permit* the execution of a motor package, based on nonvisual (motor and proprioceptive) information.

Figure 1B shows that a Δ cue in the direction of the triggering saccade S_0 (an "uncrossed" cue) is not always effective in eliciting a saccade during blanking. A proportion of the briefer uncrossed cues are actually *missed*. This phenomenon is the only sign that we see of anything resembling the mislocation and suppression effects found in perceptual studies by other workers. More typically, however, both uncrossed and crossed cues (Figs. 1C, 1D) elicit saccades toward unlit targets, even when the cues are so brief as to be intrasaccadic (Δ = 1–50 msec). Note that allowance is made for the size of the saccadic movement S_0 that intervenes between the Δ cue and its response S_1.

In Fig. 1 the Δ cues are "true cues" which indicate where the target will be when it is finally relit. In the experiment illustrated by Fig. 2A, this is not so, but the responses to the cues seem to be the same. In Fig. 2B the triggering saccade S_0 blanks out the target for 10 msec and then exposes it as a true cue for Δ = 20 during the peak velocity of S_0 when the velocity is in excess of

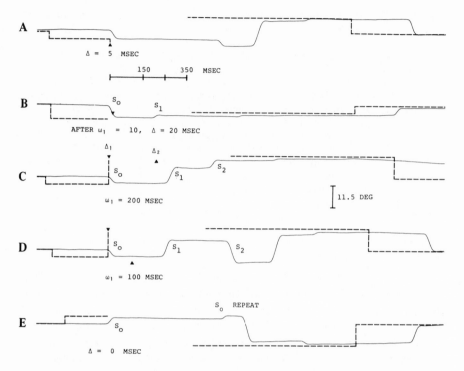

FIG. 2. (A) In this experiment (16 major varieties of position pattern), the brief cue is sometimes "true" and sometimes "false." Nevertheless, there are typically saccades toward the position of the currently unlit cue, even when, as in this case, the response is clearly inappropriate. (B) After a delay of 10 msec the cue is exposed for 20 msec at the peak velocity of triggering saccade S_0. Nevertheless, there is still a response toward the physical position of the target. (There are four major varieties of pattern.) (C, D) Saccade S_2 to cue Δ_2 is modified to allow for size and direction of the intervening saccade S_1. (There are 16 major varieties of position pattern. ω_1 is the time interval between the Δ_1 and Δ_2 cues.) (E) $\Delta = 0$ experiment. In a proportion of trials the S_0 saccade is apparently repeated after a delay. (There are 5 major varieties.)

$290°/\text{sec}$: the S_1 saccade is typically toward the physical position of the target. In Fig. 2C and 2D, a second cue Δ_2 occurs prior to the S_1 response to cue Δ_1. In Fig. 2C the retinal image positions of the Δ_1 and Δ_2 cues are nearly the same but the amplitude of saccade S_1 to cue Δ_1 is increased to allow for saccade S_0, and the amplitude of S_2 to Δ_2 is reduced to allow for S_1. In Fig. 2D the retinal distance of Δ_2 from the fovea is quite small, but S_2 is very large because of the allowance made for the intervening saccade S_1.

The fact that the size of a saccade is not determined by retinal position alone may seem surprising, given that the known visual pathways are on retinal coordinates. However in "feedback experiments" with various gains in which eye position drives the continually lit target, we find, as have others (e.g., Robinson, 1964), that humans (but not monkeys, Fuchs, 1967b) can gain control of the target by modifying their saccade amplitudes; and there is other evidence (e.g., McLaughlin, 1967) that saccade size can be conditioned—these types of experiments suggest considerable perceptual analysis which is, however, largely frustrated by the present conditions of extensive randomization and brief trials.

Figure 2E shows a special $\Delta = 0$ experiment in which the target is blanked out immediately at the beginning of the S_0 saccade, and in a proportion of trials the S_0 saccade is repeated after a delay. It is as if the situation is temporarily "open loop," with the eye chasing some faint retinal memory trace that has not been quenched because of the absence of visual inflow subsequent to the start of the S_0 saccade. Finally one may note in Figs. 2A, 2D, and 2E that saccades still occur despite the fact that they are quite inappropriate, given newer information as to target position. The latent processes are clearly ballistic in at least the latter half of the latent period (as is well known).

The present conclusions are obvious enough on inspection of several trials, but can be supported by measurement of saccade latency and amplitude in about 2,000 trials for a wide variety of substantially different target patterns (on the order of 30–40, not counting mirror-image patterns and minor variations). The important question does arise, however, as to how it is possible for the oculomotor system to behave as if it knows the physical position of the target, given the evidence from perceptual experiments that flashed targets are perceptually mislocated (e.g., Matin & Matin, 1972) and that perceptions influence eye movements (e.g., in illusory situations: Festinger, 1971). There are three main possibilities.

1. Visual navigation. Given a continually lit target or a continually lit landmark against which positions of flashed targets can be reckoned, then some form of "visual navigation" might be possible. There is then no need to postulate use of motor outflow or proprioceptive feedback. The only possible "landmark" in our experiments is the very remote, dim parasitic light from our near-infrared source which is invisible for much of the time because of the Troxler (1804) fading effect. This possibility seems very unlikely.

2. Continuous correlation of eye and retinal image position. If one's philosophy is that the visual pathways show an ill-defined "duality" between largely perceptual (cerebral) and largely nonperceptual paths (brainstem and cerebellum) one may argue that the fixation reflex is a very early orientational response that is a *prelude* to perception. If perceptual studies are not relevant to present experiments, one can go so far as to postulate continuous correlation of eye and retinal image position at (say) "brainstem levels" so that the *approximate* physical position of the target is always known to the oculomotor pathways, although it is not readily accessible to the more remote and more sluggish perceptual processes. This idea offers no explanation for "missed" cues (Fig. 1B) and is not easy to test by neurophysiological techniques; nevertheless it is the idea we favor.

3. Static eye position plus associative pairing of retinal image and response. If one's philosophy is that eye movements depend on perception it is possible to develop different arguments. There are good reasons for believing that static eye position is known between saccades, when the eye is operating in the purely "saccadic mode." For example, Skavenski (1972) concludes from difficult experiments that static eye position in the dark is known both perceptually and at the oculomotor level. Robinson and Keller (1972) show that static eye position is well coded at the motorneuron level in the monkey. One can conjecture that slightly mislocated targets can be associated with proper responses, provided that static eye position is known. If mislocation is very serious for some cues (e.g., Fig. 1B) then this may account for these cues' being useless on occasions. We cannot exclude this more psychological explanation. However, the association of retinal image and response would need to be built up rather rapidly, to be resistant to "false-cue" situations and to cope with a wide variety of target patterns and timings.

In summary, for our experiments, it is clear that there is important visual inflow from the retina to oculomotor pathways during saccades. Retinal image position alone is not the stimulus for saccades but, on average, allowance is made for any saccadic eye movement that intervenes between the target flash and its response. Saccade size is proportional to the error that needs correcting, not to whatever retinal information existed in the past. Whatever the mechanism is for this, it does seem important that the saccadic system be able to allow for its own prior actions. Successive saccades are not independent of each other.

DISCUSSION

ROBINSON: I am wondering if there is, or is not, a conflict between your oculomotor results and Dr. Pola's perceptual findings. If the target is presented in the *middle* of a saccade, it is mislocated in one direction or the other. If saccades are dependent on perception, it is conceivable that the average saccadic response to a midsaccadic cue *might* be accurate, but the response would be crude, there would be considerable spread, and it is more likely that the average response would be idiosyncratically inaccurate from subject to subject.

HALLETT: No, I think that that explanation is wrong. Lightstone and I used a wide variety of timing arrangements, including flash targets presented before, during, and after saccades. Perceptual mislocation effects vary with timing, but our result is always simple. Saccades are toward the physical positions of previously lit targets—mean saccade size being a *fixed* portion of what needs to be corrected, irrespective of the lighting conditions. The spread in saccade size is normal, about SD/mean = 16%, and inspection does not suggest that scatter is related to the various lighting conditions.

ROBINSON: If we assume that mislocated cues are associated with proper responses, wouldn't you expect better performance with longer duration cues?

HALLETT: Possibly. Actually our findings are that mean saccade size is not affected by cue duration in the range 1–300 msec. The amount of light energy in the retinal image should not have much effect on the retinal coding of image position.

POLA: I think that an individual could learn to adjust his saccadic behavior to allow for perceptual mislocation.

HALLETT: I am undecided as to the best explanation of our findings. Although the more psychological hypothesis of associative pairing of mildly mislocated cues with appropriate responses has some plausibility, as a physiologist my bias is more toward the view that the fixation reflex is an early orientational response utilizing a coarse representation of the physical world at lower brain levels.

YOUNG: I bear some responsibility for the idea of sampling by the saccadic system, and this idea is often misunderstood and oversimplified. I believe that visual inflow for a given saccade occurs over a period of time but ceases to be capable of modifying a given saccade some 50 msec prior to the saccade. The saccade is calculated and launched in a ballistic fashion, and subsequent visual information is used in launching the next corrective saccade. All too often people treat the notion of sampling as though there is a snapshot taken of the retina to calculate the next saccade.

Afterthoughts

SENDERS: I participated as a casual subject, in the study of W. B. Templeton & Tania Anstis at York University, and pointed with my finger at the apparent positions of light sources emitting short flashes during saccades.

One sees the place where the light is going to be, and knows it is going to be there. As the eye moves across, the light flashes, and it is seen as being at the end point or sometimes at the beginning point of the saccade. Being of a turn of mind that makes me like to see these things in the real world, I went out and looked at the CN Tower (that is in Toronto and will be the tallest building in the world). There is a flashing beacon on it which emits very short flashes.

I asked myself whether I could get the lights off the tower. It is remarkably easy. I spent a little time making saccades, looking at clouds, and searching, and every once in a while that beacon was way up in the middle of the sky. I was reminded that when one is dealing with flashing lights of similar intensity-duration characteristics on aircraft, it is sometimes very difficult to find an airplane that you think you have just seen.

It occurred to me that there may very well be circumstances in which during search the light source might be displaced sufficiently far from its true position to guide the search behavior into a nonproductive area of the visual field and possibly lead to problems in air-to-air detection and collision avoidance.

HALLETT: Perhaps. The illusion can be dramatic, but in our experimental situation the eye movements are ordinary.

IV.6

A Psychophysical Model
of Visual-Movement Perception

Ronald A. Kinchla

Princeton University

Dr. Mackworth has already suggested that it is possible to learn useful things about the eye-positioning system even with rough measurements of eye movements. I would like to make the even more-radical suggestion that it is possible to learn useful things about the eye-positioning system without measuring eye movements at all. I would suggest that the direct study of the eye-positioning system could be influenced by purely psychophysical studies in much the same way that direct physiological studies of retinal mechanisms were guided by the *earlier* psychophysical analyses of such phenomena as "acuity," "spectral sensitivity," and "dark adaptation."

I am going to describe a simple psychophysical model of visual-movement discrimination which I have described in more detail in several earlier papers (e.g., Kinchla, 1971; Kinchla & Allan, 1969). The model is used here to characterize the *discrimination of linear, fixed-velocity movement of a point of light, viewed in the dark, for durations of from .5 to 2 sec.* While these may seem like strong constraints on the applicability of the model, I think you will agree that many, if not most, of our judgments concerning whether or not a target is moving are made within such time periods. Furthermore, by considering an apparently basic and theoretically tractable type of movement discrimination it seems possible to utilize a very simple but quantitatively precise model.

Let me begin by describing the types of *stimulus patterns* I've used in my research. You will probably recognize that they are similar to those employed in some experiments described earlier at this meeting. The stimuli are represented graphically in Fig. 1. Note that each of the four graphs in Fig. 1 represents *lateral position* on the ordinate and *time* on the abscissa. Lateral position is defined in degrees of visual angle displacement, along an imaginary left–right

264   RONALD A. KINCHLA

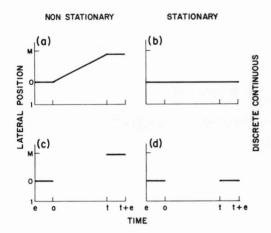

FIG. 1. Four representative stimulus patterns defined by the position of a point of light at various times. Confusing patterns a and b, or c and d, is a failure of "movement discrimination" (mistaking b for a, or d for c, is the "autokinetic illusion," mistaking b for d is "flicker fusion," and mistaking c for a is the "phi phenomenon").

dimension, from some arbitrary point directly in front of an observer, with positive displacements to the right and negative ones to the left. Time, on the ordinate, is expressed in seconds. Thus the solid lines on the graphs denote the lateral position of a point of light at various times. For example, in Fig. 1a the point of light is illuminated at time $-e$ at position zero where it remains stationary until time zero, then moves to the right at a constant angular velocity of $v°$/sec arriving at position m at time t (i.e., $v = m/t$), remaining stationary there until it is extinguished at time $t + e$. In all the experiments we shall consider, e will be equal to .5 sec, although this duration does not seem critical so long as it is sufficient to make the point of light visible. Notice that Fig. 1b is essentially the same type of stimulus pattern except that m equals zero, that is, the light remains stationary from time 0 to time t. Thus I shall refer to patterns in which $m \neq 0$ as *nonstationary* and those in which $m = 0$ as *stationary* (as indicated in Fig. 1). Actually, I will speak first about some experiments involving stimuli of a slightly different sort, the type which are illustrated in Figs. 1c and 1d. Note that they differ from the previous stimuli (in Figs. 1a and 1b) in only one respect, the light is extinguished during the t-sec period from time 0 to time t. For obvious reasons I shall refer to patterns in which the light remains on continuously as *continuous patterns,* and those in which the light is off during its t-sec transition from position 0 to position m as *discrete patterns.* In either case, however, the central concern here is with an observer's ability to *discriminate* (respond differentially to) *stimulus patterns that differ only in the value of m.* For example, the ability to discriminate between the patterns shown in Figs. 1a and 1b, or between those shown in Figs. 1c and 1d. I will refer to this ability as *movement discrimination.* This should be carefully distinguished from one's ability to discriminate the patterns in Figs. 1a and 1c (the tendency to confuse the pattern in Fig. 1c with that in 1a is the so-called *"Phi illusion"*), or to discriminate the patterns in Figs. 1b and 1d (a tendency to confuse the pattern in Fig. 1d with that in 1b is *"flicker fusion"*).

It is important to stress that our main interest is *not* in an observer's general tendency to report movement (report $m \neq 0$), but in his ability to distinguish patterns which differ only in the value of m. For example, it has long been known that an observer's tendency to mistake a stationary pattern for a nonstationary one (the so-called "autokinetic" illusion) can be influenced by many factors. "Social-pressure" experiments (e.g., Sherif, 1936) show how the report of a "dummy" subject can influence a real subject's tendency to describe a stationary point of light as moving. However, such studies say nothing about one's ability to *discriminate* between a stationary and nonstationary stimulus pattern, since they do not assess the subject's *relative tendency* to report movement, given each type of stimulus (in fact such experiments normally employed *only* a stationary pattern).

The *theoretical model* to be considered can be defined by two statements, the first indicating how a *stimulus* evokes a *subjective impression of movement,* and the second indicating how this *impression* is translated into a *response.* While the first statement embodies the central assumptions of the model which are invariant in all of its applications, the second varies somewhat with the specific response options. Thus it will be useful to define a particular discrimination task before specifying the model.

Suppose an observer was asked to discriminate between a stationary stimulus pattern, denoted by S_0, and one involving movement to the right, denoted by S_1, i.e., if the m parameter of stimulus S_i is denoted by m_i, then $m_0 = 0$, and m_1 is some positive value. Let A_1 denote a report of movement to the right, and A_0 a report of no movement. Then an observer's performance can be summarized by the proportion of A_1 responses to S_1 stimuli, denoted by $\hat{P}(A_1 | S_1)$, and the proportion of A_1 responses to S_0 stimuli, denoted $\hat{P}(A_1 | S_0)$, i.e., so-called "hit" and "false-alarm" rates, respectively.

A model for this task can now be defined as follows:

1. Each presentation of stimulus pattern S_i having parameters m_i and t_i evokes a "subjective impression of movement" x, that is a value of a Gaussian random variable X, having variance ϕt_i and an expected value of m_i.

2. The decision process is such that movement to the right, A_1, is reported only if the subjective impression of movement x exceeds a judgmental criterion β, otherwise no movement, A_0, is reported.

Note the first statement indicates that the most probable subjective impression of movement, given S_i, is the actual displacement m_i, although the variance or "noise" in this impression is directly proportional to the duration of observation t, the theoretical parameter ϕ being the constant of proportionality. Thus ϕ

could be interpreted as the *constant* rate at which noise in the position-sensing system accumulates over time (this constant accumulation of variance is a basic property of a mathematical "random walk" or "Weiner process" which I shall mention later in the talk).

The assumptions embodied in the model imply that, *for any fixed judgmental criterion* β, an observer's tendency to report movement to the right, given S_1, $P(A_1|S_1)$, will exceed that for given S_0, $P(A_1|S_0)$, so long as m_1 exceeds m_0; however, the greater the variance in X the smaller the difference between $P(A_1|S_1)$ and $P(A_1|S_0)$. In other words, the larger the variability in X relative to the displacement the observer is trying to detect (m_1), the poorer will be his discrimination. If he adopts a very liberal judgmental criterion for movement to the right (a very small or negative value of β) he will report movement very often whether it occurs or not; i.e., he will make not only many hits but many false alarms (autokinetic reports). He can reduce the number of false alarms by adopting a more conservative judgmental criterion (a larger value of β) but only at the cost of also reducing his tendency to report movement when it actually occurs; i.e., reducing his hit rate $P(A_1|S_1)$.

Thus, the particular hit and false alarm rates exhibited by an observer depend both on the physical-stimulus parameters m_1 and t (t_0 and t_1 are always identical so the subscript is dropped) and on the two theoretical parameters ϕ and β. However, the observer's *ability to discriminate movement* (his "movement sensitivity") is really characterized by the rate at which noise accumulates in the visual-position-sensing system, that is, the parameter ϕ; since the judgmental criterion β is essentially an arbitrary and easily modified aspect of his performance (e.g., by instructions to be more, or less, "conservative" in reporting movement). Fortunately, and this is the primary advantage of the model, there is one aspect of the observer's performance which is theoretically independent of (invariant under) changes in β; specifically,

$$d' = Z_0 - Z_1 \tag{1}$$

where Z_i is that value of a standard normal variable (Z-score) exceeded with a probability equal to $P(A_1|S_i)$, for i equals 1 or 0. Furthermore it can be shown that this *discriminability measure* d' is simply the expected subjective impression of movement given S_1, $E(X|S_1)$, minus the expected value given S_0, $E(X|S_0)$, all divided by the standard deviation of X, the square root of Var (X):

$$d' = \frac{E(X|S_1) - E(X|S_0)}{[\text{Var}\,(X)]^{1/2}}$$

$$= \frac{m_1}{(\phi t)^{1/2}} \tag{2a}$$

or, in terms of the *angular velocity* $v_1 = m_1/t$,

$$d' = \frac{v_1 \, t^{1/2}}{\phi^{1/2}}$$

(2b)

Note that d' is a type of signal-to-noise ratio of the sort employed in other signal-detection analyses (e.g., Green & Swets, 1966), since it characterizes the systematic difference in the expected impression of movement, m_1 or $v_1 t$, relative to the noise unit, root Var (X).

These relations allow one to obtain an *estimate* of the noise parameter ϕ, denoted $\hat{\phi}$, using the observed proportions of A_1 responses to S_1 and S_0, denoted respectively by $\hat{P}(A_1|S_1)$ and $\hat{P}(A_1|S_0)$, since they can be considered estimates of the corresponding conditional probabilities; specifically, an estimate of d', denoted $\hat{d'}$, follows directly from Eq. (1) as

$$\hat{d'} = \hat{Z}_0 - \hat{Z}_1$$

(3)

where $\hat{Z}_i$ is that value of a standard normal deviate exceeded with a probability equal to $\hat{P}(A_1|S_i)$, for $i = 0, 1$. Thus appropriate rearranging and substituting in Eq. (2) yields

$$\hat{\phi} = \frac{m_1^2}{(d')^2 \, t}$$

(4a)

or, in angular velocity,

$$\phi = \frac{v_1 m_1}{(d')^2}$$

(4b)

Figure 2 presents data from four subjects (Keller & Kinchla, 1968) which illustrate a simple application of the model. This experiment utilized discrete stimulus patterns of the sort shown in Figs. 1c and 1d, with each subject's discrimination evaluated using a single value of m_1, .44°, and four different values of t, .5, 1.0, 1.5, and 2 sec. The fact that the noise parameter ϕ estimated under each duration of observation t was invariant for a given observer is indicated by the "fit" between the estimates of d' at each t value [using Eq. (3)] and the theoretical function defined by Eq. (2a) given a single "optimal" value of $\hat{\phi}$ for each observer. These optimal estimates of the noise parameter $\hat{\phi}$ for observers 1 through 4, respectively, were .11, .15, .17, and .17 deg²/sec.

These data are highly reliable since each datum point represents something like 2400 observations (trials). This probably seems like an inordinate amount of data to fix these four curves. In fact there were other variables manipulated in the study which we thought might have a strong influence on a subject's accuracy, but didn't. The major one was whether or not we stabilized the

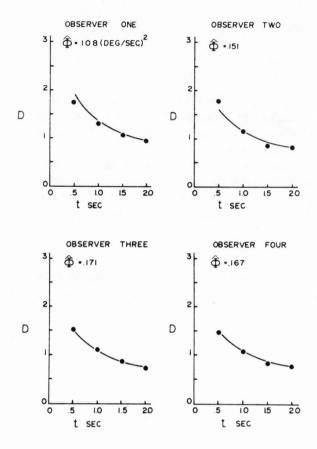

FIG. 2. Data from Keller and Kinchla (1968) showing how the discriminability (D) of a .44° movement diminishes as the time interval (t) over which that movement occurs is increased. The theoretical curve is based on a single estimate of ϕ for each observer.

observer's head with a biting block, as opposed to letting him sit naturally without any constraints. Surprisingly there wasn't any increase in accuracy when the head was stabilized even though it seemed reasonable a priori to assume that the unsupported head would provide an unstable platform for the eyes and therefore contribute to the noise parameter ϕ. While there may be such a head-movement component of noise in some viewing situations, it appears to be a negligible consideration in measurements of this sort. Another variable that had no discernable effect was monocular or binocular viewing.

Figure 3 presents data from a similar experiment (Kinchla & Smyzer, 1967) in which both t and m_1 were varied from one testing session to the next: $t = .5$, 1.0, 1.5, or 2 sec; while $m_1 = .38°$ or .76°. There is more variability of the observed $\hat{d}$ values about the theoretical functions than in Fig. 2, although no more than could be attributed to random sampling, given the fewer trials in this study, and no systematic deviation.

It should be noted that the discriminability measure d' is positively, but *not linearly,* related to the proportion of correct responses, since the probability of correct responses is partially determined by β, whereas d' is independent of β. In any case, the data in Fig. 3 represent performances ranging from about 95% correct at t equal .5 sec for observer One, to about 55% correct at t equal 2 sec for observer Four. The model predicts [Eq. (2)] that the discriminability measure d' will be doubled when m_1 is doubled, thus the theoretical function for $m_1 = .76°$ has ordinate values which are twice those for $m_1 = .38°$ at each observation duration. Again, a single estimate of ϕ provides a good account of each observer's data, although there are individual differences in the noise level, with $\hat{\phi}$ equalling .19, .22, .27, and 1.56 for observers One through Four,

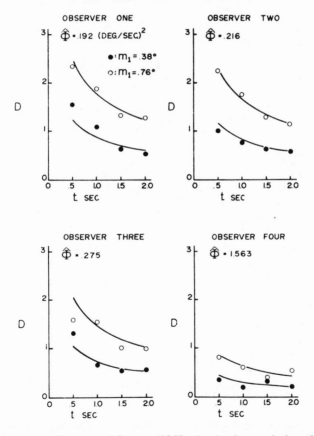

FIG. 3. Data from Kinchla and Smyzer (1967) showing how a single estimage of ϕ can account for the discriminability (D) of either a .38° or .76° movement occurring over an interval of t sec.

respectively (observer Four was an unusually poor, but theoretically consistent, discriminator).

Figure 4, presents an interpretation of some data reported by Matin and Kibler (1966). They used a task similar to the one just considered, except that instead of the displacement on each trial (m) being either 0 or some positive value, there were *nine possible displacements* ranging from a $1°$ movement to the left ($m = -1$) to a $1°$ movement to the right ($m = 1$), in increments of $.25°$. Each of these nine patterns will be denoted by S_m, with $m = -1°, -.75°, \ldots, .75°, 1°$. Furthermore, the observers had three (rather than two) response options: no movement, movement to the right, or movement to the left. These will be denoted, respectively, A_0, A_1, and A_2. This requires a slight modification of the

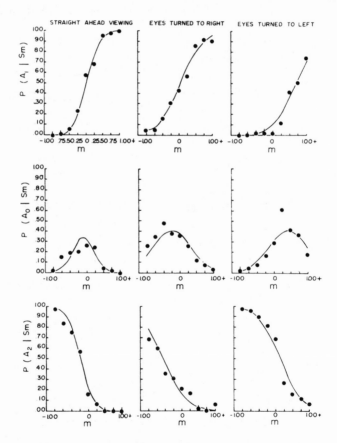

FIG. 4. A reanalysis of data from Matin and Kibler (1966) indicating how judgments of "no movement" (A_0), "movement to the right" (A_1), or "to the left" (A_2), given actual movements of from $-1°$ (left) to $1°$ (right) can be interpreted with the model (see Table 1 for theoretical parameter estimates).

response rule defined earlier in statement 2, which can be restated here as follows:

2. The decision process is such that the observer reports movement to the right, A_1, if x exceeds a response criterion β_1, and reports movement to the left, A_2, if x is smaller than a response criterion β_2; otherwise he reports no movement, A_0.

In other words, the observer is now seen as dividing the range of X values into three parts: those large enough to warrant reporting movement to the right, those negative enough to warrant reporting movement to the left, and an intermediate range $(\beta_2 < X < \beta_1)$ which he labels as no movement. This means there are a total of three theoretical parameters required to fit the data: ϕ, β_1, and β_2. Estimates of these three parameters were chosen to provide the "best-fitting" theoretical functions shown in Fig. 4. This was done separately for the three conditions of observation employed in the study: the data in the leftmost three graphs in Fig. 4 were obtained under normal "straight-ahead" viewing conditions with the observer's head fixed in a bite block; the data in the middle column of three graphs were obtained with the eye "strained" to the right by fixing a bite block so that the observer had to rotate his eyes 34.5° to the right to view position zero; and the data in the graphs on the right were obtained with the eyes similarly "strained" 34.5° to the left. As can be seen from inspection of Fig. 4 the model does a pretty good job of accounting for the observed proportions of each type of response, given each displacement. More importantly, it allows one to consider two quite different aspects of the observer's performance under the three viewing conditions. The estimates of the three theoretical parameters used to fit the data in each condition are presented in Table 1. In the straight-ahead viewing condition the observer's noise parameter was .17 square degrees per sec and he seemed to require a subjective impression

TABLE 1

Estimates of Theoretical Parameters[a]

Viewing condition	$\hat{\phi}$	$\hat{\beta_2}$	$\hat{\beta_1}$
Ahead	.17 deg^2/sec	−.60°	.04°
To the right	.56 deg^2/sec	−.135°	.13°
To the left	.56 deg^2/sec	.30°	1.66°

[a]Based on horizontal-movement judgments of Observer GEM in the Matin and Kibler (1966) study. Note that in addition to altering "judgmental criteria," β_1 and β_2, straining the eyes to the left or right almost tripled the "noise" levels, ϕ.

of movement greater than .04° to report movement to the right, or less than −.60° to report movement to the left, describing anything in between as no movement. When his eyes were strained to the right or left his criteria for reporting movement seemed to change in a manner specific to the direction of strain. Quite distinct from this aspect of the data, however, is the fact that *the noise parameter φ appears to be almost three times as great in the eye-strained conditions than in straight-ahead viewing.* This seems to reflect a very different feature of the data than the judgmental criteria, since those can easily be modified by instructions (e.g., telling him he is being too careful about reporting movement to the right).

Figure 5 presents data from a study (Kinchla & Allan, 1969) in which *continuous movement patterns,* of the sort shown in Figs. 1a and 1b, were employed; that is, the point of light is not extinguished during the period from time 0 to time t, but may be viewed continuously. This t-sec observation period

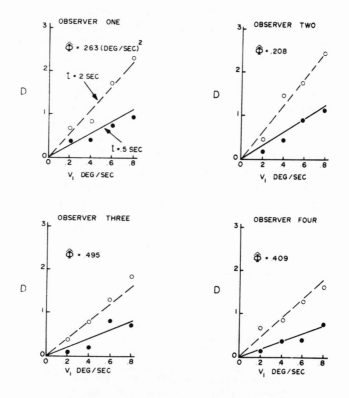

FIG. 5. Data from Kinchla and Allen (1969) showing how the discriminability (D) of a continuously illuminated point of light varies with the angular velocity of the light (v_1), for a duration of observation (t) of either .5 or 2 sec. All 8 combinations of t and v_1 are consistent with a single $φ$ value for each observer.

is indicated to the subject by a tone which is on only during that period (in order to distinguish it from the .5-sec periods before and afterwards when the light is on but always stationary). The observer's task is the same as in the first experiment in that there were only two response options on each trial, movement to the right, A_1, or no movement, A_0. There were eight different experimental conditions defined by two durations of observation, t equal 1 or 2 sec, and four angular velocities of movement to the right, v_1 equal .2, .4, .6, or .8° per sec. The prediction of the model is defined by Eq. (2b); specifically, that discriminability (d') is directly proportional to v_1. Again, a single estimate of ϕ for each observer provides a good fit of his performance in all eight experimental conditions. Furthermore, the noise levels $\hat{\phi}$ are similar to those obtained using discrete stimulus patterns.

A direct comparison of one's ability to discriminate displacements defined by discrete, rather than continuous, patterns (see Fig. 1) was obtained by testing each of three observers using discrete patterns during some sessions and continuous patterns during others (these results are reported here for the first time). The observer's task was always to distinguish between a movement to the right $(m_1 > 0)$ and no movement $(m_1 = 0)$. The specific value of m_1 during any one session was 0, 1/3, or 1° with the viewing period t a constant 1 sec; thus the angular velocity on "movement" trials was simply m_1. The principal features of the data obtained in this fashion can be summarized as follows. Although all three observers evidenced a small but statistically significant $(P < .01)$ tendency to report movement more often when continuous stimuli were employed, as compared to the tendency for corresponding discrete stimuli, there *were no significant differences in the estimates of $\hat{\phi}$* (a more detailed report of these data is in preparation). In other words, "movement" was discriminated no better when the observer could see the test stimulus during the t-sec interval from time 0 to time t, than it was when the "target" light was extinguished during this period. These results seem to have important implications for theories about how an observer interprets the small eye movements which maintain a target on the fovea. There is no question that many such movements occur during one's observation of a continuous pattern. Far fewer, if any, occur during the t-sec period of total darkness when a discrete pattern is presented, since there can be no retinal signals for maintaining fixation. However, our results suggest that an observer has little basis for distinguishing refixations, necessitated by an actual displacement of the target, from those required simply to compensate for "drifts" in eye position, since our estimates of ϕ were the same using discrete and continuous patterns: about .2–.3 deg^2/sec.

In an earlier edition of this model (Kinchla & Allan, 1969) I discussed the concept of "position memory" in more detail, suggesting how one might conceive of a subject as utilizing such memory processes in visual-movement perception. One suggestion that seemed rather appealing at the time was that an observer's overt eye drift was something like a mathematical "random walk" during the t-sec dark interval in a discrete stimulus pattern. The discrete stimulus patterns I have utilized involve t values ranging from about .5 sec to no more than 2 sec, and the model seems to work quite well within that range. Matin, Matin, and Pearce (1970) suggested that eye drift during dark intervals of this magnitude did approximate a random-walk process. (There were also systematic drift components, but these are not inconsistent with the linear increase in variance associated with a random walk.) However, another line of work reported by Skavenski and Steinman (e.g., Skavenski & Steinman, 1970; Skavenski, 1971) clearly indicates a limit to the similarity between "eye drifts in the dark" and a random-walk process. At the very least there appears to be an upper bound to the amount of drift which accumulates, since an observer seems able to orient his eyes within $3°$ of an initial target, no matter how long he remains in the dark. One might still argue that early in the drift process, before eye movements exceed $3°$, the process is something like a random walk, and contributes to the *psychophysically* defined value of $\hat{\phi}$. However, even if one accepted the Matin, Matin, and Pearce (1970) data as reflecting a random-walk process, the eye drift would account for no more than one-half to one-third of the noise ($\hat{\phi}$) suggested by the psychophysical data. So in any case there must be more to the psychophysical noise than overt eye drift.

Again let me emphasize that the model is a psychophysical one which explains in relatively simple terms how one can characterize a subject's ability to discriminate movement, over a fairly wide range of stimuli, with just a single theoretical constant $\hat{\phi}$ ranging between .2 and .3 deg^2/sec. Whether overt eye drift represents a major component of this psychophysical noise is difficult to say at this point; however, *the psychophysical data are not going to change.* It seems clear that the model does a good job of characterizing what an observer can do, and the burden of accounting for this on a physiological level should be one goal of any physiological investigation.

Before concluding let me elaborate the problem of movement discrimination one step further. Up to this point, the model has been applied to detecting the movement of a single point of light seen in a totally dark field (and I assume one would obtain similar effects if the target stimulus were moving in any type of Ganzfeld, such as a black dot moving in a totally homogeneous white field). However, suppose one introduced a second point of light into the field which remained entirely stationary $r°$ to the right of position zero (the initial position of the target light). Clearly, if this second light were located close enough to the test stimulus it could serve as a sort of reference point, and the observer could judge whether the target point moved or remained stationary by deciding whether the *distance between* the "test" and "reference" points changed over time or not. This seems like a very different type of perceptual process in which you would be judging the *relative* position of two lights rather than the *absolute* position of a single light.

I have compared absolute and relative judgments of this sort (Kinchla, 1971). An interesting aspect of my findings is that in order for the absolute-judgment model to apply, the area around the test stimuli need only be homogeneous (devoid of discernible reference points) for $10°$ or so. Thus, while our simple model can be elaborated so as to deal with relative movement perception, it seems possible to ignore other reference points in the visual field so long as they are more than about $10°$ away from the target stimulus. If the target is within such a local Ganzfeld, the observer discriminates its movement no differently than in a total Ganzfeld (at least for the range of m and t values we have considered). This is much like trying to discern the movement of a cloud in an otherwise clear blue sky. Only if you can introduce a fixed reference point, such as a telephone pole or rooftop, fairly close to your view of the cloud will it be possible to improve your perception of the cloud's motion.

Obviously there are more complex types of movement, in more complex visual fields (Kinchla, 1970), and I won't try to say anything further about them here. However, I do feel that the basic types of movement discrimination I have considered are well characterized by the very simple, but mathematically precise, model presented in this paper. And furthermore, that the theoretical constant $\phi \cong .3$ deg^2/sec emerges as a basic constant characterizing "noise" in the visual positioning system.

IV.7

The Nature and Role of Extraretinal Eye-Position Information in Visual Localization[1]

Alexander A. Skavenski

Northeastern University

It is well known that organisms accurately locate visual stimuli while they move about in their environments. Since their eyes move with respect to the head, these determinations cannot be based solely on the behavior of the image of the stimulus on the retina. Following Helmholtz's (1962) suggestion more than a century ago, many believe that such judgments are based on a combination of signals indicating target position on the retina with nonvisual information indicating eye position with respect to the head. The accuracy of retinal position and velocity information is well documented and is compatible with this notion (see Matin, 1972, for a discussion of the precision of retinally based position information). However, some investigators (Festinger & Easton, 1974; MacKay, 1972; and Matin, 1972) have found that both the accuracy of extraretinal signals and their temporal correspondence with eye movements is so poor that they have questioned the adequacy of this model and others like it as explanations of spatial perception. I would like to review some work I did in collaboration with Steinman and Haddad (e.g., see Skavenski, Haddad, & Steinman, 1972) which examined the nature and accuracy of extraretinal eye-position information and which, I think, suggests an alternative to this view. In particular, our work suggests that there is, in fact, an accurate and easily remembered extraretinal

[1] Recent experiments on control in the dark and this report were supported by Grant EY1049 from the National Eye Institute to the author. Earlier work on control in the dark and perception was supported by Grant EY325 from the National Eye Institute to R. M. Steinman.

indication of eye position, and further, that studies which demonstrate that this signal is sloppy may have been confounded by a procedural problem.

One way to directly examine the accuracy of extraretinal eye-position information is to record attempts to maintain the eye in a defined position in the absence of visual information about eye position. Skavenski and Steinman (1970) and Skavenski (1971) found that such control was reasonably good. Figure 1 shows typical recordings of horizontal and vertical eye position during attempts to maintain the eye in several positions in the dark.

All three records illustrate the good control of eye position that we typically observe in the dark. Detailed statistical analyses of such patterns (e.g., see Skavenski & Steinman, 1970; Skavenski, 1971) indicated that this control was characterized by a slow movement of the eye away from the defined position, coupled with a remarkably small and uniform short-term variability in eye position. In addition, a correlational analysis of the eye-movement pattern (Skavenski, 1971) revealed significant departures from expectations based on a random-walk model and indicated that there was a corrective eye-movement pattern in the dark. These findings, combined with the proposals of Helmholtz (1962), von Holst (1954), and others suggest that control in the dark could be represented schematically as shown in Figs. 2 and 3. The process is broken into two parts for simplicity.

Figure 2 illustrates one way the subject could obtain and store the location of the target in memory during the period when it was visible. The upper boxes show image position with respect to the eye ($\theta_{T/E}$) being used by various visuomotor systems to produce eye position directly. The lower paths show that

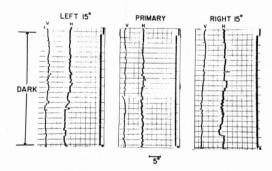

FIG. 1. Representative recordings showing horizontal (H) and vertical (V) eye position during attempts to maintain eye position in the dark. Each record begins at the top and repetitive horizontal stripes indicate 1-sec periods of time. Position-defining targets were presented in the primary or 15° arc to the left or right of primary position and were briefly visible for the first 1.5 sec of each record. Targets were switched off for the remainder of each record (labeled *dark*) during which time the subject attempted to keep his eye in the position defined by the target when it was visible. The length of the bar at the bottom indicates a 5° arc rotation on both meridians. Movements of traces to the left correspond to down in V and left in H.

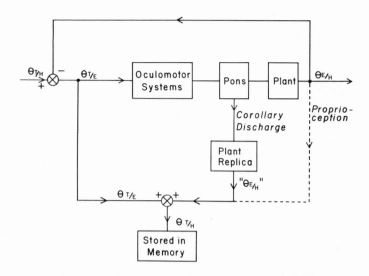

FIG. 2. A block diagram schematizing a method by which the nervous system could determine the spatial location of a seen object and store its position in memory. Upper paths show the position of the image with respect to the head ($\theta_{T/H}$) combining with eye position in the head ($\theta_{E/H}$) to yield retinal image position ($\theta_{T/E}$). This information is used by various *oculomotor systems* to produce eye position through neural mechanisms in the *pons* and the mechanical properties of the orbital contents (*plant*). See Robinson (1971; 1973) for models of the contents of these boxes. Lower paths show target positions with respect to the eye being added to extraretinal eye-position information ("$\theta_{E/H}$") to yield information regarding the spatial location of the target with respect to the head ($\theta_{T/H}$). This information is stored in memory. Details about corollary discharge and proprioceptive sources of "$\theta_{E/H}$" are described later in the text.

a central representation of target position with respect to the head is obtained by simply adding eye-position information to retinally based image-position information. Target position is stored in memory.

Figure 3 shows how remembered target position can be used to control eye position in the dark. Remembered target position is shown to deteriorate following a time course and extent similar to the movement of the eye away from the target in the dark (Skavenski & Steinman, 1970; Skavenski, 1971). In this diagram, eye-position information is subtracted from remembered target position to yield signals used by the saccadic system to control eye position in the dark. The assumption made is that central knowledge of eye position is exact and compared accurately to remembered target position. In fact, short-term standard deviations of eye-position measures in the dark suggest that the accuracy is better than 20 min arc (Skavenski & Steinman, 1970). Therefore, the majority of error in controlling eye position in the dark is assumed to arise from the subject's poor memory for the spatial location of the target.

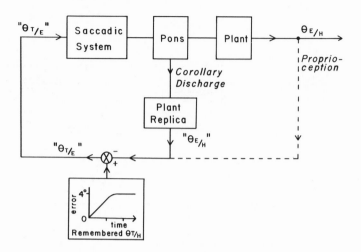

FIG. 3. A block diagram illustrating one way remembered target position would be used to maintain eye position in the dark. The lower paths show the extraretinal eye position signal ("$\theta_{E/H}$") being subtracted from remembered target position with respect to the head (*remembered* $\theta_{T/H}$) to provide an error signal "$\theta_{T/E}$" that bears similar properties to the visual error signal $\theta_{T/E}$ of Fig. 2. "$\theta_{T/E}$" is used by the saccadic system to control eye position in the dark. Other features of this diagram are the same as those described in Fig. 2.

Other features of the schematics in Figs. 2 and 3 are also consistent with our experiments. For example, a proprioceptive source for the extraretinal signals was included because subjects can use inflow signals from orbital mechanoreceptors to control eye position in the dark (Skavenski, 1972). However, quantitative replications of Helmholtz's (1962) observations (Skavenski, Haddad, & Steinman, 1972) indicate that the extraretinal signals used in spatial perception are derived from the outflow commands sent to the extraocular muscles. Two experiments were done. In the first, known external forces were applied to a subject's right eye while he was required to fixate a target. Vision in the other eye was obscured. In this experiment the target remained on the same retinal locus so that its perceived direction depended only on the state of the extraretinal indication of eye position. When the load was applied to the right eye, the subject had to change outflow to increase the force on the eye by an amount exactly equal to the load, but in the opposite direction, to continue fixating the target. This change would normally rotate the unencumbered eye and extraretinal signals based on outflow would indicate that the eye moved opposite to the load. If perceived target direction depended solely on outflow, then the target would be perceived to move *opposite* to the applied load.

Since the eye remained in the same position in the orbit, inflow would predict that the target would not appear to move when the load was applied. Actually, the inflow prediction is somewhat complicated because the activity of the muscle spindle, the presumed source of inflow, is known to depend directly on activity in the gamma efferent system (Granit, 1955). If the gamma efferent system for the eye behaved as it does elsewhere in the body, then the level of activity of the gamma efferents in the agonist muscle for the load should have increased along with alpha motoneuron activity when the load was applied. Such changes in innervation to intrafusal muscle fibers via the gamma efferents would result in an increase in the discharge from the annulospiral endings. This increase would correspond to inflow signals that the eye rotated *in* the direction of load application if the activity of the gamma efferents was disregarded by the nervous system (Matin, 1972).

A more likely possibility would be that proprioceptive signals from stretch receptors were combined with gamma efferent activity to provide a hybrid inflow signal. Specifically, absolute extraocular muscle length could be determined by simply subtracting gamma efferent activity from muscle spindle activity if both were properly scaled. Although such a combination has not been previously proposed as a means of obtaining eye position from stretch receptors, it is a straightforward computation to make and can easily be done with neural elements. In the present experiment, the inflow prediction based on such a hybrid combination of inflow and gamma efferent outflow would be that the eye did not change position when the load was applied. An example using the agonist muscle with respect to the applied load will serve to illustrate. On load application, alpha–gamma cocontraction would cause gamma efferent activity to increase. However, this increase would be exactly canceled by the return barrage from the muscle spindle, so that the output of the hybrid circuit would yield no net change in eye position. This prediction follows whether one views the muscle spindle as a length transducer or as a "misalignment detector" (Granit, 1955).

Therefore, increases in proprioceptor activity resulting from changes in gamma efferent activity would indicate that the eye did not change position if the gamma efferent activity was taken into account by the nervous system or that the eye moved toward the load if the nervous system disregarded gamma efferent activity. Finally, if there were no change in the gamma efferent system, proprioceptor activity would remain uniform because the loaded eye remained in the same position and the nervous system would be so informed. Thus, inflow would predict that perceived target direction would remain unchanged or shift in the direction of the load and there is a clear difference between inflow and outflow predictions.

The results shown in Fig. 4 support the outflow prediction because the shift in perceived direction was always opposite to the direction of the load.

In this experiment subjects indicated the perceived direction of the fixation target by placing a second movable target in their "subjective" straight-ahead position; a task that they could perform quite reliably.

Figure 4 shows mean shifts in the perceived direction of the fixation target for various loads applied to the left and right of subject RS's right eye. Perceived shifts were obtained by calculating the difference between the mean straight-ahead position when no load was applied to the eye and the mean straight-ahead position when the eye was loaded. Perceived shifts in the direction of the target that would be predicted from outflow are shown as oblique lines. The slopes of these lines are equal to the measured spring constants for the subject's eye. These lines indicate that, based on outflow, the fixation target should be perceived to shift opposite to the load by an amount equal to the applied load divided by the spring constant. Inflow would predict no shift in the perceived direction of the fixation target (a vertical line) or that the target would shift in the direction of load application (roughly orthogonal to the outflow prediction). Figure 4 shows that the perceived direction of the target always shifted opposite

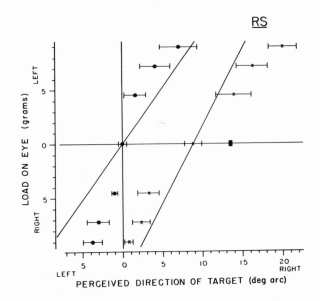

FIG. 4. Mean perceived direction (abscissa) of a fixation target for various loads (ordinate) applied to the *left* and *right* of RS's right eye. Subject RS's mean straight-ahead position (when no load was applied to the eye) is plotted at the intersection of the axes. Circles (●) represent mean shifts in perceived direction of the fixation target when it was straight ahead, and crosses (x) indicate mean shifts when the target was placed 13.5° arc to the right of primary position. Each datum point is the mean of 10 position measures, and error bars indicate one standard deviation on each side of the mean. Diagonal lines indicate perceived shifts predicted from outflow theory. The rectangle (■) at the right shows the objective position of the target when it was placed 13.5° arc to the right. The datum point just to the left of the rectangle indicates that the subjective straight ahead was biased toward the fixation point when it was displaced. The present experiments did not reveal the cause of this bias. After Skavenski et al. (1972).

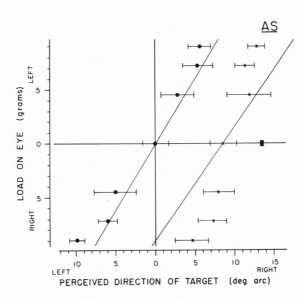

FIG. 5. Mean perceived direction of the fixation target for various loads applied to the left and right of subject AS's right eye. All features of this plot are the same as those shown in Fig. 4. After Skavenski et al. (1972).

to the applied load and that the amplitude of the shift increased monotonically with load magnitude. Figure 5 shows that similar results were obtained from a second subject.

These results support the conclusion that perceived target direction is proportional to the magnitude of the outflow signals. In addition, this finding is also first-hand evidence that extraretinal eye-position information is directly involved in visual spatial perception.

In the second experiment we searched for evidence for the contribution of inflow to the perception of direction by keeping outflow constant while systematically varying inflow. The results indicated that systematic changes in inflow had no effect on the perceived direction of a fixation target (Skavenski et al., 1972). Combined with the results of the preceding experiment, these data formed the basis for the suggestion that eye-position information, of particular importance for perception, is largely outflow in nature. It must be noted that the possible contribution of inflow to our visual spatial perceptions has not been completely ruled out on the basis of these experiments because the inflow messages from one eye have been placed in conflict with the outflow to both eyes as well as the inflow from the eye that was not encumbered.

The diagrams in Figs. 2 and 3 also suggest that the outflow extraretinal signals originated in the pons near the final common path. This speculation arises jointly from considerations of the types of eye movement for which there must be accurate position information as well as the neural structures producing these movements. For example, there is mounting evidence suggesting that accurate extraretinal signals indicating eye position seem to be available no matter what system produces the eye movement. Skavenski and Steinman (1970) showed that a subject could return to within 2° arc of a previously seen fixation target after making 30 large voluntary saccades in randomly chosen directions during a dark period. In addition, we noted the occurrence of a noisy drift that moves the eye toward the primary position when subjects attempt to maintain the eye in any eccentric position in the dark. We found that subjects were able to correct the errors introduced by these drift movements by making a saccade in the opposite direction. Becker and Klein (1973) have since confirmed this observation in other subjects.

Preliminary data from my own laboratory indicate that, in the dark, a subject can also correct errors in eye position caused by natural stimulation of the vestibular system. In this experiment the subject viewed a single target presented in one of four positions evenly distributed along the horizon and covering a 45° arc range. The target was switched off and the subject continued to maintain eye position in the dark for 2 sec. Then, on half of the trials the eye was driven 20 to 35° arc away from this position by rotating the subject at various velocities about the vertical axis in a randomly selected direction. On the other half of the trials the subject made a large horizontal saccade in a randomly selected direction to a new position about 30° arc from the position of the fixation target. Five seconds after the onset of each movement the subject was instructed to return his eye to the position, with respect to his head, that was originally defined by the fixation target. The subject attempted to maintain the return position for an additional 7-sec period in total darkness. We measured error (the distance between mean eye position in the head when the target was visible and mean eye position during the 7-sec period following the return movement). On the horizontal meridian, mean error was 2.0° arc following the saccades and 1.8° arc following the slow phase of vestibular nystagmus. The small difference between these two error measures was not statistically reliable. Therefore, the extraretinal signals appear to be as accurate indicators of eye position driven by the vestibular system as they are for rapid saccades.

Combined, these data indicate that accurate extraretinal eye-position information is available following at least three major classes of eye movement. This finding leads to the speculation that the origin of these signals might be near the final common path. To illustrate, our understanding of the motor systems producing various types of eye movement suggest that they share few neural structures in common except those brainstem structures forming the final common path (Robinson, 1971). In addition, the ways in which they drive the eye is thought to differ (Robinson, 1971). The consequence of this is that the activity of some brainstem structures would seem to be the only correlates of eye position regardless of movement type in the motor system and would be the most likely source of the eye-position signals. Alternatively, the commands to the eye would have to be passed through neural replicas of the various structures imposed between the source of the command and the eye to accurately indicate eye position for all types of movement. Although it is less likely, the possibility of an inflow source for the extraretinal signal must be left open. This third source is the most parsimonious and requires no neural replicas of oculomotor mechanics or premotor neural elements.

In conclusion, the data from these studies indicate that there is accurate extraretinal eye position information for several types of eye movement that can be used to control eye position in the dark. According to this view the extraretinal signal would appear to be sufficiently accurate to explain perceived stability during eye movement as well as our visual spatial perceptions. This interpretation is notably at variance with the view expressed by others at this symposium and probably arises because prior investigators have assumed that the quality of our spatial memory is better than it really is.

Most studies of extraretinal signals have deprived the subject of visual cues about the direction and motion of the target by showing him a reference target and then removing it from view. After some delay in a featureless field, the subject is presented with a second target whose position and motion is to be judged with respect to the subject's memory of the location of the first target. The result is that localization of the second object with respect to the first is somewhat poor and most conclude that the extraretinal compensation for eye movement is defective (Matin, 1972). The view I have presented would suggest that the defect, if we can call it that, lies in the subject's memory for the spatial location of the first reference target: a possibility that has been mentioned in the past by Matin and his co-workers (*e. g.*, Matin, Pearce, Matin, & Kibler, 1966) and by Skavenski and Steinman (1970) but has been largely neglected. This view is compelling but admittedly has no direct supporting evidence. However, the alternative is much weaker. No one has explicitly measured the fidelity of the subjects' memory for the spatial location of a reference target under conditions in which the accuracy of the extraretinal signal was not a contaminating variable. Thus, the quality of visual spatial memory, as well as the kinds of variables that may influence it, are unknown. One hint that spatial memory is poor and deteriorates with time may be found in Posner's (1967) demonstrations of subjects' poor abilities to reproduce movements or positions after brief delays using the arm: a limb whose position sense is not questioned. In addition, it is well known that comparisons of all stimuli are much better when done simultaneously than when done successively when a delay occurs between comparison and test stimuli. It is unlikely that visual spatial perception is an exception.

DISCUSSION

FRY: How did you apply loads to a human subject's eye?

SKAVENSKI: A stalk was cemented to a contact lens which was held on the subject's eye by suction. Two threads were attached to this stalk and were placed over pulleys on either side of the subject so that the downward force of a weight attached to the end of the thread would produce a lateral force on the eye.

POLA: I have a few comments to make in order to indicate that the extra-retinal signal which L. Matin and I measured is perhaps not merely an artifact of the situation we used.

First, I have asked a large number of people how visual space appears to them in a normally illuminated environment when they turn their eyes from one location to another. Most of them have had nothing to do with visual direction experiments. They responded that there are noticeable jumps in the environment which would be consonant with the viewpoint that there is perhaps a sloppy extraretinal signal. Either the time course of the extraretinal signal or its final magnitude could be nonveridical.

In addition, I notice that when I make a saccade over a dimly lit window in a dark room, the window often seems closer to my fovea than it ought to be after I have made the saccade. This would be consistent with the fact that I typically have an extraretinal signal which overcompensates for my eye movement.

Finally, in pilot experiments with E. Matin, it was found that during saccades away from a fixation target, the target could be shifted as much as $3°$ arc in the direction opposite to the eye movement without the subject's noticing that shift at all. Shifts of the target in the direction of the eye movement were fairly easily discriminated. This finding is also consonant with a viewpoint that the extra-retinal process is overcompensating for the eye movement.

Afterthoughts

SKAVENSKI: The amount of perceived movement of the visual field during saccades that subjects casually report must be viewed with caution because such subjective reports are known to be biased by whims or expectations of the subject. To illustrate, I never notice "jumps" in the visual field when I make saccades despite the fact that I have specifically searched for them. But then few would have confidence in this statement when viewed in light of my bias expressed above. Similar biases can be easily communicated to "naive" subjects. There may, in fact, be some failure of veridical extraretinal compensation for retinal image motion during saccades. However, a sluggish compensatory extra-retinal signal, which begins its change 200 msec before a saccade and continues its growth for up to 1500 msec after a saccade (Matin, 1972), would cause apparent movement of visual objects for a period of nearly 2 sec and would preclude accurate visuomotor coordinations. Since typical saccade rates are on the order of 1 to 2 per sec, a sluggish extraretinal signal could never "catch up" to eye position and consequently visuomotor coordinations would be poor. How are we to explain the relatively good localizations that we routinely make? The phenomenon of saccadic suppression which leads to a dimming of visual objects during saccades may account, in part, for perceived stability during rapid movement but is of no help to an organism faced with the need for accurate visual localizations. Therefore, the single known mechanism that would account for accurate localization is that described earlier in Fig. 2; viz. a combination of retinally based image-position information with a veridical extraretinal eye-position signal.

Acknowledgments

I thank R. M. Steinman for his collaboration on all aspects of most of the experiments described in this manuscript and for his valuable suggestions regarding the manuscript itself. I also thank R. Hansen, L. Kiorpes, and G. Timberlake for their technical assistance and comments on this paper and M. M. Figueiredo for typing the manuscript.

IV.8

Pursuit Eye Movements and Visual Localization[1]

Frank Ward

University of Rochester

I would like to describe a few experiments on pursuit eye movements that we are currently doing at the University of Rochester. These experiments assess an observer's ability to localize a briefly presented target during the act of pursuit.

It has been argued (Festinger & Canon, 1965) that the pursuit eye-movement system does not have access to extraretinal information as does the saccadic system. However, there is a series of experiments in the literature that suggests that localization is possible during pursuit movements.

I am referring to some work done in Germany several decades ago (Hazelhoff & Wiersma, 1924) and in Japan (Mita, Hironaka, & Koika, 1950). The experimental paradigm has been called "the localization method." Basically, an observer tracks a predictable target and, during this act of pursuit, a brief pulse is delivered—say, directly below the tracking target. This test pulse is then localized by reference to a pointer or some object in the visual field. In general, it has been found that the apparent location of the test pulse is displaced in the direction of pursuit.

For example, if one were to track a small spot of light from the left to the right, and a test pulse were presented while the eyes were tracking, the pulse's apparent location would be shifted to the right.

One explanation for this phenomenon has to do with the visual latency of the test pulse. It takes a finite amount of time for the visual system to transmit information about the pulse. During this time interval, the eyes continue to pursue the target. When the pulse is finally perceived, the eyes will have moved in the direction of pursuit. Perhaps the pulse is localized to the position where

[1] Presently at Wright State University, Dayton, Ohio.

the eyes are pointed in physical space at the instant that the pulse is perceived. If this were the case, then one could infer that the brain keeps a continuous record of eye position *during* pursuit and that it is the interaction of the pulse information with this eye-position record that accounts for displacement of localization in the direction of pursuit.

We have done several experiments to try to support this hypothesis. But before I tell you about them, let me describe the apparatus shown in Fig. 1.

Our apparatus consists of an optical system that projects a 6-min tracking spot onto a curved tangent screen. The optics are located above the subject's head such that the axis of rotation of a mirror galvanometer is located directly above the subject's eyes. With a suitable signal generator and amplifiers, the galvanometer (actually an oscillograph pen motor) can be driven with a triangular waveform so that the projected tracking spot moves at a constant velocity across the screen. The total excursion is about 37°. A brief xenon pulse (<200 μsec) is delivered 3' below the tracking spot at the predetermined position on the screen. This test pulse is optically locked to the tracking spot through the mirror galvanometer optics.

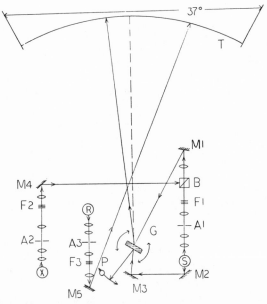

FIG. 1. A schematic diagram of the optics used to project the stimuli for the EZ experiments. The tracking stimulus originated at source S, was reflected from mirror M1 to the galvanometer mirror G, and was then reflected to the tangent screen T. The brief test pulse, from source X, was reflected from M4 and combined with the tracking stimulus at beam splitter B, so that the test pulse was optically locked to a point 3' below the tracking stimulus. The light path from S to M2, M3, G, and P was used for electronic timing of the test pulse. (Source R was not used in the present series of experiments.)

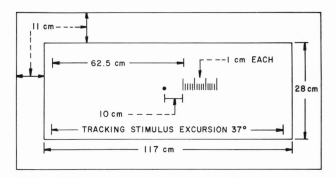

FIG. 2. Details of the scale and stimulus display. Stimuli were projected on a diffusely reflecting screen that was surrounded by a black border. The hatch-mark scale (shown enlarged) was displaced to the right to enable *Ss* ample time to acquire the tracking stimulus. Since data were always gathered as the eyes tracked from left to right, *Ss* had 1.8 sec (at 12°/sec) to acquire the target before the eyes were directed at the scale. The distance between the smallest scale divisions is approximately .35°.

Figure 2 shows the stimulus display screen with the scale. Notice the hatch marks on the screen. These are reference points in the visual field, so that the observer can localize the test pulse. In a typical trial, the subject tracks the moving spot from left to right. Somewhere in the region of the hatch marks, the test pulse is delivered. The observer then calls out, or signals, the particular mark on the screen beneath which the spot appeared. The physical location of the test pulse is varied from trial to trial.

During these trials, we monitored eye movements on an oscilloscope and recorded some trials from most experimental sessions.

The eye-movement monitoring system provides diffuse IR illumination in the area of the iris, and the reflected light from the iris–scleral junction is picked up by two detectors and differentially amplified. This system is especially convenient for us because it allows the use of both eyes *and* it can be used with subjects wearing normal eyeglasses.

In our initial replication of the "localization method" paradigm, it seemed that we should first establish that localization—or the inferred visual delay—does *not* depend upon the tracking velocity. There is no theoretical reason to expect that it should; however, previous studies had not shown any velocity effect, and we wanted to be sure we could replicate those findings.

Figure 3 shows the results of our delay or localization-versus-velocity experiment. The vertical bars are 95% confidence limits, not standard errors. Each point represents at least 60 observations.

In general, the curves are flat. And we conclude that, for moderate velocities, the speed of pursuit does not influence localization.

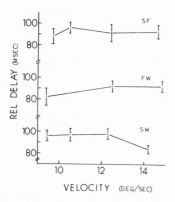

FIG. 3. The influence of pursuit velocity upon the relative visual delay for 3 *Ss*.

Note that for subject SW (on the bottom) the highest velocity does produce a shorter delay. This subject was our poorest tracker—and her eye-movement records showed many corrective saccades during her attempts to pursue at velocities above 14°/sec.

We wanted to demonstrate that the localization we measured has a latencylike function, so we attempted three more experiments to show some of the same visual latency effects that are obtained from reaction time and Pulfrich studies (see, for example, Rogers & Anstis, 1972; Mansfield, 1973).

In the first of these experiments, we varied the background luminance while keeping the pulse intensity constant. The results are presented in Fig. 4. You will note that for very dim backgrounds from −1.0 to −2.0 log foot-Lamberts (ft-L). the curves are essentially flat. At brighter backgrounds, there is some tendency toward increased visual latency for the test pulse, although these differences are not statistically significant. Our study, then, is in agreement with the findings of Rogers and Anstis that moderate adaptation levels do not affect visual latency.

To obtain further verification that background luminance had virtually no effect on delay, we also did a reaction-time study with results as shown in Fig. 5.

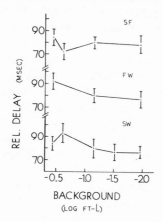

FIG. 4. The influence of background luminance upon relative delay for 3 *Ss*.

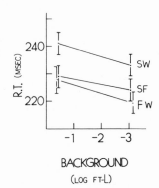

FIG. 5. The influence of background luminance upon reaction
time for 3 *Ss.*

Again, a brighter background produces only a very slight and nonsignificant
increase in reaction time.

Most studies of visual delay show that luminance of the *test* stimulus is the
major variable in determining how long it takes to perceive the test pulse.
Although the energy in our test pulse limited the range we could explore, you
can see from Fig. 6 that an attenuation of only .3 log unit produced a noticeable
although insignificant, increase in relative delay for SF. A .6-log unit attenuation
produced a significant increase in delay for subject SW. Subject FW produced a
significant increase in delay for only a .3-log unit attenuation. Thus, we are in
general agreement with the findings of other workers: that the luminance of the
test stimulus is a principal determinant of visual latency.

Some of our most interesting data come from the eye-movement records.
Figure 7 shows a typical pursuit trial, with delivery of the pulse at P and
cessation of tracking at T; the calibration marks indicate 5° displacement and

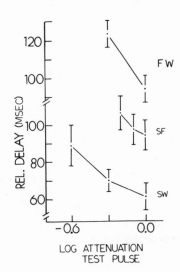

FIG. 6. The effect of test luminance upon relative visual delay.

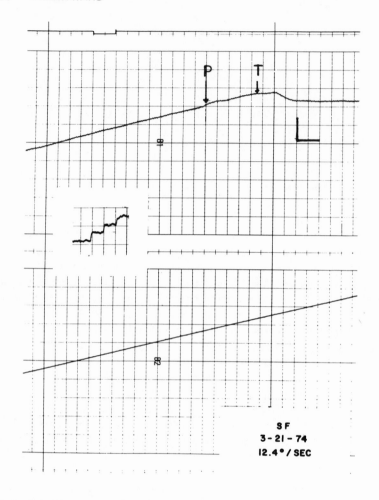

FIG. 7. Sample eye movement record of subject SF. The scallop just after point T is a saccade. Electrical dampening in the eye-movement monitor slowed its responses slightly.

100 msec. The insert shows a calibration trace for targets 1.75° apart. The bottom trace is the signal to the galvanometer. Note that after the subject stops tracking, he then saccades back in the direction of the pulse. This will be discussed later.

Again, Fig. 8 shows pursuit up to, and past, the pulse, and a cessation of tracking followed by a very small saccade back in the direction of the pulse. Calibration marks are as before (5° and 100 msec.). I should point out that this subject rarely executed detectable saccades back toward the pulse. He usually just stopped tracking.

Figure 9 shows our third subject. Her records are very much like those of the first subject. Note the small perturbation just past the point where the pulse was delivered. This is an electrical artifact caused by the xenon discharge. It is not a saccade. Calibration is the same on the others.

We have further analyzed our eye-movement records to show that the actual act of saccading does *not* seem to be related to localization judgments. We correlated the length of the interval from the pulse to cessation of tracking *with* the difference between the pulse's judged position and the position to which the eyes actually saccaded. Product moment correlations were .09, .22, and .19 for our three subjects. None of these correlations is significantly different from zero.

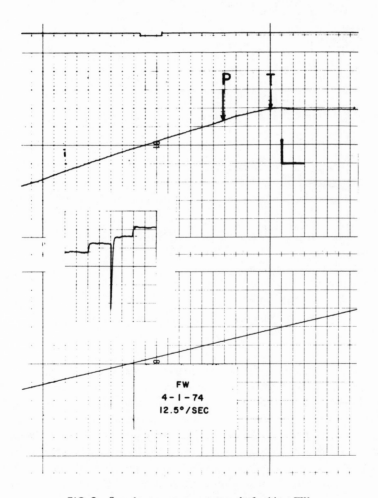

FIG. 8. Sample eye-movement record of subject FW.

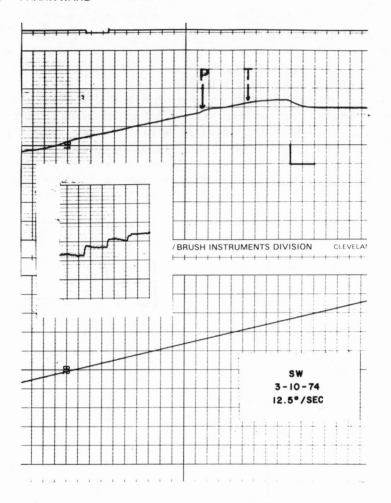

FIG. 9.   Sample eye-movement record of subject SW.

These pulse-to-cessation of tracking intervals covered a wide range of times (120–350 msec) and their distributions showed no particular trends.

The differences (in visual angle) between the pulse's judged position and the position to which the eyes saccaded also covered a wide range. However, individual differences among the subjects were very noticeable. One subject consistently failed to saccade much at all, and had a mean difference of 1.25° to the right of the judged position. Another was fairly accurate and had a mean position of .27° to the right. Our third subject consistently saccaded too far back toward the pulse and her mean difference was .27° to the left of the pulse's judged position. Thus, we conclude that the time from the pulse delivery to cessation of tracking *and* the magnitude of a saccade, if any, are unrelated to the judged position of the pulse.

It is important that the pulse's judged position not be associated with the act of saccading. If it were, one could, of course, argue that localization is mediated by the saccadic eye-movement system—however, we do not find any such association. Consequently, we believe that our data support the original hypothesis—that localization during tracking is a function of the pursuit eye-movement system, and that this system must, therefore, have access to some type of eye-position signal.

DISCUSSION

ROBINSON: Would you please remind me of what the subject is required to do.

WARD: The subject calls out the hatch mark under which he saw the pulse. There are three large ones and some smaller ones, so he might say "1.2" and that would indicate where he saw the pulse.

ROBINSON: He is not instructed to look at the flashing point, but he has to look at the marks?

WARD: No, he can get the scale position however he wants. We monitor each trial on the CRT and if we saw that he was not tracking, we would not accept his response. He has to be tracking at the moment that the pulse is delivered. That's the crucial thing.

Afterthoughts

SENDERS: The explanation of the displacement of a pulse during pursuit in the direction of tracking seems to assume that knowledge of eye position is instantaneously known whereas processing the pulse information takes time. What evidence or theory would support a zero latency perception of eye position?

IV.9

References

Bartlett, J. R., & Doty, R. W. Influence of mesencephalic stimulation on unit activity in striate cortex of squirrel monkeys. *Journal of Neurophysiology*, 1974, 37, 642–653.

Becker, W., & Fuchs, A. F. Further properties of the human saccadic system: Eye movements and correction saccades with and without visual fixation points. *Vision Research*, 1969, 9, 1247–1257.

Becker, W., & Klein, H. Accuracy of saccadic eye movements and maintenance of eccentric eye positions in the dark. *Vision Research*, 1973, 13, 1021–1034.

Bowen, R., Pola, J., & Matin, L. Visual persistence: Effects of flash luminance, duration, and energy. *Vision Research*, 1974, 14, 295–303.

Brindley, G. S., & Merton, P. A. The absence of position sense in the human eye. *Journal of Physiology*, 1960, 153, 127–130.

Brooks, B. A., & Jung, R. Neuronal physiology of the visual cortex. In R. Jung (ed.), *Handbook of sensory physiology*. Vol. 7, Pt. 3. Berlin: Springer–Verlag, 1973. Pp. 325–440.

Buttner, U., & Fuchs, A. F. Influence of saccadic eye movements on unit activity in simian lateral geniculate and pregeniculate nuclei. *Journal of Neurophysiology*, 1973, 36, 127–142.

Cornsweet, T. N., & Crane, H. D. Accurate two-dimensional eye tracker using first and fourth Purkinje images. *Journal of the Optical Society of America*, 1973, 63, 921.

Cynader, M., & Berman, N. Receptive-field organization of monkey superior colliculus. *Journal of Neurophysiology*, 1972, 35, 187–202.

Doty, R. W., Wilson, P. D., & Bartlett, J. R. Mesencephalic control of lateral geniculate nucleus in primates. I. Electrophysiology. *Experimental Brain Research*, 1973, 18, 189–203.

Evarts, E. V. Relation of pyramidal tract activity to force exerted during voluntary movement. *Journal of Neurophysiology*, 1968, 31, 14–27.

Festinger, L. Eye movements and perception. In P. Bach-y-Rita, C. C. Collins, & J. E. Hyde (Eds.), *The control of eye movements*. New York: Academic Press, 1971.

Festinger, L., & Canon, L. K. Information about spatial location based on knowledge about efference. *Psychological Review*, 1965, 72, 373–384.

Festinger, L., & Easton, A. M. Inferences about the efferent system based on a perceptual illusion produced by eye movements. *Psychological Review*, 1974, 81, 44–58.

Fuchs, A. F. Saccadic and smooth pursuit eye movements in the monkey. *Journal of Physiology*, 1967, 191, 609–631. (a)

Fuchs, A. F. Periodic eye tracking in the monkey. *Journal of Physiology*, 1967, **193**, 161–171. (b)

Goldberg, M. E., & Wurtz, R. H. Activity of superior colliculus in behaving monkey. I. Visual receptive fields of single neurons. *Journal of Neurophysiology*, 1972, **35**, 542–559. (a)

Goldberg, M. E., & Wurtz, R. H. Activity of superior colliculus in behaving monkey. II. Effect of attention on neuronal responses. *Journal of Neurophysiology*, 1972, **35**, 560–574. (b)

Granit, R. *Receptors and sensory perception.* New Haven: Yale University Press, 1955.

Green, D. M., & Swets, J. A. *Signal detection theory and psychophysics.* New York: Wiley, 1966.

Hallett, P. E. Disturbances of rod threshold forced by briefly exposed luminous lines, edges, disks, and annuli. *Journal of Physiology*, 1971, **215**, 449–476.

Hallett, P. E., & Lightstone, A. D. Corrective saccades and visual inflow during the prior saccade. *Journal of the Optical Society of America*, 1973, **63**, 1311.

Hallett, P. E., & Lightstone, A. D. Saccadic eye movements towards stimuli triggered during prior saccades. *Vision Research*, 1976, **16**, 99–106. (a)

Hallett, P. E. and Lightstone, A. D. Saccadic eye movements to flashed targets. *Vision Research*, 1976, **16**, 107–114. (b)

Harris, C. S. Perceptual adaptation to inverted, reversed, and displaced vision. *Psychological Review*, 1965, **72**, 419–444.

Hazelhoff, F. F., & Wiersma, H. Die Wahrnehmungszeit. *Zeitschrift für Psychologie*, 1924, **96**, 171–188.

Helmholtz, H. von *Handbuch der physiologischen Optik.* Leipzig: Voss, 1909. [English translation from 3rd ed., J. P. C. Southall (Ed.), *A Treatise on Physiological Optics, Vol. III.* Unabridged reprint by Dover Publications, New York, 1962.]

Hubel, D. H., & Wiesel, T. N. Receptive fields and functional architecture of monkey striate cortex. *Journal of Physiology* (London), 1968, **195**, 215–243.

James, W. *The principles of psychology,* Vol. 2. New York: Holt, 1890. Reprinted: New York: Dover Publ., 1950.

Johansson, G. *Configurations in event perception: An experimental study.* Uppsala: Almquist and Wiksells Boktryckeri AB; 1950.

Keller, W., & Kinchla, R. A. Visual movement discrimination. *Perception and Psychophysics*, 1968, **3**, 233–236.

Kinchla, R. A. Visual movement perception: A comparison of sensitivity to vertical and horizontal movement. *Perception and Psychophysics*, 1970, **8**, 399–405.

Kinchla, R. A. Visual movement perception: A comparison of absolute and relative movement discrimination. *Perception and Psychophysics*, 1971, **9**, 165–171.

Kinchla, R. A., & Allan, L. G. A theory of visual movement perception. *Psychological Review*, 1969, **76**, 537–558.

Kinchla, R. A., & Smyzer, F. A diffusion model of perceptual memory. *Perception and Psychophysics*, 1967, **2**, 219–229.

Lightstone, A. D. Visual stimuli for saccadic and smooth pursuit eye movements. Doctoral Thesis, University of Toronto, 1973.

MacKay, D. M. Elevation of visual threshold of displacement of retinal image. *Nature*, 1970, **225**, 90–92.

MacKay, D. M. Visual stability and voluntary eye movements. In R. Jung (Ed.), *Handbook of sensory physiology.* Vol. 7, Part 3. Berlin: Springer-Verlag, 1973. Pp. 307–331.

MacKay, D. Visual stability. *Investigative Ophthalmology*, 1972, **11**, 518–524.

McLaughlin, S. C. Parametric adjustment in saccadic eye movements. *Perception and Psychophysics*, 1967, **2**, 359–362.

Mandl, G. The influence of visual pattern combinations on responses of movement-sensitive cells in the cat's superior colliculus. *Brain Research*, 1974, **75**, 215–240.

Mansfield, R. J. W. Latency functions in human vision. *Vision Research*, 1973, **13**, 2219–2234.

Matin, E., Clymer, A., & Matin, L. Metacontrast and saccadic suppression. *Science*, 1972, **178**, 179–182.

Matin, E., Matin, L., Pola, J., & Kowal, K. The intermittent-light illusion and constancy of visual direction during voluntary saccades. Paper Presented at the 10th Annual Meeting of the Psychonomic Society, St. Louis, 1969.

Matin, L. Measurement of eye movements by contact-lens techniques: Analysis of measuring systems and some new methodology for three-dimensional recording. *Journal of the Optical Society of America*, 1964, **54**, 1008–1018.

Matin, L. Eye movements and perceived visual direction. In D. Jameson & L. M. Hurvich (Eds.), *Handbook of sensory physiology*, Vol. 7, Pt. 4. Berlin: Springer-Verlag, 1972. Pp. 331–380.

Matin, L., & Bowen, R. Measuring the duration of perception. Unpublished manuscript.

Matin, L., & Kibler, G. G. Acuity of visual perception of movement in the dark for various positions of the eye in orbit. *Perceptual and Motor Skills*, 1966, **22**, 407–420.

Matin, L., & Matin, E. Visual perception of direction and voluntary saccadic eye movements. In J. Dichgans & E. Bizzy (Eds.), *Cerebral control of eye movements and motion perception. Bibliotheca ophthalmologica*, No. 82. Basel: S. Karger, 1972.

Matin, L., Matin, E., & Pearce, D. G. Visual perception of direction when voluntary saccades occur: I. Relation of visual direction of a fixation target extinguished before a saccade to a flash presented during the saccade. *Perception and Psychophysics*, 1969, **5**, 65–80.

Matin, L., Matin, E., & Pearce, D. G. Statistical characteristics of eye movements in the dark during the attempt to maintain a prior fixation position. *Vision Research*, 1970, **10**, 837–857.

Matin, L., Matin, E., & Pola, J. Detection of vernier offset, eye movements, and autokinetic movement. Paper presented at *Eastern Psychological Association*, Washington, 1968.

Matin, L., Matin, E., & Pola, J. Visual perception of direction when voluntary saccades occur. II. Relation of visual direction of a fixation target extinguished before a saccade to a subsequent test flash presented before the saccade. *Perception and Psychophysics*, 1970, **8**, 9–14.

Matin, L., Matin, E., & Pola, J. Visual perception of direction when voluntary saccades occur. III. Relation of visual direction of a fixation target extinguished before a saccade to a flash presented after the saccade (in preparation).

Matin, L., & Pearce, D. G. Three-dimensional recording of rotational eye movements by a new contact-lens technique. In W. E. Murry & P. F. Salisbury (Eds.), *Biomedical sciences instrumentation*. New York: Plenum Press, 1964. Pp. 79–95.

Matin, L., & Pearce, D. G. Visual perception of direction for stimuli flashed during voluntary saccadic eye movements. *Science*, 1965, **148**, 1485–1488.

Matin, L., Pearce, D. G., Matin, E., & Kibler, G. Visual perception of direction in the dark: roles of local sign, eye movements, and ocular proprioception. *Vision Research*, 1966, **6**, 453–469.

Matin, L., Pola, J., & Matin, E. Changes in visual direction with voluntary saccadic eye movements: Influence of visual persistence. *American Academy of Optometry*, 1972, **49**, 897 (Abst.).

Mita, T., Hironaka, K., & Koika, J. The influence of retinal adaptation and location on the "Empfindungszeit." *Tohoku Journal of Experimental Medicine*, 1950, **52**, 397–405.

Mohler, C. W., Goldberg, M. E., and Wurtz, R. H. Visual receptive fields of frontal eye field neurons. *Brain Research*, 1973, **61**, 385–389.

302 REFERENCES

Noda, H., & Adey, W. R. Retinal ganglion cells of the cat transfer information on saccadic eye movement and quick target motion. *Brain Research,* 1974, **70,** 340–345.

Pola, J. The relation of the perception of visual direction to eye position during and following a voluntary saccade. Doctoral dissertation, Columbia University, New York, 1973.

Posner, M. I. Characteristics of visual and kinesthetic memory codes. *Journal of Experimental Psychology,* 1967, **75,** 103–107.

Rizzolatti, G., Camarda, R., Grupp, L. A., & Pisa, M. Inhibition of visual responses of single units in the cat superior colliculus by the introduction of a second visual stimulus. *Brain Research,* 1973, **61,** 390–394.

Robinson, D. A. The mechanics of human saccadic eye movement. *Journal of Physiology,* 1964, **174,** 245–264.

Robinson, D. A. Models of oculomotor neural organization. In P. Bach-y-Rita & C. Collins (Eds.), *Control of eye movements.* New York: Academic Press, 1971. Pp. 519–538.

Robinson, D. A. Models of the saccadic eye movement control system. *Kybernetik,* 1973, **14,** 71–83.

Robinson, D. A., & Keller, E. L. The behavior of eye movement montoneurons in the alert monkey. *Bibliotheca Ophthalmologica,* 1972, **82,** 7–16.

Rogers, B. J., & Anstis, S. M. Intensity versus adaptation and the Pulfrich stereophenomenon. *Vision Research,* 1972, **12,** 909–928.

Schiller, P. H., & Koerner, F. Discharge characteristics of single units in superior colliculus of the alert rhesus monkey. *Journal of Neurophysiology,* 1971, **34,** 920–936.

Sherif, M. *The psychology of social norms.* New York: Harper, 1936.

Sherrington, C. D. Observations on the sensual role of the proprioceptive nerve-supply of the extrinsic ocular muscles. *Brain,* 1918, **41,** 323–343.

Singer, W., & Bedworth, N. Correlation between the effects of brain stem stimulation and saccadic eye movements on transmission in the cat lateral geniculate nucleus. *Brain Research,* 1974, **72,** 185–202.

Skavenski, A. A. Extraretinal correction and memory for target position. *Vision Research,* 1971, **11,** 743–746.

Skavenski, A. A. Inflow as a source of extraretinal eye-position information. *Vision Research,* 1972, **12,** 221–229.

Skavenski, A. A., Haddad, G. M., & Steinman, R. M. The extraretinal signal for the visual perception of direction. *Perception & Psychophysics,* 1972, **11,** 287–290.

Skavenski, A. A., & Steinman, R. M. Control of eye position in the dark. *Vision Research,* 1970, **10,** 193–203.

Sprague, J. M., Berlucchi, G., & Rizzolatti, G. The role of the superior colliculus and pretectum in vision and visually guided behavior. In R. Jung (Ed.), *Handbook of sensory physiology.* Vol. 7, Part 3. Berlin: Springer–Verlag, 1973, 27–101.

Sweet, A. L. Temporal discrimination by the human eye, *American Journal of Psychology,* 1953, **66,** 185–198.

Troxler, D. Über das verschwinden gegebener, gegenstande innerhalb unsers Geisichtskreises. In K. Himly & J. A. Schmidt (Eds.), *Ophthalmologische Bibliothek,* 1804, **2,** 51–53.

von Holst, E. Relations between the central nervous system and the peripheral organs. *British Journal of Animal Behavior,* 1954, **2,** 89–94.

Wilson, M. E., & Cragg, B. G. Projections from the lateral geniculate nucleus in the cat and monkey. *Journal of Anatomy,* 1967, **101,** 677–692.

Wilson, M. E., & Toyne, M. J. Retino-tectal and cortico-tectal projections in *Macaca mulatta. Brain Research,* 1970, **24,** 395–406.

Wurtz, R. H. Visual receptive fields of striate cortex neurons in awake monkeys. *Journal of Neurophysiology,* 1969, **32,** 727–742. (a)

Wurtz, R. H. Response of striate cortex neurons to stimuli during rapid eye movements of the monkey. *Journal of Neurophysiology*, 1969, **32**, 975–986. (b)

Wurtz, R. H. Comparison of effects of eye movements and stimulus movements on striate cortex neurons of the monkey. *Journal of Neurophysiology*, 1969, **32**, 987–994. (c)

Wurtz, R. H., & Goldberg, M. E. Superior colliculus cell responses related to eye movements in awake monkeys. *Science*, 1971, **171**, 82–84.

Wurtz, R. H., & Goldberg, M. E. Activity of superior colliculus in behaving monkey. III. Cells discharging before eye movements. *Journal of Neurophysiology*, 1972, **35**, 575–586. (a)

Wurtz, R. H., & Goldberg, M. E. The primate superior colliculus and the shift of visual attention. *Investigative Ophthalmology*, 1972, **11**, 441–450. (b)

Wurtz, R. H., & Mohler, C. W. Selection of visual targets for the initiation of saccadic eye movements. *Brain Research*, 1974, **71**, 209–214.

Wurtz, R. H., & Mohler, C. W. (in preparation).

Part V

TARGET DETECTION, SEARCH, AND SCANNING BEHAVIOR

As the preceding parts may suggest, we seem to be crawling up the brain stem from physiology toward cognitive processes. In a sense, as we go from Part IV to Part V, we will cross over a little bridge. We have been looking at fundamental processes of fixations, saccades, pursuits, and so on. The ways in which these are controlled by neural mechanisms have been clarified, their interactions at the retinal and perceptual levels have been extensively explored. Now we are concerned with the question of what people do with eye movements.

It is an important question. We spend our time, as Steinman has pointed out, sometimes voluntarily selecting places in the visual field to look at, and at other times allowing a process to go on that one is nearly unaware of, in which the eye successively fixates different parts of an apparently nicely stabilized visual field. From these "looks" we continually reconstruct, renew, and refresh some internal map of what is "out there."

There has been continuing study over the last 25 years of how people look at dynamical things, for example, dials on an aircraft instrument panel, or faces if one is engaged in conversation or lecturing. They change when one is not looking at them; sometimes they change while one is looking at them. Certain rules can be established relating the content of dynamic displays to the distribution of visual attention across these displays.

Another aspect of the visual world is the static aspect. We look at a landscape and things mostly stay where they are. Trees don't get up and walk around; paintings and cast-iron eagles in particular tend to stay exactly as they have been. Yet the eye does come back from time to time to look once again at a piece of the visual field which it has just recently visited and from which it has departed. A very interesting problem is that of the relationship between the content and structure of a visual field and the way in which one distributes visual attention over that field.

Attention, in particular visual attention, has again become a topic of great interest to psychologists. It has been the object of many intense investigations even though there is still disagreement about exactly what it is. One way of defining it is as the act of looking at something.

Norman Mackworth has said, "Sometimes one looks without seeing." True enough, but more often it is the case that if one doesn't look, one doesn't see. We should, therefore, be willing to forget for the moment about that small percentage of cases where one looks and does not see, and to be concerned almost entirely with looking and seeing.

Because the points that we discuss here are speculative, it is very much harder to establish meaningful relationships between the outside world and what it is that one does toward it.

The chairman of the fifth session was Professor John W. Senders of the University of Toronto.

V.1

Stimulus Density Limits
the Useful Field of View [1]

Norman H. Mackworth

Stanford University

The *useful field of view* is defined as the area around the fixation point from which information is being processed, in the sense of being stored or acted upon during a given visual task. The main question is: Why is this useful field of view or effective fixation area often limited in size, as compared with the physiologically possible field of view? Mackworth (1965) found useful fields of view reduced to 2° in tachistoscopic studies involving visual noise and small objects. Three letters were shown for 100 msec, and the distance between them was varied. Even at separations of 10° the subjects could easily compare the letters, but when extra "noise" letters were added to the same displays, the target letters had to be as close as 2° before they could be recognized. Even in a situation with only two dials, the subject could not detect an infrequent signal on one dial when he was looking at the other one, although the distance between the dial centers was only 6° (Mackworth, Kaplan, & Metlay, 1964).

These findings are quite different from the requirement to detect a single large object in the peripheral vision. When there is no time limit, the subject may detect the object at distances ranging from 50 to 90° from the fixation point. Edwards and Goolkasian (1974) of Iowa State University have reported that objects can be detected at 58° from the fixation point and can be identified at 10–15° from the fixation point. They dispute the conclusion put forward by Mackworth and Morandi (1967) that the peripheral retina screens off predictable

[1] The author is supported by Research Scientist Award K5-36477 from the National Institute of Mental Health. The research was supported through the Cooperative Research Program of the Office of Education, U. S. Department of Health, Education and Welfare, Contract No. OE-4-10-136, to Professor Bruner at Harvard University, Center for Cognitive Studies.

features, leaving the fovea to process the unpredictable and unusual stimuli. Senders, Webb, and Baker (1955) also report that there is a very wide field of view when large objects are displayed at low rates.

The situation is quite different, however, when the subjects are searching for a needle in a haystack. In the two experiments described here, they are asked to identify a small black square in a set of black circles. The first experiment is mainly a physiological study; the *peripheral-discrimination task* measures the visual acuity limits for the discrimination of the square from the circle at increasing peripheral angles from the fixation point. The second experiment is mainly a psychological study; this *strip-search task* examines the effect of increasing the number of unwanted or background circles on the scan path of the subject, who is searching for a target square.

It has long been known that a small target can make such demands on visual acuity that the cone of visual acceptance around the line of sight is restricted despite good lighting and vision. But even this physiological limit is often not achieved in real life because of the pressure of events. As the objects become crowded together more closely in space and time, the brain must reduce the useful field of view to a size at which each visual input can be processed by the brain. The brief glimpse obtained during scanning, limits the useful field of view to an area smaller than the visual acuity limit.

In the *peripheral-discrimination task,* the subjects were asked to monitor a vertical window which showed a slow steady stream of black circles. Occasionally a black square appeared and moved slowly down the window. This was the target to be detected. A second vertical window was placed on one side of the central display. This window might also show target squares, which were to be detected by peripheral vision, since the eyes were to be kept fixed on the central window.

Twenty subjects were tested individually. The lighting was 20 ft lamberts. Each window always showed 10 items. The nontarget black circles were .2° in diameter, (.1 in.), sharply printed on white paper. Each item took 10 sec to move down the 2-in. vertical window. During the 5 min of the test run for each display, five square targets appeared in the central window and five in the peripheral window. Each subject was tested with eight different separations of the two windows. In these eight runs, the windows were 2, 4, 6, 8, 10, 12, 14 or 16° apart. The position of the peripheral window was alternated from left to right in successive runs for each subject. Half the subjects received the right position first, and half the left. A check was kept on the position of the gaze by the use of an eye camera, to ensure that the subject was in fact monitoring the central window continuously. He was asked to report immediately when he saw a square in either window.

The results have been expressed in terms of the probability of detection of the *peripheral* targets. All the central targets were detected. Figure 1 shows the percentage of targets reported at each window separation. There were 10

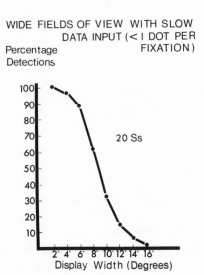

WIDE FIELDS OF VIEW WITH SLOW DATA INPUT (< I DOT PER FIXATION)

Percentage Detections

20 Ss

Display Width (Degrees)

FIG. 1. The peripheral-discrimination task: the percentage of peripheral targets detected at each window separation.

peripheral targets at each display width. At the 6° display width, 19 of the 20 subjects located all the targets, but at 8° display width only 11 subjects achieved a perfect score. It appeared, therefore, that the *useful field of view for these subjects was about 6° on either side of the central fixation point.* The limit was set by the small size of the targets and by their similarity to the nontarget circles. The rate of data input could hardly have been a factor (unlike the second study) since the rate was held constant at less than one item per fixation.

In the *strip-search task* the situation was quite different. Here the subject was asked to search a strip of several rows of circles in order to locate a target square which might be present. The question here was on the length and direction of eye movements that would be made in order to obtain adequate coverage of the display.

The number and the density of the rows of circles were varied in the different displays. Unknown to the subject, 12 of the displays contained no target at all. The other 12 each contained one square among many circles. Analysis of the eye tracks was made only with the displays that contained no target, because when the subject found a target his routine search pattern was altered.

Figure 2 shows a sample of the material. Each display showed rows of circles in a pattern that was either *dense* or *sparse.* In the dense display, shown in Fig. 2, there were about 20 circles per square inch, while in the sparse displays there were only about two circles per square inch. The vertical width of the displays varied from 1 to 6°. All displays were 10 in. in horizontal length, subtending 20°. Pilot studies had shown that there were no differences between vertical and horizontal displays. Therefore, all displays were presented with the maximum dimension horizontal. The displays were lighted from both sides at 20 ft lamberts.

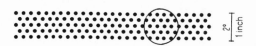

FIG. 2. Sample of test material
for strip-search task: 2° vertical
width of dense display, with schematic example of typical limiting
useful field of view enclosing 23
items.

The subjects were asked to scan the display from left to right, without
stopping or looking back over the material. They were instructed to sit back and
close their eyes when they had reached the right-hand end of the display. They
were told that there might be one or more squares present in a display, although
in fact there were never more than one. The task was to report whether or not
there was a target present.

There were 20 male and female Harvard University students who served as
subjects. They were shown 24 randomly ordered displays. The display remained
in view until the subject closed his eyes, as instructed. The material was viewed
from a distance of 28 in. in the Mackworth Stand Eye Camera (Mackworth,
1967), so that 1 in. on the display covered 2°.

The analysis of the eye tracks concentrated on the displays without targets
because the subjects tended to fixate the target when they found one. Usually
they had no great difficulty in detecting the target, but with the widest 6° dense
display, 13 of the 20 subjects missed their target square. This was quite unlike
the perfect score the same subjects made with the 6° sparse strip. Indeed, none
of the subjects missed any targets with the sparse displays. With the dense
displays, no subject missed the target in the 1° width and only three of the 20
subjects missed targets in the dense displays 2–5° wide (Table 1). Thus the
finding that *two-thirds of the subjects missed the target in the dense 6° width
indicates a cognitive limit in the ability to recognize a target in noise.* This failure
of detection clearly results from the large number of unwanted circles, since no
such failure of detection occurred with the sparse 6° display.

An even more sensitive measure was the *mean fixation time.* The duration of
each fixation increased with the amount of material within the display. Figure 3
and Table 1 show that the duration of the mean fixation time was increased by
about 50 msecs by widening the sparse displays from 1 to 6°. With the dense
displays, the fixation times were about 100 msec *longer than* with the sparse
displays. The increased times represent the extra cognitive demand added by the
need to process more nontargets.

The third and best measure for the effects of cognitive control on the scan
path proved to be the *number of circles* that the subjects attempted to process in
each visual fixation. Figure 4 was obtained by dividing the total number of
circles in the display by the mean number of fixations per display. Table 1 shows

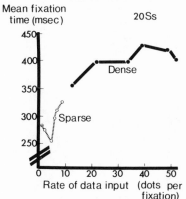

DENSER DISPLAYS NEED LONGER FIXATIONS

FIG. 3. Strip-search task: the relation among the mean fixation times, the nature of the display, and the rate of data input.

that widening the sparse displays had some effect on the number of items processed per fixation; widening the dense displays gave a huge increase in the number of circles that subjects tried to process per fixation. The increase in the number of fixations was affected very little by the number of circles in the display. For instance, the actual incidence of these items per strip increased about 50-fold from the narrowest sparse display to the widest dense display; Yet the number of fixations was only doubled, from eight fixations on the 1° sparse display to 17 fixations on the 6° dense display. Table 1 and Fig. 4 show that as a

TABLE 1

Data from the Strip-Search Task

	Quantity per vertical width (degrees):											
	Sparse displays						Dense displays					
Description	1	2	3	4	5	6	1	2	3	4	5	6
Items per display	16	22	40	45	63	70	140	270	420	500	700	840
Fixations per display strip per subject	8	8	10	10	13	13	10	12	12	13	14	17
Items per fixation per subject	2	3	4	5	5	6	14	23	35	40	50	49
Side steps per display per subject	1	2	3	3	6	8	2	4	4	7	9	11
Missed targets (max. 20)	0	0	0	0	0	0	0	1	3	0	3	13
Average fixation durations (msec)	278	272	255	293	313	327	355	401	401	434	406	427

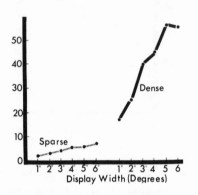

WIDENING DENSE DISPLAYS INCREASES
ITEMS ATTEMPTED PER VISUAL
FIXATION

20 Ss

Items attempted
per fixation

Display Width (Degrees)

FIG. 4. The relation among the rate of data input, the display width, and the nature of the display. The width of the display has a much greater effect when there are more dots per square inch.

result, the number of items "attempted" per fixation increased from 2 to 50, a 25-fold increase. The duration of the average fixation, however, increased only from 278 msec with the 1° sparse display to 427 msec with the 6° dense display, an increase of ~150 msec. It is not surprising that the subjects missed so many targets at the widest dense display. They were trying to process too many items per fixation and, therefore, failed to identify a target within the 50 items that were included in each fixation.

Finally, we consider the concept of the *useful field of view*. This is the area around the central fixation point that is being effectively processed in a single fixation. Two quite different procedures give the same estimate of the size of the useful field of view. The size varies with the density of the material which is being processed. With the dense displays, the useful field of view appears to be about 1° across (half an inch at 28 in). Chaikin, Corbin, and Volkmann (1962) suggested that the width of the useful field of view is probably greater than its height.

One measure of the limit of the useful field of view is the point at which detection begins to fail. One subject failed to detect a target with the 2° dense display, so we may consider this as the limiting point. Here the fixation times increased to 400 msec. An average of 23 circles was included in each fixation with this display (Table 1). Figure 2 shows how 23 circles subtend the limiting useful field of view which is only about 2° wide. No such breakdown occurred with any of the sparse displays, so it is clear that the limit was set by the number of items that had to be processed in one fixation.

Since the useful field of view is defined as the largest field at which performance is perfect, this field must be regarded as smaller than that found with the 2° dense display. Therefore, the minimum useful field of view for all subjects lies somewhere between the 14 items processed per fixation with the 1° dense display and the 23 items per fixation processed with the 2° dense display. The intermediate level of about 18 items would require about 380 msecs, that is, about 21 msec per item. The six items processed with the 6° sparse display would require only 126 msec and, therefore, it is not surprising that detection was perfect with all sparse displays.

The foregoing analysis assumes that the subject placed his successive fields of view edge to edge along each display strip without any overlapping. The fields of view are thought to be strung out along the display strip like beads along a necklace, when the subjects are processing simple materials. Support for this view comes from Table 1 where we see that the average subject took about 12 fixations to sweep his gaze along the 10 in. of the 2° dense display. It may be concluded that people literally inch their way along this dense material. In fact, however, they would have done better to move along in half inches to be certain of noticing all targets.

The useful field of view can also be estimated by recording the number of marked changes in direction of the individual eyetrack (*side steps*). Each person has his own specific and characteristic size for the useful field of view, but we will begin by discussing the average case. If the subject judges that the display is too wide for one fixation to cover the entire vertical width, then the eye track must move up and down the strip. There was an appreciable increase in the number of such side steps or direction changes between the 1° and 2° dense displays. The subjects could encompass the 1° width in a fixation, but needed more than one to cover the 2° width.

A side step is defined as a change in the direction of movement of the eye track which is greater than a 20° angle away from the horizontal axis of the display strip. Figure 5 indicates how the number of side steps can be measured for each subject. Figure 6 shows how a subject was able to process the 1° dense display without making any side steps, but when he was working with the 6° dense display, he made 26 side steps. (Not all the records were as dramatic as this one.)

Figure 7 and Table 1 give the quantitative data for the whole group of subjects. These show the percentage of all eye movements that were side steps for each density level and each vertical display width. At all widths there were relatively fewer side steps with the sparse displays than with the dense displays,

FIG. 5. The method of measuring side steps. Each side step is an eye movement greater than 20° away from the horizontal axis.

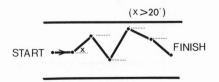

EYETRACKS WITH DENSE DISPLAYS

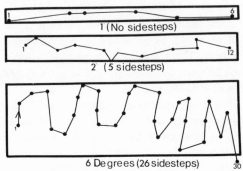

FIG. 6. The effect of the vertical width of the dense display on the incidence of side steps. Note also the smaller interfixation distances.

even though the side steps were expressed as a percentage of all eye movements on that display.

Analysis of variance for these side-step data showed that there were highly significant differences ($p < .01$) between the sparse and dense displays, and between the different widths of display. The interactions between density and width were particularly interesting. The subjects adopted a much smaller field of view for the dense displays than for the sparse ones. There were reliable increases in the number of side steps between the 1° and 2° dense displays ($p < .01$). There was, however, no such significant difference between the 1° and 2° widths for the sparse displays. This was taken to mean that the useful field of view was 1° wide for the dense, and 2° wide for the sparse displays. The useful field of view might, therefore, be regarded as the size of a dime for the dense displays

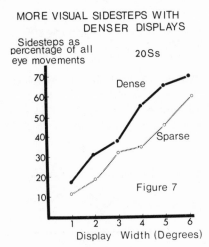

FIG. 7. The relation among the percentage of eye movements that were side steps, the density of the display, and the width of the display. Width has a greater effect than density with this measure.

and the size of a quarter for the sparse displays, if these coins were held at arm's length.

These data suggest two major findings. The first is that five different measures can be obtained from one simple experiment. The second is that these yardsticks allow us to study the interaction between the nature of the display and the cognitive control of the visual coverage. The five measures are: (1) mean number of circles attempted per fixation; (2) mean visual fixation times; (3) mean percentage of side steps or bends in eye track; (4) mean number of fixations per display strip; and (5) incidence of missed targets.

These five measures indicate how much more difficult it is to search for a needle in a haystack than to search for the same needle among only a few distracting straws. The measures are listed in rank order of sensitivity to the effects of visual noise. The best measure is the number of items that the subject tries to process in each fixation (see Fig. 4). Since he is entirely free to take as long as he wishes and to make as many fixations as he wishes, the fact that he fails to make sufficient fixations with the widest dense display is surprising.

1. The mean number of items attempted per fixation increases as the density and width of the display increases (Table 1). The rate of increase is much greater with the dense display than with the sparse display. The subjects did not miss any of the targets on the sparse display, which was really too easy for them.

2. The mean visual fixation times also increased as the number of items in the display increased. But the increase was only 50 msec for the sparse displays, from 1° width to 6° width, and for the dense displays the increase was only 70 msec. Moreover, an increase in the number of items from 70 to 840, going from the 6° sparse display to the 6° dense display, only gave an increase of 100 msec; although there were eight times as many items processed per fixation with the dense display, the fixation time increased by merely one-third.

3. The mean percentage of side steps or bends in the scan path (see Fig. 7) increased from 11 to 59% with the sparse displays from 1° to 6°, and from 18 to 68% with the dense displays. These differences between the two densities with regard to the percentage of all eye movements that were side steps were significant, although not large.

4. The mean number of fixations per display strip showed little difference between the two densities; Table 1 shows that at 5° width there were 13 fixations with the 63 items of the sparse display and 14 fixations with the 700 items of the dense display.

5. The only display that gave a real problem in detection of the target was the 6°-wide dense display. Here there was a serious breakdown in detection, since 13 of the 20 subjects missed the target at this width.

Studying the *individual* useful fields of view is also important. This can be done by determining the average visual interfixation distance for each subject. Figure 8 shows the close relationship between the individual interfixation

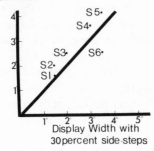

SIDE STEPS BEGIN WHEN DISPLAY
WIDTH APPROACHES INTERFIXATION
Mean Interfixation   DISTANCE
Distance

FIG. 8. Side step incidence of at least 30% of all eye movements for individual subjects related to their mean individual interfixation distances.

distance and the display width at which the subject began to make side steps on 30% of all his fixations. The data shown in Fig. 8 were based on a random sample of six subjects out of the 20 who were tested. The interfixation distance for each subject was determined by averaging across all widths, both dense and sparse. These data were then plotted against the display width at which that particular subject made about 30% of all eye movements as side steps. This was taken as the limiting width at which the subject was unable to cover the whole width in one fixation.

Figure 8 shows that some subjects had long visual steps, and also had wide useful fields. Others moved their eyes in short steps, and had narrow useful fields of view. The two measures of interfixation distance and display width gave about the same number of degrees for a particular subject, about 4° for the wide scanners and about 1–2° for the narrow scanners. In other words, the wide scanners were able to search the display by a relatively horizontal scan until the width reached 3 or 4°, while the narrow scanners were more sensitive to the width of the display; their useful fields of view were limited to 2° in diameter.

The practical implications of this evidence suggest that it is possible to select people who can use their peripheral vision more accurately if the task requires such wide intake of visual information. Scanners with narrow useful fields of view will take four times as many fixations to cover a given area, and therefore will take four times as long to make a search. Airborne radar sometimes imposes a time limit of a few seconds for a scan of a highly detailed and changing picture. In such circumstances the ability to take in information rapidly is basic. Radiologists also may benefit from a wide scan, since they have to work fast to get through the day's set of pictures. There is, however, a happy mean between speed and accuracy.

Discussion of such representational material underlines the fact that the size of the useful field of view depends on the nature of the stimulus display and the task involved. Figure 9 compares the strip-search task with results from 20 adults who were studying a well-focused close-up photograph of a street scene with relatively few but scattered details (Mackworth & Bruner, 1970). The task here was to recognize the major object, a fire hydrant, in the photograph. Figure 9 shows that the size of the useful field of view was very different in the two situations. It can be seen that there were many more very short eye movements with the requirement to make a detailed search for a small target than there were when the only requirement was an easy recognition of a large object. There were many more eye movements, with the easy recognition task, that were greater than 6° in length than there were with the difficult search task. The useful field of view is clearly much larger with the easy recognition task than with the difficult visual-search task.

The representational photograph allowed the subjects to use a wide acceptance angle (> 6°) four times as often (21% of all eye movements) than they could do with the strip-search task (5% of all eye movements). For such detailed work the subjects used what may be called tunnel vision. Figure 9 shows that this narrowing of the useful field of view is like a zoom lens that looks closely at a

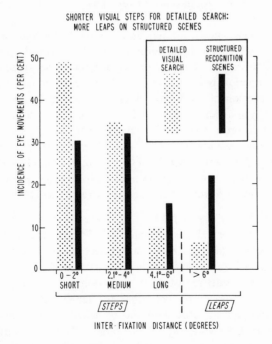

FIG. 9. The distribution of different eye-movement lengths with two different kinds of visual material, the strip-search task and visual recognition of a picture.

few items in order to see them more clearly. The ratio of very small visual *steps* (up to 2°) to *leaps* of 6° or more can give a measure of the narrowing of the gaze when detailed study is required. This *zoom ratio* is high for the strip-search task, which gives a ratio of 10 to 1, while for the visual-recognition task the ratio is only 3 to 2. There is a need to follow up this ratio finding to see how other tasks may rate with regard to the useful fields of view. It does not necessarily follow that a careful searcher, using very small fields of view, would show a similarly restricted field with a different kind of visual task. In brief, the size of the useful field of view can be expected to vary in size between *different kinds of tasks* as well as between *different kinds of people*. This is true even when the physiological factors such as lighting and viewing distance are held constant.

It is also important to determine whether the useful field of view varies within subjects while they are performing tasks requiring much attention. Subjects who attend carefully to the task will probably vary their useful field of view considerably, depending on the moment-to-moment requirements of the task. They will zoom in on details when this is necessary, and take the broader view when an understanding of the general situation is necessary. The less-careful worker might be content with a steady middle-distance look. Thus the careful worker would have a higher zoom ratio (of very small visual steps to visual leaps) than the inattentive one.

In general, much new knowledge has been gained during the last few years about the ways in which the brain initiates the physiological mechanisms of attention rather than wait for the environmental input to set these mechanisms in action. The interaction between the brain and the environment is two-way, and the set or motivation of the subject is as important as the physical input in determining the physiological responses. For instance, the pupil contracts reflexly when light falls on it, but it also changes according to the cognitive state of the brain. Similarly, *the useful field of view sharply constricts when there is high density of detail to be processed by eye and brain.* Both behavioral changes are attempts to prevent the processing mechanisms from being overloaded.

The adjustments to visual overload can be considered under six headings:

1. *Narrowing the size of the useful field of view* is the main adjustment made to deal with visual overload. Figure 1 and Table 1 show the narrowing of the angle of acceptance that takes place with such factors as the presence or absence of irrelevant details such as the black circles. The data for the sparse displays can be compared with the results reported on the peripheral-discrimination task. In both cases there is a nearly perfect score for target detection when a 6° acceptance angle is required. But with the 6° width of the dense strip, the subjects failed to detect two-thirds of the targets. This great difference was entirely due to the greatly increased number of irrelevant items through which search must be made. The same effect can be seen in a vigilance task, where a

simple increase in nontarget events causes a marked decrease in detection of the targets (Mackworth, 1970).

2. *The visual step size is reduced* as a result of the narrowing of the field of view. The best way to measure this effect is by employing the zoom ratio of the number of very small visual steps to the large leaps of at least 6° (Fig. 9).

3. *An increase in the number of side steps* is a further effect of the narrowed useful field of view. Figures 6 and 7 demonstrate this increase in side steps with wider displays, or with increased density of nontargets.

4. *Trying to include more stimuli in each fixation* is an adjustment that is useful with the smaller numbers of nontargets but breaks down when there are too many stimuli for adequate recognition within a single fixation. An increase from 2 to 50 items per fixation indicates that the subjects are not adjusting their fixation density according to the difficulty of the task (Fig. 4).

5. *Lengthening the visual fixation time* is an attempt to accommodate the increasing numbers of items that must be encompassed in a single fixation. However, such lengthening is quite limited; Table 1 and Fig. 3 show that fixation times increased by only about one-third in going from the easiest to the most difficult display. This increase, however, does indicate the increased cognitive difficulty in processing such complex visual material (Mackworth & Bruner, 1970; Mackworth, 1974).

6. *Failure of adjustment to increasing complexity* finally resulted in missed targets. Table 1 and Fig. 4 show that targets began to be missed with the 2° dense display. Here there were, on the average, 23 stimuli that were being processed in 400 msec, showing a limiting rate of about 18 msec per stimulus circle. In a somewhat similar task, Mackworth (1965) required subjects to search for target letters among other nontarget letters. Here, too, accuracy broke down when the subject processed five letters at about 20 msec per letter., with a tachistoscopic presentation of 100 msec. With three letters recognition was high, 33 msec being allowed for each letter. Travers (1974) has reported nearly perfect performance on tachistoscopic words at rates of 48 msec per letter.

In the Mackworth letter-recognition task, the target letters could be easily matched with the central one even when they were placed 5° on either side of the center, provided that there were no unwanted letters present. This 10° useful field of view was the same as that found by Edwards and Goolkasian (1974). However, their claim that all tasks can be performed with a 10° useful field of view is only true when the visual field is uncluttered. Mackworth (1965) found that when the same arrangement of target letters was embedded in a line or page of unwanted letters, detection of the target letters was reduced to less than 17% at widths greater than 2°. At the 2° width, there was 67% detection with the extra unwanted letters. Thus the detection of the target letters in a cluttered field was possible only within a useful field of view of 2°. This is very close to the 1° display width we have found for the strip-search task with dense displays.

In conclusion, the main finding of this study was that the *size of the useful field of view is critically determined by the density of irrelevant items in the display.* There is a marked difference between looking for a needle in a haystack and trying to find the same needle on a billiard table. In the first case the useful field of view is much smaller than in the second. In brief, we scrutinize densely crowded visual details very narrowly, but when there are only a few scattered details the gaze can process a much wider area.

DISCUSSION

FISHER: Did you analyze regressive movements as a function of load, or were they included in the side steps?

MACKWORTH: They are included in the side steps.

MOURANT: Did you do any correlations between the size of the field of view and the number of errors and the mean fixation duration for each subject?

MACKWORTH: No, I think this is an important suggestion and it is the kind of thing that I very much agree should be done now.

HALLETT: Didn't the well-known scanning of a radiograph (Llewellyn-Thomas & Lansdowne, 1963) show that the lung bases are totally ignored in the search? They are so full of detail as to be virtually undecipherable. I wonder whether there is an exception here, whether very densely crowded details may be avoided as a result of peripheral inspection rather than receive a lot of attention.

MACKWORTH: Well, I would agree with you if the person is a highly expert radiologist who knows the history of the case and is looking for things in the upper part of the lungs and knows that they are unlikely to occur in the lower part of the lungs. You do use the periphery of the visual field and you are able to know what not to look at directly.

GOULD: I have two comments. First, on the point you just made, it seems to me that people are really adaptive, and true visual search is, too. At IBM we looked at how expertly trained visual inspectors of very complicated integrated circuit chips dealt with them. They really conformed to the restraints of the problem. They were constrained to go at some fixed rate. They adapted; they didn't look at every place and they made errors, but they looked at the places, on the basis of experience, where they'd most likely find an error.

Second, if I understood you right, I thought you said that if you increased a display to nearly four times as many items, search time might go up to four times.

MACKWORTH: No, what I meant was that if person A has a useful field of view which can encircle the whole search area, he makes one fixation. However, if his friend has a useful field of view which is half the diameter, it is going to take him longer.

SENDERS: It will take him at least four times as long.

MACKWORTH: It is just a point that the useful field of view doesn't seem to vary very much between subjects. But if you work.it out in terms of the time taken to cover a given area, then it could be very important.

Acknowledgments

Thanks are due to Joyce Hiebert who undertook much of the testing and data analysis, and to Jane Mackworth who edited the presentation.

V.2

Looking at Pictures[1]

John D. Gould

IBM Thomas J. Watson Research Center

In this paper on how people look at pictures, I want to consider two questions:

1. Why do people look at pictures the way they do?
2. How do people integrate a series of eye fixations into a meaningful, stable percept?

Looking Behavior

The first half of my paper will be on the first question, namely, why people look at pictures the way they do. We know some first-order variables about *where* and *how long* people look when they look at pictures, and this has allowed us to make some inferences about *why* people look at pictures in the ways they do.

Some of the evidence comes from experiments that did not even involve pictures of natural scenes, but that used artifical stimuli, such as simple forms and dot patterns, in the context of visual search problems. One general result is that the geometric features of objects in a visual stimulus determine where a person fixates. The more nearly alike a particular stimulus object is to one that a person is looking for, the more likely it is that the person will foveally fixate that object.

Gould and Dill (1969) demonstrated this by showing subjects stimuli like those in Fig. 1. A subject's task was first to fixate the central or standard pattern, and then to determine how many of the eight comparison patterns, located in the periphery of the stimulus, matched the central standard pattern. The comparison patterns were about 7–8° from the center of the display. The

[1] I thank Curt Becker, Steve Boies, Brian Madden, Lance Miller, James Schoonard, and John Thomas for their helpful suggestions.

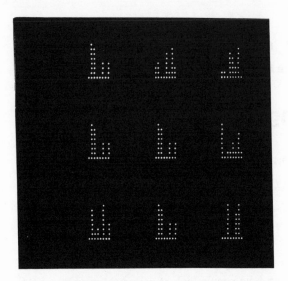

FIG. 1.   Example stimulus. (After Gould & Dill, 1969.)

"probability" of a person's fixating, or looking directly at, a comparison pattern was related to various measures of similarity between it and the center standard pattern. Figure 2 shows one of these similarity relations. The higher the percentage of dots in common between a standard pattern and a comparison pattern, the more likely that the comparison pattern would be fixated foveally. (The so-called "probability" in Fig. 2 exceeds 1.0 because refixations are included.) Peripheral vision was sufficient for subjects to determine that a comparison pattern, which differed greatly from the standard pattern, did indeed so differ. Subjects were instructed to search rapidly, and these peripheral discriminations minimized the number of eye fixations.

Williams (1967) showed how the color, shape, and size of objects on a display affected whether or not the objects would be fixated. A key result was that color greatly influences subjects' fixation patterns, whereas size and shape do not. Color provides a good cue for subjects to perform grouping operations (cf. Kahneman, 1973) on figure–background relations, whereas shape or size of objects evidently are not as effective. More generally, color coding is an effective means for people to locate targets quickly.

The length of time a person fixates a part of a picture is related to the amount of cognitive processing that he is required to do during that eye fixation. For example, Gould and Schaffer (1965) showed subjects stimuli like Fig. 3. Their task was to fixate the center three digits, add them up, and then determine how many corners of the stimulus contained digits that summed to the same value. We found that subjects' average fixation duration was 1.1 sec, which was about three times as long as fixation durations in the pattern-comparison task shown earlier. As shown in the right panel of Fig. 4, in this arithmetic task, subjects' fixation durations on a set of three digits depended upon the magnitude of their sum. The left panel shows that fixation durations on a set of three digits also depended upon the similarity of their sum to the sum of the standard, center digits.

The length of time a person fixates an object can be used to infer mental processes. When a person looks simultaneously for multiple targets on a visual stimulus, he must mentally compare each item he fixates with those he is looking for, or has in mind. Is this comparison process the same throughout a series of eye fixations? Or, for example, does it become faster later on in the sequence? Eye-movement recording provided a direct way to test this. Gould (1973) showed subjects displays in which items (alphabetic characters) were arranged in the clock positions of a circle. The subjects were instructed to fixate

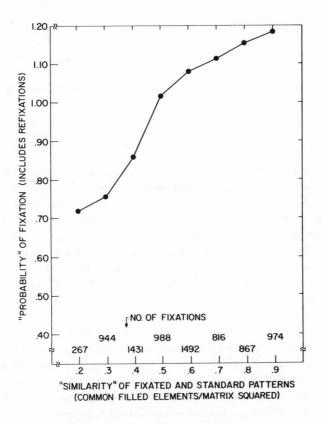

FIG. 2. Relationship between the number of eye fixations on a comparison pattern and its similarity to the standard pattern. The so-called "probability" includes refixations, which is the reason it exceeds 1.0.

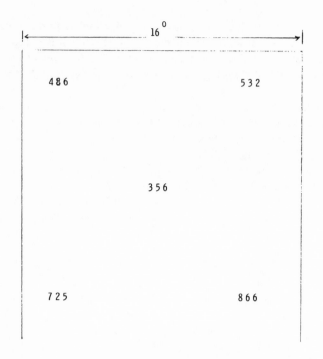

FIG. 3.   Example stimulus. (After Gould & Schaffer, 1965.)

each item in a clockwise order. Subjects looked simultaneously for one, two, or three different targets, and terminated their search when they found one of them. The duration of each successive eye fixation was recorded. Each curve in Fig. 5 indicates the fixation durations on successive items. Using Sternberg's (1967) interpretation that the slope of each curve reflects matching or comparison times, the key result was that this comparison process seems to be about the same throughout a series of eye fixations. That is, most curves had about the same slope, and there was no systematic change in slopes throughout the series of eye fixations.

Now what can studies that have used pictures themselves as stimuli tell us about why people look at a picture the way they do? One general result has been that people fixate on contours much more frequently than they fixate on homogeneous areas of a picture. This is true, of course, because contours carry more information than do homogeneous areas, as both information theorists and visual neurophysiologists have pointed out. Another general result is that motion in a picture is attention getting and will attract eye fixations.

Some objects in pictures are fixated more often than other objects, not just because they carry more information in the information theory sense, but because they convey more meaning to the looker. For example, Buswell (1935) showed that people's faces and people's hands are the most fixated areas of pictures that contain, among other things, people. Mackworth and Morandi (1967) showed that parts of pictures that were rated as being most informative by one group of subjects were fixated most often by another group of subjects. Loftus (1972) showed that objects that are reported as being remembered in a picture are fixated by the third fixation (in 95% of the cases) and are then refixated several times. Thus, in looking at pictures we fairly quickly fixate the key objects in them, and these are retained in long-term memory. Alternatively, and less likely, we simply better remember the first couple of objects that we fixate.

But we cannot understand how people look at pictures by merely being concerned with stimulus characteristics of the pictures. A person's intention or motivation in looking at pictures is important. Generally, people search pictures for meaning and not for specific targets. Consequently, the results of visual

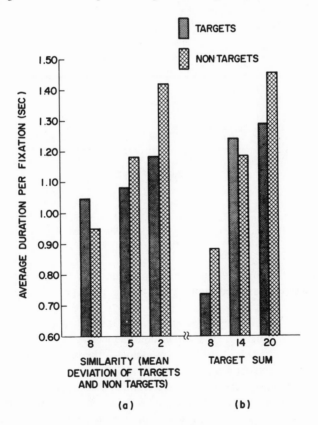

FIG. 4.   Average fixation duration on a set of three digits as a function of (a) the similarity of their sum to that of the standard sum, and (b) the size of their sum.

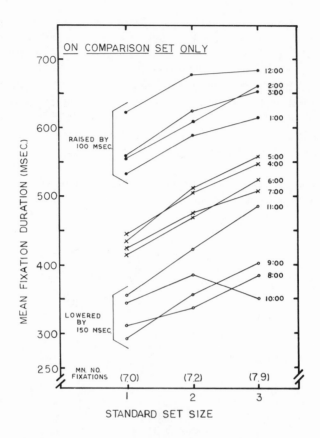

FIG. 5. Average fixation duration on successively fixated items arranged in the clock positions of a circle. Parameter is the clock position. (After Gould, 1973.)

search studies that involve repetitive examinations of many, many similar displays can have only limited implications for the more general case of looking at pictures for meaning.

Yarbus (1967) convincingly demonstrated how a person's intention affects the way he looks at a picture. He showed subjects pictures like the one in the upper left panel of Fig. 6. Panel 1 is free examination of the picture. Panel 2 is a search pattern when the subject was asked to estimate the material circumstances of the family. Many fixations are on women's clothing and on furniture. Panel 3 is the search pattern when a subject is asked to determine the ages of people. Here most fixations are on faces. Panel 4 is the search pattern when a subject was asked to surmise what the family had been doing before the arrival of the "unexpected visitor." Panel 5 is the search pattern when a subject was asked to remember the people's clothing, and most fixations are on clothes.

Clearly, then, the intensions or strategies governing fixation patterns are under the voluntary control of subjects. One strategy choice available to subjects when they have limited time to look at a picture is whether to make many brief eye fixations, or fewer but longer-duration eye fixations. Boynton (1960) pointed out that good searchers make many brief eye fixations, whereas relatively poor searchers make fewer, but longer-duration eye fixations. At IBM, we (Schoonard, Gould, & Miller, 1973) studied five highly trained visual inspectors who

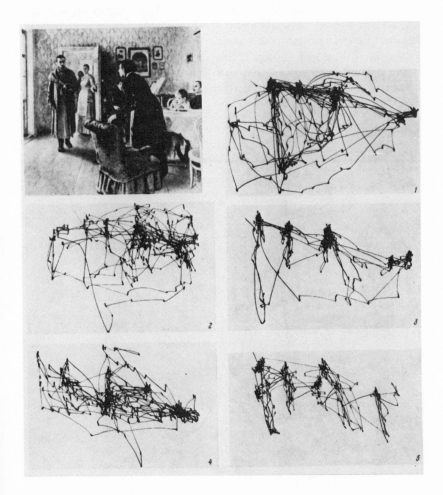

FIG. 6. Eye fixation patterns on the painting shown in the upper left-hand panel when the subject was looking at it for different reasons. (After Yarbus, 1967, with permission.)

were reported to be among the very best of a larger number of inspectors who every day searched thousands of complex integrated circuit chips for several different targets at once. As shown by the dotted curve in Fig. 7, these five inspectors had modal fixation durations of only 200 msec, which is brief compared to those found for less-well-trained subjects in simpler tasks. They fixated on areas of the chip that were likely to have targets and they seemed to ignore less likely areas. Since we did not collect data from other groups, we cannot be sure whether this strategy reflected experience or expertise, or both. Boynton's observation suggests at least the expertise.

Loftus (1972) found that the more fixations a person makes on a picture during a fixed viewing time, the higher the probability that he will correctly recognize it later. The duration or sequence of fixations did not affect how well a picture was remembered. Perhaps additional information (but not necessarily a constant amount) is taken in during each eye fixation. Alternatively, perhaps refixations are part of a rehearsal plan (Shontz & Kanarick, 1970). This positive

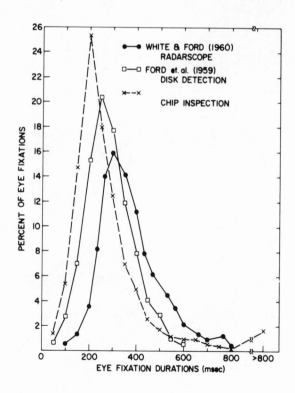

FIG. 7. Distributions of fixation durations for different tasks. (Graph taken from Schoonard, Gould, & Miller 1973.)

correlation between the number of eye fixations and memory does not hold for all pictures (Tversky, 1974). Loftus (1972) reported no difference in the number of eye fixations made by good and by poor rememberers. This result indicates, for now, that good and poor rememberers do not show the same differences on the number of eye fixations that good and poor searchers do.

There is one final consideration I would like to raise about why people look at pictures the way they do, and this has to do with the *movement* part of an eye movement. Noton and Stark (1971) proposed a theory of pattern recognition in which memory for a pattern is thought of as an alternating sequence of a sensory image, followed by motor instructions about where to fixate or attend next, followed by the next expected sensory image, etc. This raises the question of how predetermined a sequence of eye fixations is. Are there prestored programs for saccadic eye movements that may control several successive fixations? Certainly there are general scanning tendencies, such as scanning from left to right in our culture, as well as tendencies that are specific to individuals.

A recent report by Zinchenko and Vergiles (1972) certainly suggests that *movement* between eye fixations is critical for cognition. They had subjects perform several different tasks ranging from simple visual search to visual problem-solving tasks, while the displays for these tasks were stabilized on their retinas. They prevented the stabilized image from disappearing by varying its color. They reported that subjects performed correctly in all tasks, even though the displays subtended 15–30°. Searching a stabilized image required a much longer time than that under ordinary conditions, they reported, and fixation durations were about 1 sec. A more amazing result was that when the image was stabilized and when subjects were not allowed to move their eyes, they could not solve most of the problems. A subject could solve the problems only when he moved his eyes (even though the retinal image, of course, did not move). Although this result could be due to the other factors—for example, the attention required to prevent one's eyes from moving—it certainly provides for interesting speculation. Zinchenko and Vergiles hypothesize that there exists a "'functional fovea" that is controlled by eye movements and moves or scans the retinal image. Eye movements organize the movements of attention in the visual field. This theory builds upon earlier Russian developmental work cited by Zinchenko and Vergiles and upon Piaget's theory in which it is assumed that earlier overt motor responses in the child become an internalized vestigial but critical aspect of perception.

In summary of why we look at a picture the way we do, we know in general terms how eye fixations are influenced by physical parameters, such as color and geometric features of the picture, the task requirements, the relationships of the objects in the pictures, and the viewer's intention and strategies. But we know little about the role eye movements play in picture processing and in memory. What, for example, are the syntax and semantics of pictures? What is the role of eye movements here? If we knew the so-called "deep structure" of a picture, could we predict how a person would look at it? Is the process by which we gather, synthesize, and perhaps store pictorial information fundamentally different from the way we gather, synthesize, and perhaps store sentences that we read or hear?

Integrating Successive Glimpses

This takes me to the speculative question of how a person integrates a series of eye fixations when looking at a picture. How can a series of foveal and parafoveal snapshots, each about $\frac{1}{3}$ sec in duration, be integrated with each other in real time?

Asking the question in just this way may be misleading, for it may suggest that gradually an empty mental skeleton or map outline is filled in with the retinal images from each successive eye fixation, each image being placed in its proper spatial location in this outline. This suggests that we look at pictures to recreate their spatial compositions in our heads, just as we might put together the pieces of a torn photograph or a jigsaw puzzle.

Let's ask the question somewhat differently. How does a person *construct*—for surely he constructs or synthesizes—a stable, meaningful mental representation of the environment that he is successively sampling with his eyes. This representation, heavily influenced by expectancies, is updated by differences between it and new, incoming information. Processing differences or discrepancies reduces the information load. In this view, the person is an active perceiver designed to extract a meaning, not just a mental picture, from the visual environment he is looking at. Extracting this meaning does not await the complete mental recomposition of a picture.

Both Gibson (1966) and Hochberg (1968) have written about the problem of integrating successive glances. In looking for differences between these two views, I think that Hochberg lays more stress on cognitive factors, whereas Gibson emphasizes the role of stimulus invariants.

Gibson has argued that the perception of a unitary, constant picture over time can be explained by the assumption that *unchanging visual information* underlies the changing sequence of retinal images. It is this unchanging information that gets attended to. "The data for perception, the invariants of available stimulus information," writes Gibson, are "quite independent of the data for sensation, the retinal images considered as pictures" (p. 237). What are these invariants or underlying information? According to Gibson, they are higher-order variables, not open to conscious introspection. They include object overlap between the successive visual images, optical gradients and discontinuities, differences and ratios between light intensities, and rates and directions of environmental movement.

Hochberg (1968) has suggested that cognitive expectancies play the key role in integrating a series of glimpses. He proposes that a person generates a schematic map through which inputs from successive glances are related and stored. Schematic maps are thought to be a composite of what has already been seen and what is expected to be seen, both stored in a visual code. A schematic map, writes Hochberg, is "the program of possible samplings of an extended scene, and of contingent expectancies of what will be seen as a result of those samplings." Schematic maps are generated both on the basis of previous knowledge stored in long-term memory and, in real time, on the basis of what the person has just seen.

I would like to mention four general factors that may be involved in integrating a series of glimpses, some research on each, and some research that might be done to provide additional understanding. These four factors are (1) peripheral vision; (2) efference copies; (3) short-term memory; and (4) knowledge of the world.

Peripheral vision.   Whereas a person usually attends to what he views foveally, an image of what he will look at next is almost always in the peripheral retina. What role does the peripheral image play in the process of fixation integration? Does it add anything beyond what we know either foveally or from knowledge of the world? We know that peripheral vision guides subsequent eye movements (e.g., Gould & Dill, 1969). It seems probable that it provides information useful for integrating successive eye fixations, although it may not be absolutely necessary.

At Carnegie–Mellon University (under the direction and support of Professor Lee Gregg) we have built a computer-controlled system that can use eye movement and looking behavior to modify a displayed picture. One way to investigate the role of peripheral vision is to present a picture on such a computer-controlled display. Only that part of the picture around the fixation point of the subject would be shown to him. Whenever he moves his eye, a different part of the picture, corresponding to where he is now looking, is then shown. The diameter of a view could be systematically varied, say from $2°$ to $15°$. This apparatus also offers the opportunity to test Gibson's (1966, p. 262) suggestion that successive eye fixations are integrated because the retinal image from each successive glance overlaps with a previous one. The display could be so programmed that the amount of overlap of the picture from one glance to another could be systematically studied. This study would establish the degree to which peripheral vision is ordinarily used in integrating successive glimpses, and the manner and degree to which people adapt, through adjusting fixation parameters (e.g., number, direction, sequence, interfixation distance), to systematic modifications of the peripheral image. Eye movements would probably not, however, directly reveal cognitive changes in expectancies, encoding, and synthesis. That eye movement recordings are limited in this regard was shown by Tversky (1974) who found no difference in how people looked at pictures when they had to recall them and when they had to recognize them.

A zoom lens analogy is an attractive, albeit speculative, model for considering the role of peripheral vision in how people look at pictures. The key assumptions are, first, that a person has the ability to regulate the size of his field of focal attention. Zinchenko and Vergiles (1972) showed that visual resolution is sufficient over large retinal areas (15–20° for many tasks), and they postulated that a "functional fovea" scans wide areas of the retinal image. Second, there is a reciprocal relationship between the size of the effective field of view and the attentional or cognitive resolution (not retinal resolution) within it. That is, size of effective field of view times (attentional) resolution within that field is a constant. For example, the first one or two eye fixations on a picture might be quite global in nature, each merely seeking important areas to zoom in on subsequently. Suggestive support for this comes from Mackworth and Morandi (1967) and Loftus (1972) who reported that informative areas of a picture are identified early in a sequence of eye fixations, in the first one or two seconds. In terms of spatial frequency analysis, global, gross recognition could be done on the basis of low-frequency information, and attentional analysis would require access to higher frequencies for more details.

One way to test these speculative assertions, and to assess the size of the field being examined during each fixation, is to superimpose subtly and unpredictably a small simple target on a picture that a subject is actively examining. Assuming computer control of the experiment, the target would systematically appear at different times and at different distances from the point of fixation. Subjects, while searching the picture on some other pretext, would indicate if they saw the target.

Prestored efferent signal. The second factor that I want to mention as probably being involved in how people integrate eye fixations is the general belief that a signal is emitted at the time a person intends to move his eyes, which is about 150–200 msec before he actually moves them. This signal, which appears to indicate the direction and magnitude of the intended eye movement, is stored and then nulled by the afferent visual feedback from the eye movement. This is, of course, von Holst's (1954) efference-copy notion. Efference copies are generated expectations.

There are several fundamentally interesting questions about this mechanism as it relates to synthesizing successive eye fixations. Is the information contained in this prestored signal *coordinate information* about direction and magnitude of the intended movement (e.g., "the next movement will be 6° South")? Or is it *visual information* gleaned from peripheral vision and/or expectancies (e.g., "the next movement will be on the fire hydrant")? Or does it contain both types of information, with one perhaps being derived from the other? In any form, the information is a displacement signal in a feedback system, and the process that generates it needs to be understood.

When the match occurs, which is probably not an exact match, must the newly acquired, incoming information be in the same form as the prestored information? And what is the relation between schematic maps (Hochberg, 1968), which may contain a set of expectancies, and the efference copy, which contains an expectancy of at least where the next eye fixation is going to be? Could not this "efference-copy" expectancy be for a *series* of eye fixations, rather than for just a single eye fixation, especially if evidence is found to indicate eye-movement motor programs containing the instructions for several successive eye fixations?

If the efference-copy expectancy did relate to a series of eye fixations, rather than to a single eye fixation, then this would probably modify our present view of schematic maps suggested by Hochberg (1968). Now, for example, they would have a motor component—one that might be preprogrammed and lack some flexibility. In addition, now the schematic maps would have a relation to the model proposed by Noton and Stark (1971) to account for pattern recognition, in which memory for a pattern is thought of as an alternating chain of sensory images and motor instructions for where to fixate or attend next.

The computer-controlled system I mentioned previously would be useful in demonstrating powerful phenomenal effects of moving one's own eye to the right but then having the picture move, for example, to the left. Decoupling the usual relations between the intended direction of eye movement and actual eye movement, through drugs, paralysis, or mechanical means, is known to cause the world to phenomenally lose stability (von Holst, 1954).

Computer-yoked, computer-modified visual feedback would cause drastic disturbances in the process of integrating and extracting meaning from a series of eye fixations. Adjustment would be much more difficult than to experimental changes in peripheral vision proposed above.

Systematic exploration of this decoupling, through factorial variations in the direction, distance, dimensionality, and predictability of the interrupted feedback loop, should define the limits of the system. I would assume that only limited adjustment, guided by simple cognitive strategies and dependent upon the task requirements and the specific form of decoupling, could take place to this powerful phenomenal effect. At the level of eye movements, I would assume that subjects would generally make small-distance movements with long pauses between them, while they try to relate what they are looking at with what they believe they have already seen, and while they determine where to look next. This process is reminiscent of how people adapt to delayed auditory feedback, and probably is phenomenally much more difficult than piecing together a jumbled picture (which always remains stationary) as seen in Fig. 10.

Short-term memory. Extracting the meaning from a picture is a cognitive process, not just a sensory-motor one. The last two factors to be discussed are cognitive, with all the attendent complication, adaptability, flexibility, and parallelism that characterize cognitive systems and limit our understanding of them today. There have been many, many studies of human memory, and some general properties have been identified. Results of the last 15 years suggest that a fixated visual stimulus is initially encoded in visual features (angles, lines, contours, brightness, spatial frequencies) through several mechanisms, including feature detectors and spatial frequency analysis. These mechanisms can be thought of (although they usually are not) as comprising parts of long-term memory which, in turn, can be thought of as a distributed, associative network. The part of long-term memory made active by the visual representation of the fixated object interacts with other parts of long-term memory associated with the meaning and interpretation of that visual representation. The encoded visual icon is affected by expectancies, knowledge, previous experience, task demands, and is probably recoded into another type of internal representation (but one which allows visual codes to be regenerated). Some of this resulting activity provides the contents of a limited-capacity short-term memory, which can be thought of as the active part of long-term memory. There are probably multiple short-term memories, some not open to conscious introspection (cf. Anderson & Bower, 1973; Kahneman, 1973, Chapter 7, for some properties that must be held temporarily).

Many fundamental questions relate to the nature of the active memory or memories that hold the generated expectancies and that hold the information continually coming in while a person looks at successive parts of a picture. Although some research has been directed toward these questions, they remain unresolved. One general question relates to the structural characteristics of memory responsible for fixation integration. One aspect of this question on which almost nothing is known is what are the properties of the memory system that stores the temporarily generated expectancies (e.g., articulatory expectancies described by Hochberg).

What are the properties of the memory system that stores the incoming information from each eye fixation? If Sperling's conclusion (1960; 1963) is right, then iconic memory (or very-short-term visual memory, or visual-sensory-information store, or sensory buffer) is not the memory locus, for this memory has a persistence of only about the duration of a single eye fixation. Whereas Sperling used interference techniques, Mackworth (1963) measured the time course over which briefly presented objects could be reported, and she concluded that "visual memory" lasts for about 2 sec. This seems like the required persistence for integrating several eye fixations, but it is not clear whether she was tapping the same visual memory structure that Sperling did or rather a verbally recoded one. For example, Posner, Boies, Eichelman, and Taylor (1969) showed that physically identical letter matches are faster than name identity letter matches up to 2 sec after stimulus presentation. However, as Posner et al. pointed out, these visual codes that are available for 2 sec are most likely not the trace of the original fixated stimulus, but are probably activated abstract codes that serve as an internal representation of the original visual stimulus. Indeed, he concluded that people generate visual codes even when the first letter is presented aurally. Long-term memory, as normally described (Atkinson & Shiffrin, 1968; Shiffrin & Geisler, 1973), is not the likely site for integration, for every series of glimpses is hardly stored in a permanent repository. Unfortunately, nearly all work on short-term visual memory has relied upon tachistoscopic studies of a single glimpse; consequently, we know little about the short-term memory for a sequence of glimpses.

When a set of expectancies is generated from one's knowledge of the world and from what he has already seen in the picture, are these expectations in a visual code or in a verbal code? Murphy's (1971) review of the literature on the form of the code for expectancies did not resolve the issue, and besides, there are other alternatives to these two, e.g., articulatory intentions. In addition, there is evidence to suggest, based upon what is usually meant by visual and verbal codes, that both are generated (Posner et al., 1969) and that people are facile at changing codes. (This does not imply, however, that both are actually stored in long-term memory. Maybe only "meaning" is stored.) In a visual-search study in which subjects scanned alphameric displays for 40 days, Gould and Carn (1973) found evidence that suggested to us that a visual and a verbal matching process may take place, as if in a parallel race. In future investigations about the code for expectancies, it is probably useful to distinguish between two levels of expectancies. At one level are general rules about knowledge of the world and contextual clues, which will be discussed below. At a second, more detailed level, perhaps derived from the first, are specific sensory-level expectancies e.g., efference copies.

In future investigations about the code for expectancies, it is probably useful to distinguish between two levels of expectancies. At one level are general rules about knowledge of the world and contextual clues, which will be discussed below. At a second, more detailed level, perhaps derived from the first, are specific sensory level expectancies e.g. efference copies.

Is the information gathered during each eye fixation on a picture encoded visually or verbally? Literature reviews by Murphy (1971) and by Freund (1971) indicate the generally accepted conclusion that pictures are eventually coded both visually and verbally. Coding strategies, at least verbal ones, are under subjects' control. This is true for both encoding and code generation. Since both visual and verbal codes can occur, it may be that the one utilized depends upon tasks' variables. Further, it is usually tacitly assumed that verbal encoding requires attention and visual encoding does not. For example, Freund (1971) showed that when subjects had to count rapidly backwards by threes while viewing a series of pictures, their subsequent ability to recognize correctly whether they had seen those pictures before was greatly reduced, compared to that of a control group who viewed the pictures normally. The performance of the group that counted backward was still above the chance level, however. Freund's interpretation, perhaps a reasonable one, was that verbal coding was prevented by the counting backward. Thus any ability to remember pictures correctly was due to visual coding. An alternative explanation for the poor performance of the backward counting group has to do merely with the reduction of attentional capacity for the looking task.

Hochberg (1968) reported that reversible figures such as the one in Fig. 8, when moved behind a stationary slit, appeared to undergo spontaneous depth reversals, which led him to lean toward a visual-memory code for incoming pictorial information. Here one has only *local* visual cues to constrain the interpretation of a picture segment, and global visual cues are not available. I have tried this out on a few people and have received varied opinions, all with low confidence, of how they think they obtain the depth reversals.

If verbal codes for a picture are generated by covertly saying the name of an object in the picture to oneself, it is possible that verbal encoding might not occur during every eye fixation. Some parts of a picture cannot be easily labeled. Besides this, eye fixation rate (3 or 4 per sec) is about as fast as rapid mental speech.

Results from studies of split-brain patients may be useful in thinking about this coding issue. It is known (Gazzaniga, 1970) that if the right side of the brain is shown a familiar object, a patient cannot identify it by name, although he can pick it out by hand in a bag of objects or visually reproduce it by drawing it with his left hand. If the same left-side brain mechanisms that govern overt speech production also govern covert speech production or verbal labeling, then the results suggest a visual memory in the right side of the brain that is independent of verbal processes.

Does a person continuously, throughout each eye fixation, extract visual information from a picture? Or does he do this, for example, only during the first part of an eye fixation? One way to investigate this is to display a picture only when the subject moves his eye. Then the length of time during each eye

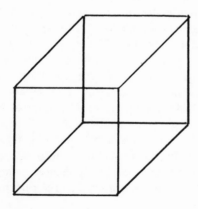

FIG. 8.   Reversible figure.

fixation that he can look at the picture on the display, and thus extract visually encodable information, can be systematically varied. For example, the picture can remain on for only 50 msec, then go off until the subject moves his eye, whereupon it comes on again for another 50 msec.

In summary, not enough is known about the short-term memory properties for fixation integration. Mackworth's (1963) results provide persistence data that seem roughly satisfactory for fixation integration, but the encoding and process characteristics of the memory structure are not determined. Passive coding, either visual or verbal, cannot explain fixation integration; active generation of cues and synthesis are probably required, as Hochberg stresses. Understanding the interaction among the incoming visual signals, their recoding, and the generated hypotheses, all of which determine the ultimate meaning of the picture, is the key issue involving short-term memory in fixation integration. Cognitive systems are characterized by flexibility and the ability to adapt rapidly and generate new interpretations, hypotheses, and strategies, facts which must be taken into account in any theory of fixation integration.

Knowledge of the world. Knowledge of the world, including expectancies, knowledge of physical laws, context, past experience, learned probabilities, and contingencies, affect the way visual information from successive glimpses is synthesized and intepreted. For example, if I fixate the chest of a person sitting at a desk, I nevertheless know that he has legs, knees, ankles, and feet below his chest, even though I may not be able to see them. If I should fixate his feet, protruding from underneath the desk, my knowledge of the world plays a part in my mentally connecting those feet with the person, rather than with the floor or desk, even though the floor and desk are actually visually contiguous with the feet and the person's body is not. Knowledge of the world operates by not only aiding the interpretation of a continual stream of otherwise ambiguous stimuli, but by providing a basis for predicting or expecting what is likely next to be seen. Whereas knowledge of the world is a very important factor in integrating eye fixations, there is less known about its role than about the previously mentioned three factors, in part because of the flexibility, adaptability, and parallelism of cognitive systems.

People always have assumptions or expectations when looking at any visual stimulus and there is no way to eliminate this. One way to assess just how important knowledge of the world is in integrating a series of eye fixations is to contradict it, however. This could be done in the laboratory by creating a situation, for example, in which a subject expects parts of a picture to be related in a particular way, but they are in fact related in very different ways. Impossible figures, such as the one in Fig. 9, are like this. We are able to process them without any drastic phenomenal effects. Behaviorally, visual cues work locally, as Hochberg (1968) demonstrated in his paper on the mind's eye. For example, when shown for the first time an impossible figure, or an Escher drawing, a person does not quickly recognize the depth contradictions. The global expec-

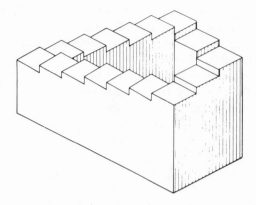

FIG. 9. An impossible figure.

tancies are so powerful that it takes several eye fixations to recognize the specific contradictions which result from comparing different spatial locations.

Experiments with "incongruent" pictures (Berlyne & Lawrence, 1964) and "jumbled" pictures (Biederman, 1972) indicate that people can rapidly adjust to significant changes in expectancies, but only in limited ways. Biederman, Glass, and Stacy (1973) showed subjects jumbled pictures like the one in Fig. 10. They found that subjects were almost as fast and accurate in finding particular objects presented in jumbled pictures as they were in finding objects presented in normal pictures (part a of figure). On the other hand, my informal observations indicate that people see the jumbled pictures as six separate pictures. It seems to take many seconds longer to be sure of the way the six panels actually fit together into the scene than it does to find an object. It's really hard to fit the six panels together if you don't look at the whole picture in the top of the figure.

Knowledge of the world has nothing to do with keeping the world stable while one looks at pictures, but it does influence over-all perception through expectancies. To the extent that knowledge of the world influences the pattern of eye fixations, it is a driving force behind the series of efference copies that are generated. Interrupting the efference-copy–afferent-feedback loop, however, not only interferes with memory but leads to a seemingly unstable world.

Knowledge of the world leads to flexible expectations that can be modified quickly, but within limits. The mental representation of a picture is constantly being constructed while one scans it; this mental representation, while being built, is flexible and modifiable. This can be demonstrated by my reading to you the following sentence, to which I would like you to pay close attention:

The stock, which the cattleman bought early on the morning of the auction, after he had checked with his foreman about the number of steers he needed, was all low-priced IBM stock.

Here one can reinterpret the meaning of "stock" rapidly and without much difficulty. Interestingly enough, whereas the meaning of the sentence seems to

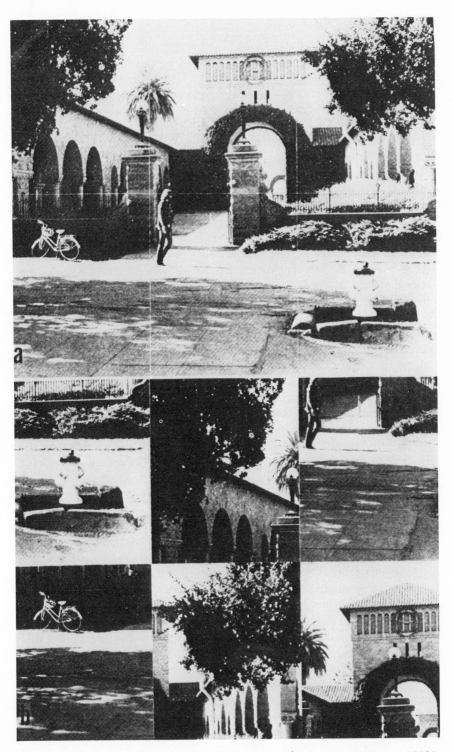

FIG. 10. Normal picture (above) and "jumbled" picture (below). (After Biederman, 1972.)

be in an active, working short-term memory, I am not sure that the individual words are now still there.

I will finish by describing a single experiment—done prior to having the computer-controlled apparatus I've described—in which, in a sense, knowledge of the world was pitted against peripheral vision. In this experiment the amount of information available in peripheral vision was varied by showing subjects five different diameters or aperture-size views of the same pictures. These views allowed subjects to see 4, 5.2, 6.6, 7.8, or 10.3° of a picture. During inspection, each of 10 subjects saw one- or another-size view of 15 different pictures taken from magazine ads. Each subject saw three pictures at each of the five aperture sizes. A picture was centered on a fixation point and flashed for 375 msec, which is about the duration of an average fixation. Subjects were told they would be tested later on their memory for the 15 pictures, but were given no specifics about the test. During the test phase, which followed a few minutes after the inspection phase, subjects were presented with a pair of different-size views of the same picture, and had to indicate which was the one they had originally seen. They were free to look at the pair as long as they wished. The results in Fig. 11 show that 25% of the judgments were erroneous. The solid curve indicates that subjects made twice as many errors in remembering the largest view than in remembering the smallest view. The dotted curve indicates that most errors on the middle three sizes were due to subjects' picking a smaller view than they actually saw. These results suggest that subjects store and retrieve information mainly from foveal and parafoveal areas. When shown a test pair they pick the smaller one, which presumably contains roughly what they had stored, even though many times they had actually seen a larger view with more detail. Subjects verbally indicated the reason for each choice, and although their reasons fell into several categories, some of them support this conclusion.

The alternative outcome—that subjects would err by choosing the larger one of the pair—was reasonable if subjects mentally filled in information predictable from the knowledge of the world, and stored this filled-in version in memory. Some pictures were chosen to provide such predictable information.

Since this exploratory experiment involved moderate-to-long-term memory, rather than a short-term memory covering a few seconds, its implications for the problem of integrating a series of eye fixations can be only suggestive. In addition we know that subjects can, within limits, control the amount and type of detail that they store from an individual eye fixation (e.g., Sperling, 1960).

To summarize, I have tried to point out some general considerations about why people look at pictures the way they do. We have considerable data describing eye-movement parameters while people look at a variety of pictures, and how these parameters are affected by task and picture variables. A fundamental problem underlying picture perception is how people integrate a series of eye fixations into a meaningful, stable internal representation of the picture. I have discussed this problem in terms of four factors that I believe to be

INSPECTION: Exposure = 375 ms.

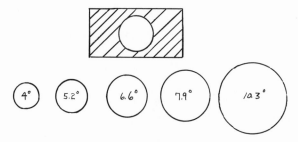

TEST: Self-paced; Two views of same picture

RESULTS:

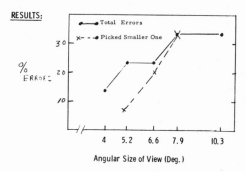

FIG. 11.   Five aperture sizes and the results.

important: peripheral vision, efference copies, short-term memory, and knowl-edge of the world. There is today little basic understanding of this problem. Some experiments were proposed, using a computer-controlled display that would be modified on the basis of where a person looks, that may provide additional understanding. Understanding peripheral vision and efference copies should be much easier than understanding the cognitive factors of fixation integration. Once the former is done, some limits of the system should be established. These should provide guidelines for subsequent cognitive studies, perhaps especially those concerned with expectancy generation which may then be the crux of the problem.

DISCUSSION

L. MATIN: How were Zinchenko's subjects (Zinchenko & Vergiles, 1972) prevented from moving their eyes?

GOULD: Three ways. One way was by instruction. The second way, I don't recall, but the third way was to have the eye with the unstabilized image fixated on a fixation point.

L. MATIN: That kind of instruction would tend to reduce the ability to pay some attention to the field.

GOULD: I should think so.

L. MATIN: If they had an eye-movement monitor on, wouldn't it, in fact, constrain them? The experimenter could tell them when they are making an eye movement, but that might, at the same time, interfere with the process in a variety of ways.

GOULD: I understand what you said, but there was no report on that. Probably it would be better than using the nonstabilized eye to fixate on a target to keep both from moving.

SENDERS: What kinds of problems were given to Zinchenko's subjects?

GOULD: One was the visual search test that I did a few years ago. It used a six-by-six array of numeric characters, and the subject had to find target characters in there. That was the simplest. Then there were some tests in which the subject had to note the orientation of Landolt rings. Then they moved on to some complicated maze problems in which the subject had to verbally indicate how he got through the maze.

SENDERS: I remember that Yarbus (1967) reports that given the task of estimating the number of times a unit square will go into a larger rectangle, both presented in semistabilized form, it becomes very difficult for the subject. Apparently, what the subject normally does is to "pick up" the unit square with his eye and put it in the rectangle in adjacent locations, and literally count how many times it goes in.

Could subjects do that with semistabilized vision in Zinchenko's study?

GOULD: I don't know.

KOLERS: Pritchard, Heron, and Hebb (1960) stabilized something like the equivalent of a matrix of letters so that the whole matrix subtended perhaps something like 30° of visual angle and the matrix contained perhaps 25 letters in some random order. You can't note internally where any particular letter is, but you can shift your attention around the matrix and report the letters in one quadrant or another quadrant. While you are attending and reporting the letters in one quadrant, you don't see the letters in, say, the opposite quadrant, so there is some sort of flexible internal scanning mechanism that can operate on a stabilized image. Pritchard et al. estimated it at something on the order of 5° of angle.

MACKWORTH: I'd like to add a point on that because it bears on what you said. There is a study by Hall (1972) who showed his subjects a matrix of alphameric characters. After the matrix was removed from view, the subjects were given a tone which told them whether the item they had to report was in the top, the middle, or the bottom row. When their eye movements were recorded after the stimulus was removed, there was a very high degree of association between where the item was and the eye movements made without the stimulus.

In other words, if they were asked for something in the top row, they started looking where the top row was. You can get a quantitative tie-up between line-of-sight searching and what Prof. Senders calls "mind's eye searching."

KOLERS: Does that mean then that they wouldn't be able to report if you obscured their line of sight?

MACKWORTH: No; it does mean, though, that if you prevent them from moving their eyes, they have difficulty. Which caused what effect is another question, but there does seem to be a very strong correlation between what you might call the mind's-eye searching and the postexposure searching.

GOULD: Yes, there is other evidence on that, too.

MURPHY: You mentioned that information theorists and neurophysiologists pointed out a tendency of subjects to fixate points of curvature and so on. I presented a paper last year showing that the oculomotor characteristics of fixation are not influenced by the shape of the visual stimulus.

I think it is important to point out that these tendencies are really reflex strategies on the part of the subjects, not constraints on oculomotor control systems on the part of the stimulus.

GOULD: Yes. I didn't know about your work, I'm sorry. I did have that kind of thing in mind, not that the eye will go there in an automatic way.

V.3
Advice to the Searcher
or What Do We Tell Them?

Edward Llewellyn Thomas

University of Toronto

The object of much of our research is to improve target detection, whether the target be a radar blip, a tank shadow in an aerial photograph, or the shadow of a tumor on an x ray. Pictures are made, often at great cost and risk; but however technically perfect they are, if the human being studying them fails to see the target, the whole process is wasted. Therefore, one of the products of our research should consist of a series of statements advising a searcher on the best way to search, and on what external and internal factors may affect his efficiency as a detector of targets.

How much of our research is relevant to this? For an example of some that is probably not relevant, Frecker and I have been studying the effects of the benzodiazepines (Librium*, Valium*) on saccadic eye movements. We can say with great confidence that these drugs reduce the acceleration and peak velocity of voluntary saccades. This is interesting to the minute population of pharmacologists interested in the effects of drugs upon the eye, and it has potential as a bioassay technique because we can develop a dose–response curve and it may help to identify the sites of action of the drugs.

But of more immediate importance is the fact that around 25% of the population of North America take these drugs at intervals. They also drive automobiles, fly aircraft, and search aerial photographs, maps, and x rays. So the question they can ask us is, "Does decreasing my saccadic velocity affect my visual performance?" My own answer at the moment is, "I don't know."

Following this line of thought I have tried to prepare a list of good advice, based on eye-movement research, which we might give a searcher to help him search better. The list is not very impressive and the fact that radiologists, for example, continue to miss some 25% of the lesions which appear in x rays should encourage us to prepare a better one. After all, most of us have our chests x rayed at intervals and the missed lesions could be our own!

If visual search is probabilistic then the best we can do is to recommend certain things that should reduce the probability of missing a signal. We should also consider dynamic as well as static images. For example, when a coronary arteriogram is taken, the dye goes through the heart with a visual "woosh" and whether the radiologist watching on a TV monitor sees something may decide whether or not they cut the chest open, stop the heart, and do things to the coronary arteries. This operation is now competing with appendectomies for popularity, so it is a question of much greater than academic interest, especially for those over 40.

The following is my own list of good advice, and I am hoping that some of you will give me items to add to it during this meeting or show that some of the advice is bad. They are excerpted from a paper (Llewellyn Thomas, 1969) dealing with the perception of the roentgen image and I recommend that issue to those interested in visual search for the value of the other papers it contains.

General

1. You cannot direct your search according to a predefined program unless you have some mechanical aid.

2. Your visual–perceptual system can add details to indistinctly perceived images, and you may believe you have searched areas of a display that you have not.

3. You have a "personal equation" for visual search, as you have for other skilled psychomotor activities. Knowledge about it may improve your performance.

4. It is natural to concentrate on areas you expect to contain information and people have been found to do this. This is permissible only when search time is limited.

5. Any clinical information you have about a case is likely to affect your initial search pattern.

6. The repeated search of a film by yourself or a colleague will reduce false negatives and increase false positives. False positives are less frequent and much less significant than false negatives.

7. Finding a lesion tends to stop further search.

8. The most important interface in the whole radiologic system is between you and the film. A poor-quality film completely searched may be worth more than a high-quality film in which signs of lesions have not been detected.

Specific

1. Arrange the best practical search environment, including illumination, viewing distances, physical comfort, and freedom from distractions.

2. Consider some "pacing" or "guiding" system to aid in securing complete search of static displays. This includes the hand.

3. Search from different distances with different illuminations, if this is possible. Use a bright spot on high-density areas.

4. Search a reduced image so that the whole display can be perceived on at least one occasion without large eye movement.

5. Carry out the initial searches, including those under different illuminations and with different visual angles, and record the results before consulting clinical reports or previous films. Concentrate on detection during the initial search.

6. Repeat the searches after studying clinical information and previous films.

7. Repeat the searches, going from specific points in the clinical reports to the display and from previous films to the film you are examining.

8. If feasible, carry out a second search session and have a comparison reading made by a colleague.

9. Because short-term human memory is untrustworthy, note detections as they are made. This applies especially to dynamic displays, such as the fluoroscopic image.

10. When time is limited, as when searching dynamic displays, try to decide on high probability areas beforehand.

11. Make a positive effort to repeat your search of smoothly textured areas, and those areas farthest from distinct edges.

12. Try to identify your personal equation by comparing the results of each search with later clinical findings and see if you have areas of roentgenograms in which your detection successes and failures are identifiable.

DISCUSSION

NODINE: I have been working with Kundel and one of the interesting things that has emerged from our recent work in the radiological lab is that, indeed, we find that radiologists make about the same number of errors without search as they do with search. Let me explain what I mean by that.

By "without search" I mean that when we present a chest film for 200 msec and ask the radiologist what he saw, very often what he tells us he saw is not much different from what he tells us after he's done a very elaborate search of the film.

LLEWELLYN THOMAS: That is something like the results of Mooney (1968) many years ago in which he said you didn't have to move your eyes to recognize all sorts of things.

NODINE: Right. I think our feeling is that the global response that Dr. Gould talked about is a pretty important factor here. Really we were starting our studies by looking at what we meant by the global response. Our first experiments were to try to see how much a radiologist saw in a single fixation, and to control that single fixation.

We have not finished our experiments yet, so I don't have very many data to talk about except the error rates, which are quite comparable to the 30% rate one finds with an extensive search.

There are other problems, of course, relating to the conspicuity of the lesion or nodule, and how one can begin to scale conspicuity or identify what one means by the "hiding of the lesion" in the very complex display the radiologist is faced with. He has more kinds of nontargets on the chest film than you might suspect: the lung area, the vessels in the lung, the ribs, the heart, and many other things distract him from finding that lesion wherever it is. Although it is a very complicated situation and I haven't got the complete story yet, I can tell you that at least as far as visual search is concerned, it may be that all the searcher is doing is confirming what he saw in the first 200 msec.

LLEWELLYN THOMAS: What was the distance of the screen from the observer?

NODINE: It was at the standard viewing distance of 2 ft, and the pictures were the regular size, 14 by 17 in.

LLEWELLYN THOMAS: That means that in order to see various areas in detail he would have to move his eyes, right?

NODINE: Yes. There were things other than lesions in these films, too. There might be an enlarged heart. That is a central problem and, therefore, should be easier to detect than a lesion, but we found that not to be the case. Peripheral viewing is another aspect of this.

LLEWELLYN THOMAS: Peripheral viewing, and whether you do indeed look at every area to get that detailed information. In reading a book you have to, and I can't help feeling that you need the same detail when reading x rays. I did a study some time ago using Rorschach cards with x rays as our control, which was interesting because in the one card you have a display that is highly informational in content even if you have to interpret it, and in the other case you have a display that has zero information content, i.e., it is an ink blot and doesn't represent anything. So the observer generates all the information that comes out. We found that the fixations got longer as people looked at these things. You could hypothesize that they were generating information because they had to give some definition to the ink blots.

I would like to know if anybody has statements which they think you could really add to help search in these situations. We'd be very grateful for them, but whether we will make the radiologists take any notice of them is another thing altogether.

MACKWORTH: I'd like to make two brief comments, one medical, one military. The medical one is the most beautiful example of the harmful effects of knowing the history of the patient. The patient was a man who had for a long time been studied for tuberculosis in one lung, but unfortunately started to develop cancer in the other lung which went undetected. The military example is one, I think, that is a more general [Freudian?, eds.] one. A long time ago I studied the problem of an expert who was overworked, e.g., someone doing 30 straight hours of inspection of aerial photographs. He was inclined to fall asleep on his sterooptical viewer. The point I think is this, and it is quite a serious one. Would you rather have your pictures, whether they are radiograms or aerial photographs, inspected by an expert who is extremely tired, who's worked for 30 hr, or would you rather have them inspected by somebody who is not an expert, but who has had an adequate amount of sleep?

LLEWELLYN THOMAS: That is a real problem for a radiologist in certain situations. It also raises the question of what instructions to give to paramedical personnel because, as you know, the doctors are pricing themselves out of the market. Not professors, I would say. For God's sake, we are not going up as fast as everybody else, but the clinicians are sort of piling it on. As you know, the tendency is to have more and more of these jobs done by paramedics. Such people are very highly skilled, but I have a nasty feeling that nobody knows what to tell them and I know that others have worried about it. They don't have the clinical training or the general background that the radiologist has, but they can be very good scanners. It has been observed that individual differences in search behavior are very large. Even if one can select scanners, we don't know what training and instructions to give them to optimize their visual search patterns.

The danger at the moment is that the people who are good don't know how they search yet they have set ideas about how they do it, and you can see their students going rib by rib down the other side exactly as the master tells them. The master doesn't scan like this, he just thinks he does.

GOULD: There are some standard training techniques that you didn't mention. One is a flicker enhancement technique in which standard defects are flickered to make them stand out.

LLEWELLYN THOMAS: There is also color enhancement, image enhancement, and computer analysis.

GOULD: Then there is the approach Professor Fry (Towsend & Fry, 1960) found useful, in which the subject is to look only at a small part of a picture at any time.

LLEWELLYN THOMAS: That is what I meant by a tracking device. I meant a device that opens up a window.

GOULD: We found that with integrated-circuit inspectors that wasn't useful. Then there is the approach of having two people look at the same thing.

LLEWELLYN THOMAS: That's strongly advised, yes. This increases your false positives but decreases your false negatives.

GOULD: Again, I think the evidence is that it varies from task to task. In some cases, people are almost independent, in other cases the same two people will miss the same defects.

LLEWELLYN THOMAS: It is like a Venn diagram, a large group would be in the intersection, but not all. Of course, there is a problem here. Who gets the money for reading the x ray if you've got two people reading it?

SENDERS: That's a serious problem, I admit.

LLEWELLYN THOMAS: Certainly these are things to advise, but they are not the sort of thing that gets done. On line computers, image enhancement, and particularly bringing color into x rays, will help and there is no doubt these will eventually be used.

We produced our EMI brain scanner, and it gives fabulous pictures of the whole brain. It's an incredible machine, a triumph of science and engineering, and yet in the end some jerk can be looking at it and miss something. In the end the computers are not interpreting it. We still need a good group of human beings, skilled and dedicated.

ANLIKER: Do you know whether or not the practice of inserting blanks or false or known x rays into the series that the scanner has to process has been studied? That would follow frequent evaluation and exercising of the searcher.

LLEWELLYN THOMAS: We have recommended that this be tried, particularly in on-line dynamic fluoroscopy. I can't say it met with any enthusiasm from the start. They still got it all mixed up with reward and punishment, and the feeling that we are trying to catch them. It is only when you got radar operators to accept the idea that such things are not gimmicks for catching them, but ways of enhancing their vigilance, that it worked.

We have talked about doing studies on false images, but it hasn't been done as a routine thing. Work in other fields suggests it would be an excellent idea.

KOLERS: I'd just like to make one point, and that is that there ought to be a fundamental difference between looking at a Rorschach plate tachistoscopically and looking at an x-ray plate. Although there may be no improvement beyond the first 200 msec of exposure from a detailed search of an x-ray plate, there is an enormous difference in output as a function of duration of exposure time of a Rorschach plate. The longer people look, beginning with, say, a 5-msec exposure and letting it go up to 30 msec or so, the amount of information that a person reads into the plate increases dramatically.

It seems to me, given this difference, that one must be doing substantially different things in achieving a recognition in 200 msec of an x-ray plate and in fantasizing some sort of perceptual representation in respect to a Rorschach.

SENDERS: I am sure that is true. My own immediate reaction when I heard of this 200 msec thing was that it was very similar to the experiments of Potter and Levy (1969). They showed a succession of unrelated pictures to the viewer fixating the projection area. He might be required to press a button when he saw a member of some previously designated class.

It is astonishing to be a subject. One is to press a button upon seeing a *game*. Ten unrelated pictures may be run off in 1 sec and one of these may be a chess game or a basketball game or what have you. Yet people respond with great rapidity. One is led to suspect that the radiologist goes into the situation with an almost infinite rather than a small set of expected images which may be verbally identified as to class and quite general. If anything gets through the filter, he stops and identifies it pretty well. Probably the ones that he misses then and the ones that he missed in his ordinary scanning use are the ones which don't really conform to any of the preconceived notions that he might have.

V.4

Speculations and Notions

John W. Senders

University of Toronto

I will make a few comments on the preceding papers, address myself briefly to some things that seem to be interesting problems, then conduct a general discussion.

Gould pointed out that good inspectors make more and shorter fixations while poor inspectors make fewer and longer fixations. A similar thing is true of aircraft pilots, even very highly skilled ones. There are important and consistent differences between pilots with 3,000 hr and pilots with 7,000 hr.

That is to say, a 7,000-hr pilot makes shorter fixations on his instruments and, therefore, is able to make more fixations. This suggests that when we do what we consider long experiments in the laboratory involving an hour or two of experience and possibly 15,000 fixations, we are not really getting at the behavior of a skilled, fully understanding subject who knows the statistics of the process and knows the geometry and the geography of the visual world that he is being asked to scan. I suspect we'd find (if we looked for them) continuing important changes in scanning behavior over very large numbers of trials. As will be seen later, this is also true of reading.

With regard to Zinchenko's "functional fovea," (Zinchenko & Vergiles, 1972), I recall that there is an experiment described by Helmholtz (1924, Vol. III, pp. 454–455) in which a stereo pair of drawings, with pinholes through them at corresponding points, are illuminated from the rear. When one fuses, in the stereoscope, the two points of light, one knows that the eyes are fixated on these points. When the scene is illuminated by a flash, stereopsis appears around the point of regard. However, Helmholtz points out that one can direct the "inner eye" to some other part of the picture. Then stereopsis appears at that part of the picture on the first flash. This also relates to Mackworth's comment about the contraction of the functional fovea (tunnel vision) with short exposures.

Since I tend to work as if tunnel vision were true, I find it easier to separate my stimuli so that a subject looking at one can't see the others. Then I don't have to worry about peripheral vision.

In most real situations, particularly in the case of looking at pictures, one is forced to some kind of foveal-plus-peripheral-input model. I like to imagine the system to be an antenna in which the total gain is fixed, but which can be directionally oriented. If one directionally orients an antenna, what one does, of course, is to concentrate the total available gain along a particular direction and thus to shorten the side lobes, or in general the radius vector, in other directions. See Fig. 1.

This would suggest that when you have a very high information stimulus at F the gain (or capacity) directed toward that stimulus is high with a consequent reduction in gain (or capacity) elsewhere as at peripheral points P_1, P_2, and P_3. Of course, we don't see out of the backs of our heads and this is merely a conceptual notion. However, the engineering–mathematical tools that are appropriate for antennas might formalize the cerebral phenomenon that Mackworth talks about.

Another problem that has interested me has been the question of when a saccade is planned. The timing of eye movements is very interesting. I don't know how long it takes to absorb the available information once the eye arrives at a new point of regard. The latency for the initiation of a saccade to an external stimulus is, depending on whom you read and what subject you have,

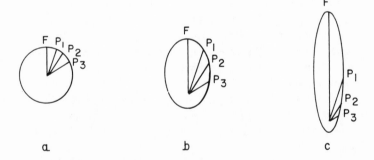

a   b   c

F = FOVEAL POINT OF REGARD

$P_{1,2,3}$ = PERIPHERAL AREAS 20°, 35°, & 60° FROM POINT OF REGARD

FIG. 1. A "directional antenna" model—unit total capacity area is the same for all figures. (a) No focusing of attention—uniform receptive field, radius vectors all equal; (b) moderate foveal attention (or attentional demand) somewhat reduced peripheral sensitivity, with greater reduction for greater angles; (c) extreme foveal attention (or attentional demand) severely reduced peripheral sensitivity. One could, of course, have lobes corresponding to the "mind's eye" or the functional fovea.

somewhere between 180 msec if you go back to Miles (1936), and 320 msec if you take some rather fatigued Navy trainees that I had in experiments I ran in Florida (Senders & Rankin, 1972). Let us take 250 msec as a fair estimate.

If a fixation F_0 has a duration of 250 msec, when is the plan made for the saccade to go to the next location? Is it made during the fixation F_0 or is it made on F_{-1}? In other words, is the succession of saccades programmed one or possibly even two or three saccade units before movement?

Like Gould, I have imagined experiments that might tell us about that. The subject is told to look at the computer-controlled scene. In one corner of this scene is a small frog approaching a puddle. At some time after enough fixations have been made on the frog, when the eye is making a saccade from the frog to the cow or whatever, we change the frog into a field mouse.

Now we wait until the eye comes back and looks at the field mouse. The question really is whether the eye will stay there soaking up this new information (and perhaps asking what happened to the frog) or will fly off to some other place or even to two before coming back. If the latter, then planning of the saccades would be accomplished on F_{-1} or F_{-2}. The process appears to the outside observer, the experimenter, like a Markoff process. That is to say, we cannot predict exactly, only probabilistically, where the eye is going to go on the next saccade even if we had an indefinite amount of prior data. We are able to make statistical summaries: people look at faces; people look at hands. We cannot say, though, that if the eye is now regarding the hand, it will go to the face (or to some other designated place). At the present time we don't seem to have any way of separating these out.

This is another thought experiment. Suppose A looks and B sees. That is, if B is presented with a picture which moves around so that the succession of visual images of B is identical to that of A, what will B see? Will B see the "Mona Lisa" or will B see a succession of unrelated garbage?

DISCUSSION

ROBINSON: Something like that was done for fun by Derek Fender at his Christmas parties. He would have two subjects wear contact lenses and measure the miniature eye movements of one. (These are all small eye movements.) The other one would have a stabilized image which would be destabilized according to the eye movements of A. Nothing violent at all happened to B's perception of the visual image or the room and B used to complain and say to A, "I want to look over to the left, will you look over?"

There was no careful verbal report but B certainly did not have any kind of fragmented appreciation of his visual surround. This was not done at all scientifically, as you know.

KOLERS: Why do you expect one? Can't you recognize a picture that is jiggled periodically in front of you?

SENDERS: It is very hard to make a picture "saccade" and not see it while it is moving, whereas if one did it using video techniques, it might be easier. It seems to me, this bears on the question of whether the eye movement is a determined sequence or a random sequence in which the observer dips into an urn full of chips marked with different coordinates, pulls one out and goes to the indicated location.

ANLIKER: I have done an experiment, a very informal one, of this sort where the display for B is generated by the eye movements of A. A looks and sees, but B is only allowed to look into the display. If the signal for B is displayed, in other words brightened up, only during the fixation of A, then B has great difficulty in seeing anything coherent by the time A's point of regard is shifted.

SENDERS: I presume that is because B has to initiate a saccade to the location which is illuminated by A's point of regard.

ANLIKER: I am saying if B looks only at patches when presented by A, then A can inspect the figure on his own saccadic maneuver, but B tries to look at what A sees simultaneously and can't see anything.

SENDERS: Presumably there is a latency of 200 msec between the termination of A's saccade and the initiation of B's saccade. Since that is not much shorter than the fixation time of A, the "target" will always be gone by the time B gets there, won't it?

ANLIKER: Well, that is one part of the problem. But the other part of the problem is that even if I start extending the exposure time for B by a considerable amount, it is as if it is being handed to him in some order he doesn't want.

SENDERS: That suggests that there *is* a plan and that the plan programs the insertion of information in a particular place in some internal map. Another question, of course, is whether A can serve as A's own guide.

We might record the eye movements of A during observation of a picture and then give A that same picture after a lapse of time and see whether or not A at time T_1 can serve as the program, as it were, for A at time T_2.

FARLEY: I think that *effective* perception is actually *directed* perception and that the goals you have will affect both where you will look and how you will see. I think we saw that in Yarbus' (1967) pictures where indeed the goal of answering a question did alter what was looked at. On the other hand, you cannot form a complete plan of where you will look, at least very far ahead, because you are interacting with the environment.

It is not like a problem-solving situation where I can plan 10 steps ahead on how to add numbers because nothing's going to change. I am constantly interacting. If I have a plan now, a goal, and I look at a place in the field, what I see may change the plan.

SENDERS: Clearly you don't set up a preplan on the first glance which then guides you through the picture, although in some of our search patterns people appeared to organize scans. There the picture was fairly uniform in informational density and content and it was a search rather than a looking operation. I am sure that there wasn't a very long chain of planned fixations.

The chain must be short and I think it is of considerable interest to consider exactly how long it is and whether it has a fixed or variable length.

LLEWELLYN THOMAS: I would like to make a point here. In studies we did some years ago with schizophrenics, we saw very different search plans, whatever this means. I think it emphasizes the point that you raised, that the internal imaging, whatever that is, is a great backdrop for the search plan and what you see when you get there has a great effect.

I remember one patient who had tried to commit suicide by slashing her wrists. She took one look at one wrist on a projected picture and from then on throughout the whole of the series of 10 full-sized projected images never looked at her wrist again. That one look was tremendously powerful in that case and I think it is similarly powerful for most of us.

SENDERS: When one is searching, there sometimes may be regular scan patterns. However, when one is monitoring, there is a powerful *illusion* of regular scan. Pilots characteristically state that they have a scan pattern. In fact, if you measure the eye movements of pilots (I am sure this will be true for radiologists and others), you find that the data seem to agree with a stochastic model.

They dip into an urn and pull out a chip labeled "altimeter," throw it back, and look at the altimeter. At any rate, such a model predicts very well the statistics of a skilled pilot's fixational behavior.

Relevant to these questions are Potter's experiments (Potter & Levy, 1969) with successive rapid presentation of unrelated pictures (see Gould). Pictures were presented at eight or ten per second so that a great deal of information was being presented to the eye in a very short time. Under those conditions there were virtually no eye movements. The eye apparently stays fixated on the place where information is presented and soaks it up. If scanning is an information-seeking or an uncertainty-reducing process, then if one provides information at the point of regard, eye movements should be suppressed.

I feel that in order to deal with these questions and with data one needs a model of the scanning process.

Assume that the selection of the next point of regard is based on all the available information from the scene given the present point of regard. In particular, assume that all possible points of regard are ranked according to the probability that each will be the next fixated. The choice of the next point will then be a random one from the total set, and so on. The probability that any point will be selected will be the result of the following process: the density distribution of information in the scene over all points is operated on by the resolution function of the eye for each point, and the outcome is compared with the residual or memory image associated with each point as a consequent of all the antecedent fixations everywhere on the visual scene. The greater the difference of this last comparison at any point, the greater the probability of a fixation at that point.

The net probability is then dependent on three things: the physical distribution of contours in the scene, the capacity of the eye to resolve contours at various distances from the point of regard, and the psychological or memorial function associated with each point of regard as mapped onto some internal representation of the scene. Such a simple system will tend not to "fixate" empty space (although it might with low probability). It will in general tend to follow contours but will depart from them after they have been "learned." Depending on the decay-time constants of its "memory," it would generate scan "patterns" or apparently random scans. I suspect that with simple adjustment of the two "internalized" functions it would do what Noton and Stark (1971) report their subjects did.

I think it will look at faces, and probably at eyes and mouths, with greater frequency than the middle of the cheek, and so on, but in a stochastic rather than a deterministic way. The model is, of course, related to earlier eye-movement models of instrument scanning which have been fairly successful in predicting pilot behavior.

ROBINSON: I wish to comment on the first point you made about when one has made up one's mind to make a saccade and then being irrevocably committed. One of the traps that many of us have fallen into is that of using small target steps. Small saccades are over with so quickly, there is little time to find out what would have happened if one wanted to cancel a saccade. Becker and Jurgens (1974) have looked at 60° saccades where a target is on one side, and suddenly it goes out, and flashes on at the other side. One hundred msec later, before anything has happened, the target jumps back again. What the subject very often does is to start the saccade, get half-way there, slam on the brakes, and without a single pause or hesitation start right off at saccadic velocity to the original target location.

I think one can say several things about this. First, there must have been parallel processing going on: what to do about this target and what to do about that target; and the calculations were going on in the brain simultaneously not serially.

Then consider the first saccade. The first saccade was clearly not preprogrammed. If a saccade can be stopped in midflight, we can no longer have the idea that saccades are ballistic, preprogrammed, dedicated, and unstoppable. They can fairly repeatably be stopped under the right conditions.

The second saccade was probably not preprogrammed either because it very cleverly took into account and subtracted from itself the eye position created by the first saccade. That probably means that it was operating on information, not on retinal sign, but on absolute target position in space.

The point I want to make that might be relevant here is that the idea of the brain as a serial programmer which can solve only one problem at a time is probably not very dependable. We should recognize that many problems, visual problems, can be solved simultaneously, leading to different programs that might conflict with each other.

STEINMAN: I would like to comment on something relevant to what Dr. Robinson said. We started doing experiments on the tracking of *small steps,* and we began to see (although very slowly at first) in the micropattern of the prestep period a minisaccade that would go 3 to 4 min of arc to the right, return to the start position, and then go a bit off to the left. In other words, it was as though the subject thought the step had occurred, sent the command, and immediately sent the opposite command.

The point is that we never saw this before beginning to work in *small-step* tracking. There are these little pulse saccades which go and come back and end up no place. I have thousands of them on paper now. There is no intersaccadic interval you can describe.

LLEWELLYN THOMAS: I think Dr. Frecker can describe this kind of thing happening also in 20° saccades. The problem that I find is in the very short time available for the processing of the information needed for this to occur. You know, one always had the comforting thought that saccades must be ballistic because there isn't time for the loop to be closed with what we knew of the speed of neural transmission. Of course, your nasty fact wrecks my theory; I must say it seems from what we have heard today, that that is indeed happening. I still am baffled by the very short times within which this all takes place. Do you have any ideas?

ROBINSON: Well, the point was that there were two programs running in the brain simultaneously so that the second saccade wasn't something that had to be totally planned and executed after the first saccade was canceled. The second program came along and canceled the first program. So there is no embarrassment about any time differences.

LLEWELLYN THOMAS: That is similar to the path curvatures which arise when another muscle comes into action and is then withdrawn again during a saccade. We did a study some years ago showing such curvature—these hooks in the path—but they are not standard, they come in sometimes and not at others, but they are there very frequently.

CORNSWEET: It worries me to hear you refer to saccadic movements as stochastic. They may be. There are some processes that apparently really are stochastic like radioactive decays and things, but most of the things that we call stochastic are those for which we just don't understand the antecedent condition.

SENDERS: The experimenter sees them as stochastic, I don't quite believe it myself.

LLEWELLYN THOMAS: "Probabilistic" is all right; the movements are not deterministic.

SENDERS: I am not sure at all.

KOLERS: I wanted to comment on the cancellation phenomenon. Difficult as it is to understand backward masking at the perceptual level, it seems to me there is backward masking at the motor level, where the subsequent command is inhibiting the execution of the antecedent, much as the subject's later visual input somewhat inhibits the perception of the antecedent input.

ROBINSON: How about sideways masking?

KOLERS: That is called lateral inhibition.

MACKWORTH: I think one of the most relevant studies relating to skilled and unskilled inspectors is by Ohtani (1972). He compared the inspection of sheet metal and laboratory inspection processes in the steel industry. The important point is that he makes a distinction between fast transport movements and movements related to identification and processing. When he plots his data on cumulative probability paper he gets two straight lines with different slopes. The line has a fairly steep initial slope—the transport movements—then there is a sudden break to a lower slope as the fixation time is increased—the inspections.

SENDERS: Not too surprising.

FRY: I just wanted to comment that Cobb and Moss (1926) at one time had a program in which they had a sequence of fixation points. The task was to go from one fixation point to a second and then bounce off that to a third point; in this way they got short fixation pauses.

SENDERS: A preprogrammed sequence.

FRY: Yes. I don't know if that is relevant to what Dr. Robinson was talking about. I'd like to ask him what times were involved in executing the movements as compared to the time required to initiate a new movement? In other words, cancellation might work with a long excursion, but wouldn't work with a short one.

ROBINSON: I don't know why you couldn't trick the eye into doing this more often for $10°$ saccades. The probability of its occurring seems to go down with small saccades. I suspect that two programs trying to reach contrary conclusions in the brain simultaneously is a thing that one doesn't really want to have happen.

I suppose these two programs are trying to inhibit each other so that only one of them gets executed. You have to get conditions just right and be very lucky to get one that can crash in while another is being executed and stop it. It is glib to say that large saccades that take 150 msec to be completed offer more time to crash probabilistically through this door and get the thing into reverse. That's the only explanation I can think of, but I am sure it is simplistic.

NICKERSON: I don't know whom this is directed to, but somebody who knows about the scanning of x rays and such things. When people miss the critical item, the lesion or the enlarged heart or whatever it is he is looking for, is there any evidence that they miss it even though they have fixated on it, or is it a failure to fixate at the appropriate place?

SENDERS: That sounds like a question for Mackworth.

MACKWORTH: Unfortunately, I don't think there is direct evidence on the radiology situation, but I did a study which showed quite clearly on a dial inspection task that when the dials were 6° apart, the missed signals very often had been directly fixated (Mackworth, Kaplan, & Metlay, 1964).

SENDERS: Well, I seem to recall that you had data showing that when people are scanning matrices of numbers for a particular target number, the eye will in fact rest upon the target number, proceed to some other place without its being reported, and then go back with a higher probability than a pure random process would predict to the target (Mackworth & Mackworth, 1958).

MACKWORTH: That is true. A point related to an earlier comment is that there was a great deal of information from D. O'Connell and J. Bruner (unpublished data) on the idea of preprogramming the sequence of pictorial areas that are presented by copying the previous tracks.

LLEWELLYN THOMAS: There are many cases where people do look at things and do not report them. Now, whether this is a failure of short-term memory or a failure of recognition, we haven't investigated. Perhaps others have; it is an obvious area that needs looking into. We were more worried when they reported things they never fixated on.

GOULD: I think that many applied inspection tasks are not like looking for a square in a background of circles where the target is well defined. Many errors are made in interpretation. A person may look at a potential defect and really see it, but decide it is not a defect.

NICKERSON: I am curious to know if you ever studied the eye movements of people trying to debug programs. I know you have been interested in that problem.

GOULD: I have done a little bit, but I don't have anything useful to say.

LLEWELLYN THOMAS: I had some films of people solving differential equations, and Mackworth and I both have some films of people looking for errors in electronic circuitry. If one has a one-shot multivibrator drawn in diagram on the board and changes a component, and has a knowledgeable engineer look at it, he would make patterns of inspection through the circuitry which look at rational kinds of things. It is as though he is asking himself what would happen with this condenser or this resistor changed.

We haven't done any more on that. It is surely one way of getting insight into the process.

NODINE: In reply to your question, Dr. Nickerson, about whether the radiologist failed to fixate missed points, I don't think the evidence is clear there. You find, as Dr. Thomas said, some do and some don't fixate on a lesion that they fail to report. These are differences that develop in the patterning of the fixation pattern from the medical student to the internist to the radiologist;

and there seems to be a faster finding of the lesion as you move up that progression. That is, they arrive at the abnormality faster and they tend to cover more area in their search.

SENDERS: Do they generally make more fixations as they become more experienced?

NODINE: No, fewer, but more appropriate ones.

SENDERS: I was interested in relating your observations to Loftus' (1972) findings about number as opposed to duration of fixations with regard to subsequent recognition.

NODINE: I think the point is that perhaps all we are seeing in the search pattern is the confirmation phase of what has already been decided is wrong with that film to begin with. A failing to fixate the lesion doesn't really tell us the whole story.

SENDERS: I think the question was whether he fixates the lesion and fails to report. Was that not it, Dr. Nickerson?

NICKERSON: Yes, that was part of it. I was wondering if you can find errors of failure to fixate and errors of failure to report in spite of fixation, and what that ratio might be.

SENDERS: Apparently there is no immediate answer forthcoming.

RUSSO: One explanation for the failure to detect, that is the nonreporting of something that is fixated, would be a sort of hypothesis-testing explanation. If the eye fixates on a new location triggered by some expectation, what it sees may not be what was expected. What you found might also have been a lesion or a kind of lesion, but if it wasn't what was expected, it would not be detected. If you went with the right hypothesis, you would have detected it, but if you view the search as sort of an active hypothesis-testing process, possessing a strong cognitive component along with the perceptual, then I think one can explain how certain things can be missed.

LLEWELLYN THOMAS: Zeidner and Sadacca (1960) in their study of photointerpreters showed this very clearly. If they knew there was an armored division in the area, they saw tanks all over the road; if they didn't, they saw puddles. I think this is what one is saying here. The observer has a template.

McCONKIE: I wanted to make a comment about your question of lag and how long it takes to set up an eye movement. We put together a system which allows us to modify the image on the screen based on eye movements and eye fixation patterns.

This has been used in the study of reading. In one of our studies, we placed in a paragraph a letter string in place of a particular target word. Then as the person was reading on that line approaching that particular word position, we replaced that letter string with the word during fixation.

SENDERS: During a fixation?

McCONKIE: I mean during a saccade. Then we looked at those fixations which landed upon that particular word location as a function of the distance to it of the previous fixation point. I will describe that in detail tomorrow, but can state now that it is true that on that fixation you get an elongated duration, so that the duration of that fixation has not been preprogrammed on the basis of some prior fixations. You hit that particular fixation and it is in fact elongated under certain conditions, so that you know that what is going on right now is being influenced by information on this particular fixation.

MONTY: It seems to me that much of this session can be summarized as follows (Fig. 2):

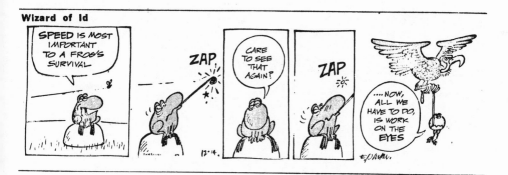

FIG. 2. (By permission of John Hart and Field Enterprises, Inc.)

V.5

References

Anderson, J. R., & Bower, G. H. *Human associative memory.* New York: Wiley, 1973.

Atkinson, R. C., & Shiffrin, R. M. Human memory: A proposed system and its control processes. In K. W. Spence & J. T. Spence (Eds.), *The psychology of learning and motivation: Advances in research and theory.* Vol. 2. New York: Academic Press, 1968.

Becker, W., & Jurgens, R. Saccadic reactions to double step stimuli. Paper presented at the *Symposium on Basic Mechanisms of Ocular Motility and Their Clinical Applications,* Stockholm, 1974.

Berlyne, D. E., & Lawrence, G. H. Effects of complexity and incongruity variables on GSR, investigatory behavior, and verbally expressed preference. *Journal of General Psychology,* 1964, **71,** 21–45.

Biederman, I. Perceiving real-world scenes. *Science,* 1972, **177,** 77–80.

Biederman, I., Glass, A. L., & Stacy, E. W. Searching for objects in real-world scenes. *Journal of Experimental Psychology,* 1973, **97,** 22–77.

Boynton, R. M. Summary and discussion. In A. Morris & E. P. Horne (Eds.), *Visual Search.* Washington, D.C.: National Academy of Science, 1960.

Buswell, G. T. *How people look at pictures.* Chicago: University of Chicago Press, 1935.

Chaikin, J. D., Corbin, H. H., & Volkmann, J. Mapping a field of short-time visual search. *Science,* 1962, **138,** 1327–1328.

Cobb, P. W., & Moss, F. K. The fixational pause of the eyes. *Journal of Experimental Psychology,* 1926, **9,** 359–367.

Edwards, D. C., & Goolkasian, P. A. Peripheral vision location and kinds of complex processing. *Journal of Experimental Psychology,* 1974, **102,** 244–249.

Ford, A., White, C. T., and Lichtenstein, M. Analysis of eye movements during free search. *Journal of the Optical Society of America,* 1959, **49,** 287–292.

Freund, R. D. Verbal and nonverbal processes in picture recognition. Unpublished doctoral dissertation, Stanford University, California, 1971.

Gazzaniga, M. S. *The bisected brain.* New York: Appleton, 1970.

Gibson, J. J. *The senses considered as perceptual systems.* Boston: Houghton Mifflin, 1966.

Gould, J. D. Eye movements during visual search and memory search. *Journal of Experimental Psychology,* 1973, **98,** 184–195.

Gould, J. D., & Carn, R. Visual search, complex backgrounds, mental counters, and eye movements. *Perception and Psychophysics,* 1973, **14,** 125–132.

Gould, J. D., & Dill, A. Eye movement parameters and pattern recognition. *Perception and Psychophysics,* 1969, **6,** 311–320.

Gould, J. D., & Schaffer, A. Eye movement patterns during visual information processing. *Psychonomic Science,* 1965, **3,** 317–318.

Hall, D. C. The effect of eye movements on the recall of information with visual imagery. Unpublished doctoral dissertation. Stanford University, Institute for Communication Research, California, 1972.

Helmholtz, H. von Physiological optics. [Translated by J. P. C. Southall.] *Optical Society of America,* 1924, **3,** 281–369, 400–488.

Hochberg, J. In the mind's eye. In R. N. Haber (Ed.), *Contemporary theory and research in visual perception.* New York: Holt, Rinehart, and Winston, 1968. Pp. 309–332.

Kahneman, D., *Attention and effort.* Englewood Cliffs, New Jersey: Prentice-Hall, 1973.

Llewellyn Thomas, E. L. Search behavior. *Radiologic Clinics of North America.* 1969, **7,** 403–417.

Llewellyn Thomas, E., & Lansdowne, E. L. Visual search patterns in radiologists in training. *Radiology,* 1963, **81,** 288–291.

Loftus, G. R., Eye fixations and recognition memory for pictures. *Cognitive Psychology,* 1972, **3,** 525–551.

Mackworth, J. F. The duration of the visual image. *Canadian Journal of Psychology,* 1963, **7,** 62–81.

Mackworth, J. F. *Vigilance and attention.* Harmondsworth, England: Penguin Books, 1970.

Mackworth, N. H. Visual noise causes tunnel vision. *Psychonomic Science,* 1965, **3,** 67–68.

Mackworth, N. H. A stand camera for line-of-sight recording. *Perception and Psychophysics,* 1967, **2,** 119–127.

Mackworth, N. H. The line-of-sight approach to children's reading and comprehension. In S. F. Wanat, H. Singer, & M. Kling (Eds.), *Extracting meaning from written language.* Newark, Delaware: International Reading Association, 1974.

Mackworth, N. H., & Bruner, J. S. How adults and children search and recognize pictures. *Human Development,* 1970, **13,** 149–177.

Mackworth, N. H., Kaplan, I. T., & Metlay, W. Eye movements during vigilance. *Perceptual and Motor Skills,* 1964, **18,** 397–402.

Mackworth, N. H., & Mackworth, J. F. Eye fixations recorded on changing visual scenes by the television eye marker. *Journal of the Optical Society of America,* 1958, **48,** 438–445.

Mackworth, N. H., & Morandi, A. J., The gaze selects informative details within pictures. *Perception and Psychophysics,* 1967, **2,** 547–552.

Miles, W. R. The response time of the eye. *Psychological Monographs,* 1936, **47,** 268–293 (Whole No. 212).

Mooney, C. M. Recognition of novel visual configuration with and without eye movements. *Journal of Experimental Psychology,* 1958, **56,** 133–138.

Murphy, R., Recognition memory for sequentially presented pictorial and verbal spatial information. Unpublished doctoral thesis, New York University, 1971.

Noton, D., & Stark, L., Scanpaths in eye movements during pattern perception, *Science,* 1971, **171,** 308–311.

Ohtani, A. The analysis of child development by eye-movement studies. *Proceedings of the 20th International Congress of Psychology.* Tokyo, Japan, August, 1972. Pp. 264–266.

Posner, M. I., Boies, S. J., Eichelman, W. H., & Taylor, R. L. Retention of visual and name codes of single letters. *Journal of Experimental Psychology Monograph,* 1969, **79,** 1–16.

Potter, M. C., & Levy, E. I., Recognition memory for a rapid sequence of pictures. *Journal of Experimental Psychology,* 1969, **81,** 10–15.

Pritchard, R. M., Heron, W., & Hebb, D. O. Visual perception approached by the method of stabilized images. *Canadian Journal of Psychology,* 1960, **14,** 67–77.

Schoonard, J. W., Gould, J. D., & Miller, L. A., Studies of visual inspection. *Ergonomics,* 1973, **16**, 365–379.

Senders, J. W., & Rankin, W. C. The effect of signal probabilities on the time required to redirect the gaze. *NAVTRADEVCEN 70-C-0234-1,* Naval Training Devices Center, Orlando, Florida, 1972.

Senders, J. W., Webb, I. B., & Baker, C. A. The peripheral viewing of dials. *Journal of Applied Psychology,* 1955, **39**, 433–436.

Shiffrin, R. M., & Geisler, W. S., Visual recognition in a theory of information processing. In R. L. Soslo (Ed.), *Contemporary issues in cognitive psychology: The Loyola Symposium.* New York: Winston, 1973.

Shontz, W. D., & Kanarick, A. F., Eye fixation recordings during information acquisition in short-term memory. Minneapolis, Honeywell Corp., Document *12177-FR.* 1970.

Sperling, G. The information available in brief visual presentations. *Psychological Monographs,* 1960, **74**, 1–29, (Whole No. 498).

Sperling, G. A model for visual memory tasks. *Human Factors,* 1963, **5**, 19–31.

Sternberg, S. Two operations in character-recognition: Some evidence from reaction-time measurements. *Perception and Psychophysics,* 1967, **2**, 45–53.

Towsend, C. A., & Fry, G. A. Automatic scanning of aerial photographs. In A. Morris & E. P. Harne (Eds.), *Visual search techniques.* Washington, D.C. National Academy of Sciences–National Research Council, Publ. 712, 1960.

Travers, J. R. Word recognition with forced serial processing. Effects of segment size and temporal order variation. *Perception and Psychophysics,* 1974, **16**, 35–42.

Tversky, B. Eye fixations in predictions of recognition and recall. *Memory and Cognition,* 1974, **2**, 275–278.

von Holst, E. Relations between the central nervous sytem and the peripheral organs. *British Journal of Animal Behavior,* 1954, **2**, 89–94.

White, C. T., & Ford, A. Eye movements during simulated radar search. *Journal of the Optical Society of America,* 1960, **50**, 909–913.

Williams, L. G. The effects of target specification on objects fixated during visual search. *Acta Psychologica,* 1967, **27**, 355–360.

Yarbus, A. L. *Eye movements and vision.* New York: Plenum Press, 1967.

Zeidner, J., & Sadacca, R. Research on human Factors in Image Interpreter Systems. Research Study *60-3,* Washington, D.C., U.S. Army, Human Factors Research Branch, TAG Research and Development Command, 1960.

Zinchenko, V. P., & Vergiles, N. Y. *Formation of visual images: Studies of stabilized retinal images.* [Translated by Consultants Bureau, New York: Plenum, 1972.] (Originally published in Moscow by Moscow Univ. Press.)

Part VI

THE ROLE OF
EYE MOVEMENTS IN READING

The possibility of keeping physical records as aids to memory by the use of spatially organized materials must have occurred very early to ancient man. The particular ways in which these materials are specially organized, however, has varied through all possible arrangements. Languages may be written from left to right or right to left and top to bottom or bottom to top, in vertical lines and in horizontal lines, and there is no particular reason to assume that any one way of organizing material is better than any other. However, some serial arrangement in one sense or another must be imposed if the written material is to be interpreted correctly. The degree, however, to which positional structure within sentences is important depends upon the degree to which the language is inflected. English is a highly positional language in which the meanings of sentences are determined both by the words within the sentence and by the positions they hold relative to the other words. This is not necessarily true of all languages.

When people read aloud, the voice may be as many as three or four fixations behind the eye. Whether this is true of comprehension and memory storing and encoding in silent reading is an interesting question.

In reading there are illusions similar to those that occur in scanning of the visual world. There is the illusion of clarity during normal reading, and the illusion of smoothness and continuity. The papers which follow present basic information about reading and eye movements derived from the early work of Buswell as well as new data obtained using sophisticated computer and eye-movement apparatus interconnected in such a way as to alter the material presented for reading on the basis of on-line measurement of eye fixations. These latter studies make clear the limited range within which reading does occur. It becomes clear that reading is a very complex high-level process involving both linguistic and memorial functions and that it possesses some of the qualities of visual space perception. The way in which the reader moves his eyes can be shown to be related to the linguistic structure of the written material and to the processes involved in its comprehension.

The chairman of the sixth session was Dr. Paul Kolers of the University of Toronto.

VI.1

Buswell's Discoveries

Paul A. Kolers

University of Toronto

Psychology, lacking a notation with which to cumulate its knowledge, reinvents its subject matter from generation to generation. A topic is worked on at some time, interest in it peaks and then wanes, the topic is set aside, and then some time later is rediscovered. Movements of the eyes is such a topic; their saccadic nature in reading was reported first only in 1878. They were studied intensively for a generation, then ignored for another, studied again, again ignored, and now are studied once again. One of those cycles caught up Raymond Dodge in the early years of this century; another, about a generation later, caught up Guy Thomas Buswell. Dodge's work has never been wholly out of the canon of the experimental psychologist, but Buswell, working in a different tradition, has not been as well known. His first important work on eye movements was published in 1920 when he was in his thirties, and he continued to publish on the subject for more than 25 years. Except for a book in 1935, *How People Look at Pictures,* his major works were published in *Supplementary Educational Monographs,* a series published by the University of Chicago, where he did his work, and were well known to educational psychologists, but not to many others.

From time to time I have looked at Buswell's monographs, and have almost always discovered that some of the best ideas experimental psychologists concerned with information processing have had can be found, demonstrated, and tested, in Buswell. I thought it would be useful and interesting to recapitulate some of these intellectual adventures of 40 and 50 years ago and relate them to our current interests. I have selected only a few works from Buswell's large bibliography (Buswell, 1920, 1935, 1937; also Judd & Buswell, 1922).

Intellectual Basis

Buswell's concern was to educate the psychological fraternity who were trying to educate school children, and in particular, teachers of reading. His main message in this respect was that reading was a cognitive process, a manipulating of symbols, not merely implicit speech. Hence in his early work he was concerned to show only a few things, but to show them clearly. One of these was that oral reading—reading aloud—was not silent reading with voice added, as many educationists held it to be. Rather, he alleged, readers were working in substantially different ways when reading aloud and reading silently. A second issue was to show that not all reading was the same, that people differed greatly from one to another in the way they read. Indeed, even the same person read in different ways on different occasions.

If these two notions seem commonplace today, they were not commonplace 50 years ago. Reading tended to be thought of as a monolithic process, performed fairly similarly by all people, and certainly it was thought to be carried out similarly by the same person on different occasions. Buswell gathered the empirical data in the 1920's and 1930's relevant to these points, and explored the range and diversity of skills that go into successful reading. In the course of his work he touched upon or studied many questions that occupy psychologists and other students of eye movements even today. I'll return to them in a moment. First a word about the style of the work.

Buswell's style was so distinctive that after a while one can identify a Buswell monograph even without titles. The style was that of the data-oriented empiricism of the Midwest in the second quarter of this century. In his monograph on the eye–voice span, which runs to 104 pages, there are 13 figures, 37 plates, and 17 tables. "Silent Reading" is 157 pages long, with more than 100 given over to 90 plates and 21 tables. "How Adults Read" is 146 pages long, with 36 plates and 46 tables, and *How People Look at Pictures* is 198 pages long, with 67 plates, 10 tables, and 3 figures. This concentration on data is a hallmark. In addition, "How Adults Read" was based on a sample of 1120 subjects and used 22,000 feet of film, and *How People Look at Pictures* used 18,000 feet of film. The film was analyzed by hand, frame by frame.

The method of measurement was a variation on Dodge's, and has been modified subsequently by Mackworth and others. One version of the apparatus is shown in Fig. 1, which Buswell (1937) described as follows:

> The selection to be read is placed directly in front of the subject's eyes at a distance of fourteen inches. . . [and] is sufficiently large so that an entire page of reading material may be presented at one time.
>
> The method of making a record of eye-movements consists in photographing a beam of light from a six-volt ribbon-filament lamp reflected first to the cornea of the eye from silvered glass mirrors and then from the cornea to a second set of mirrors through a camera lens, and thus to a moving kinetoscope film. In the present apparatus the source of light is under the table, the beam being passed through a series of condensing lenses, then up through a hole in the table to a set of mirrors which reflects the beam to the subject's eyes. The film record has one line which is the reflection from a silvered bead on a pair of spectacle frames worn by the subject. This line is used for the purpose of measuring any movements of the head. . . After the beam of light leaves the eye, it is

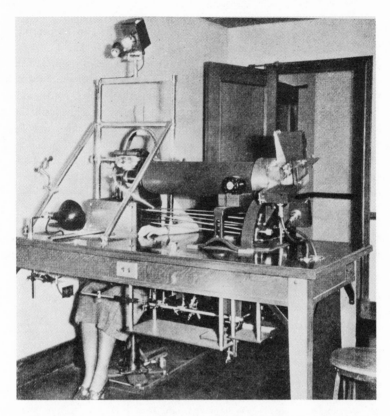

FIG. 1.   A late version of the eye-tracking apparatus. (After Buswell, 1937.)

intercepted by a revolving blade mounted on the shaft of a synchronous motor which cuts the beam of light once every thirtieth of a second, thereby giving a line of dots for measuring the duration of the pauses of the eye. While the fixations of the eyes are plotted at a given point on the line of print, . . . the plotting simply shows the center of the fixation area [pp. 22f].

In some cases the film also carried a record of the text being looked at; in some cases a voice key left a record on the film, and by various ingenious techniques sometimes the position of the eye was signaled on a voice record. The result was motion picture film which, blown up, revealed the dots of light, the interrupted beam, the number of which signaled how long the eye was fixated, and whose position showed the eye's movements from fixation to horizontal fixation. (The system could not record vertical motions.) Heroic analyses were undertaken on the frames of film. Nowadays we do an analysis of variance on several factors involving hundreds of observations in just a few seconds, but even 20 years ago a single analysis of variance required the better part of a day to compute. As the speed of operation increases, sometimes, too, does mindlessness in its execution.

With Buswell's techniques, on the other hand, one had to be careful in the analyses one undertook, for carrying one out might take weeks.

Figure 2 shows some typical data. The vertical lines define points of fixation, the numbers above them showing their sequence, and the numbers below showing their duration in thirtieths of a second. This figure is for a good reader and for prose of modest difficulty. Notice the regularity of sequence and spacing of the fixations. Figure 3 shows the results for two other readers, one good and the other fair. Greater variability in sequence, duration, and spacing of the fixations can be seen. They are even more marked in Fig. 4, comparing a fair and a poor reader. Figure 5 reveals something of the range of variation.

Reading Is Symbolic Activity

The issue is not settled yet regarding the nature of reading. One group of investigators assumes that reading is implicit speech. According to this theory,

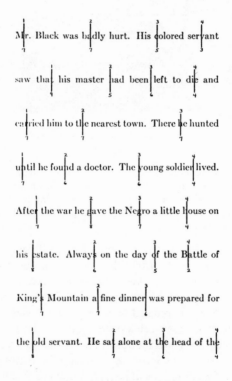

FIG. 2. A good reader on prose of modest difficulty. The vertical lines identify approximate fixation points; the numbers above show their sequence and the numbers below show their duration in thirtieths of a second. (After Buswell, 1937.)

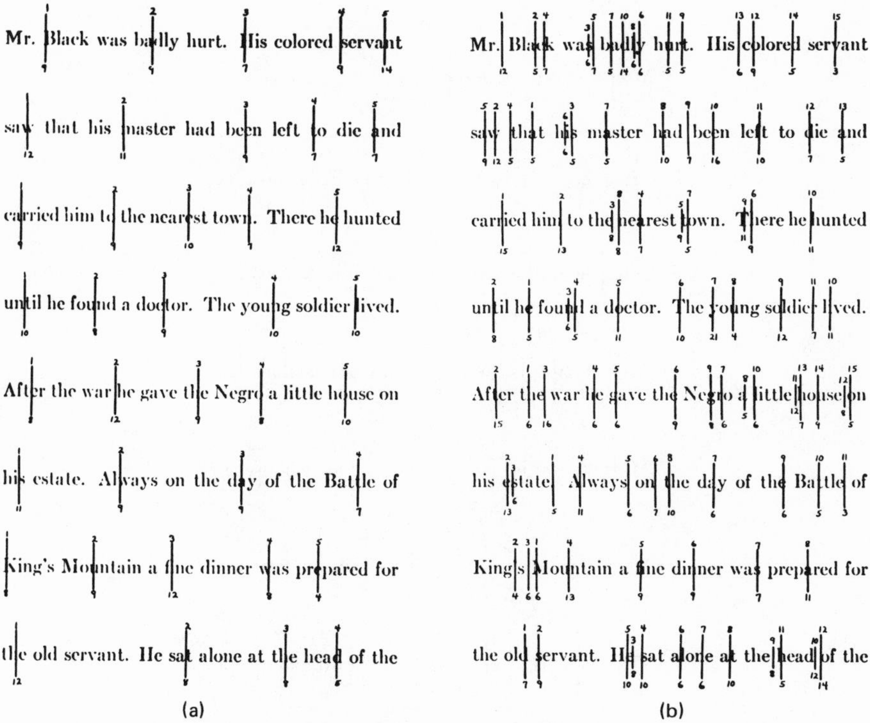

(a)

(b)

FIG. 3. Results (a) for a good reader and (b) for one of moderate skill. (After Buswell, 1937.)

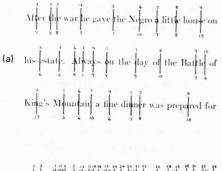

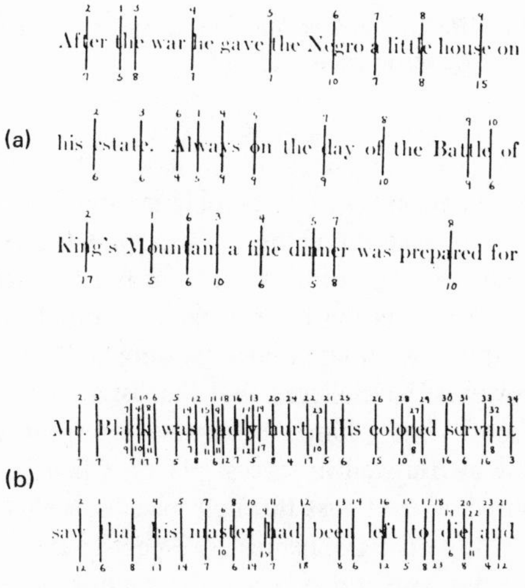

(a)

(b)

FIG. 4. (a) A fair reader and (b) a poor one. (After Buswell, 1937.)

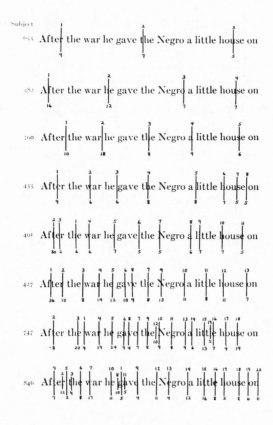

FIG. 5. Results for eight different readers, illustrating variations in performance from good (top) to poor (bottom). (After Buswell, 1937.)

the eye must have the ability to translate graphic symbols into their phonemic transcriptions, but does not have the ability to interpret the symbols in respect to their semantic content. This has often struck me as a ludicrous theory. If the visual system is capable of translation of the mark to sound, why should it not be able to go farther? And why should understanding be based only on sounds? Many psychologists, however, have alleged that the visual system can only act to translate marks to sounds but cannot otherwise interpret them. Quite the opposite view is argued by Buswell in several places, when he emphasizes that reading is usually impaired when it goes through speech, implicit or overt; that it is best when it operates upon the graphemes in respect to their characteristics as symbols possessing meaning and not as signs for sounds or as instructions to sound out. "Reading," he says, "is a process of comprehending meanings" (Buswell, 1937, p. 69). These meanings are derived from visual analysis of the visual symbols.

Eye–Voice Span

A way of studying this cognitive aspect of literacy is found in one of the earliest works (Buswell, 1920). For this investigation subjects read aloud while a record was made of where they were looking and what they were saying. The idea that one's eyes lead one's mouth in reading aloud is always hard to believe. We have the strong subjective sense that we are looking at what we are saying! Buswell showed not only that one's eye leads, but that the distance that it leads increases with an increase in reading skill, at least through the first six grades; moreover, the distance varies through the course of the sentence. Figure 6 shows the variation in eye–voice span through elementary grades. Figure 7 extends the curve to adulthood. From second grade to fourth year of college, the eye–voice span almost doubles, on average. The increment in information-processing skill varies even more, since the material read by the subjects varied with their grade level. Skill with the language, memory span, and related phenomena enter in as explanations. For example, Fig. 8 shows the relation, collapsed across all subjects, between normal reading rate and eye–voice span. People who read at faster rates, irrespective of grade level, also tend to have larger spans. The increased rate is not due to a larger span; rather, good readers both are faster and have larger spans.

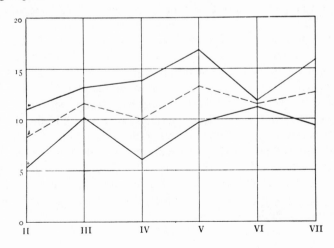

FIG. 6. Variations in eye–voice span through the elementary grades. The three lines are for best (top), poorest (bottom), and average (middle) performance. (After Buswell, 1920.)

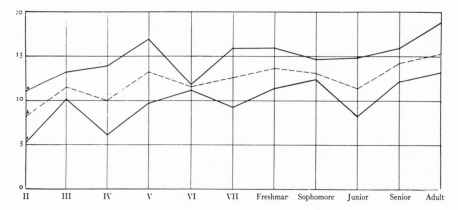

FIG. 7. Development of eye–voice span for all subjects, from grade school to adulthood: good (top), poor (bottom), and both (middle). (After Buswell, 1920.)

In studies of this kind the customary measurement was of the number of fixations in a line of print. In light of the psycholinguistic concern of the past decade regarding the proper unit of analysis for reading, it is interesting to note that even in 1920 Buswell showed that as far as eye movements are concerned, neither the word nor the line is the proper unit of analysis; the sentence itself is. In Fig. 9, the size of the eye–voice span is shown to decrease with progress through the sentence, being longest at the beginning and shortest at the end. The eye seemed to move at a regular rate in respect to frequency, Buswell found, but varied its input, taking a larger eyeful at the beginning of a sentence, and smaller portions as it progressed through the linguistic frame. This is especially curious since the subject of the sentence and the verb are usually in the earliest part of the sentence and only qualifications occur toward the end, in English. Are qualifications harder to understand than the main action? Or is the attenuation in size of span due to the upcoming full stop?

It is especially worthy of notice that Buswell found little if any relation between visual sensitivity and skill in reading. By "visual sensitivity" I mean the visual functions such as acuity, form threshold, stereopsis, and the like that the optometrist measures. In one study Buswell (1937) assessed the best 100 readers and the poorest 100 on a battery of visual tests, with the results as displayed in Table 1. Impaired visual capability, apparently, is not a necessary inhibitor of reading, nor is excellent visual capability a sure predictor of superior reading skill. The purely visual component is subservient to the cognitive one in acquiring information from the page.

Programmed Movements

How does the eye know where to go? Does it acquire some words and then decide where to go next? Does the eye perform two functions in parallel, part of it acquiring semantic information while another part assesses the cognitive terrain to decide where to go next? Are the eyes' movements preprogrammed, always marching in the same way despite variations in the signal? Buswell did not explicitly formulate a model of the control of the eye in reading; but he did seem to have some notions in mind. Their gist argues for a flexible, adaptive system rather than a preprogrammed one, and suggests an answer to these questions.

RELATION OF EYE-VOICE SPAN TO READING RATE—ALL SUBJECTS

Number of Subjects	Rate of Words per Second	Average Eye-Voice Span
	By Rate	
1	0–0.9	3.4
2	1–1.9	5.7
10	2–2.9	11.3
29	3–3.9	12.7
12	4–4.9	16.5
	By Eye-Voice Span	
3	1.6	3–5
7	2.9	6–8
10	3.3	9–11
24	3.5	12–14
4	4.1	15–17
5	3.8	18–20
1	4.8	21–23

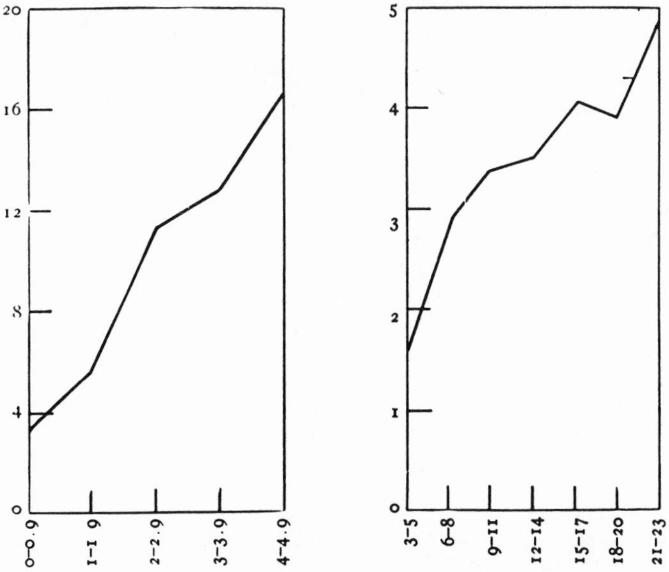

By rate **By eye-voice span**

FIG. 8. Relation between eye–voice span and reading rate. (a) By rate; (b) by eye–voice span. (After Buswell, 1920.)

TABLE 1
Number of Visual Tests Passed by 100
Adult Subjects with Lowest Reading-
Test Scores and by 100 Adult Subjects
with Highest Reading-Test Scores

Number of visual tests passed	Number in group of lowest 100	Number in group of highest 100
15	30	27
14	25	22
13	16	18
12	8	11
11	7	6
10	2	6
9	3	3
8	1	1
7 or fewer	7	1
Total subjects[a]	99	95
Median number of visual tests passed	13.7	13.6

[a]The visual tests for one subject in the low group
and for five subjects in the high group were incomplete.

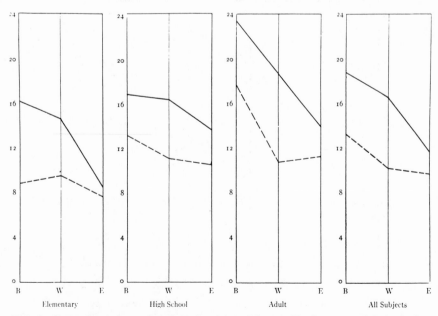

FIG. 9.   Eye–voice span as a function of position of the word in the sentence: B, beginning;
W, within; E, end. (After Buswell, 1920.)

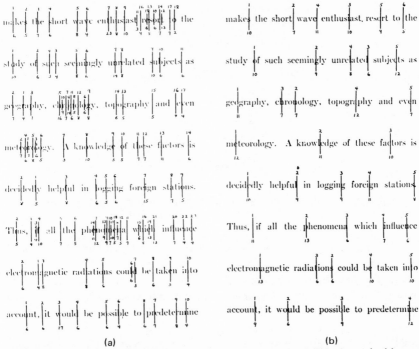

FIG. 10. Illustrating the rapid feedback that continues analysis of difficult words. (a) more limited reader; (b) more skilled reader. (After Buswell, 1937.)

One point he made several times is that reading is not a monolithic process; it is made up of constituent skills which individually contribute to performance. Thus the syntactic or semantic difficulty of a text can contribute to variation in the fixational movements, as witness the results for two readers on the same passage. In Fig. 10 one of the readers had a limited technical vocabulary, and the words *meteorology, chronology,* and *phenomena* caused this adult of limited competence a great deal of trouble. One could say there is some regularity of movement by the better reader, but not by the poorer. Notice, however, that the pattern-analyzing task the reader is performing apparently feeds its results back into the system quite rapidly, to have it continue the analysis of difficult words. With respect to sequence and duration of eye movements, Buswell reported that the likelihood of a regressive eye movement increased with an increase in the size of the eye–voice span: That is, positive deviations from some mean span value for an individual were associated with regressive movements, the eye presumably returning to pick up something the reader had missed. Parenthetically, in respect to this matter of control, Buswell reported that 39% of all regressive movements were to the second fixation on the line; the eye tended to undershoot its starting point in making a return sweep after finishing a line. I don't know whether this

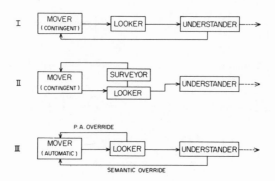

FIG. 11. Schematic representation of three models of the reader (see text).

would still hold up, or whether it was a matter of somewhat lesser literacy skills 50 years ago.

Both the number of fixations and the number of regressions varied widely among readers, but pause duration was remarkably stable. Table 2 shows that the number of fixations per line declined with an increase in reading skill, but there is less variation in the duration of a fixation. This variation, and the variation in the eye–voice span as a function of the part of the sentence being read, are votes for a model quite opposite that of a rigidly preprogrammed scanner and sampler; they are votes for a system which modifies its behavior adaptively to fit the characteristics of the text being sampled. How might such a system work?

One possibility is that each fixation determines where the eye will go next—ahead, back, above, below, and so forth—depending upon the information just acquired. This would be a cognitive semantic control system. A second possibility is that information acquired by the visual periphery acts as a ranging or guidance instrument to direct the eyes' movements. This is also a cognitive semantic control system, but with two functions being carried out. A third possibility seems to be raised by Buswell's work. The three models can be caricatured for convenience as made up of three components: a control system that moves the eyes, a system for acquiring the data the eyes are looking at, and a system concerned with its interpretation. In the cognitive model, I in Fig. 11, the mover moves the eye so that the looker is pointed at the sample, the looker acquires the sample, which is then operated on until it is understood, and that event is signaled back to the mover. The eyes' movements are thus directly contingent on the mind's understanding. Model II in Fig. 11 adds a scanner to the operations, in parallel with the data acquisition phase (that is, with the analysis of the sample being looked at), a device for assessing the terrain to determine where the eye should look next. Feedback from the scanner to the

TABLE 2
Comparative Data for 1,042 Subjects Showing Average Number of Fixations per Line, Average Number of Regressive Movements per Line, and Average Duration of Fixation Pauses

Selection read	Adult subjects grouped by last school grade attended					High-school seniors	University students	Pupils from grade VI	Remedial-reading pupils from junior high school
	VI or below	VII-VIII	IX-X	XI-XII	XIII or above				
Number of cases	122	225	201	204	152	50	38	20	30
Selection I (silent):									
Fixations	10.8	8.9	8.4	8.1	7.5	7.2	6.4	8.2	9.3
Regressive movements[a]	2.0	1.5	1.5	1.4	1.2	1.2	1.0	1.7	2.0
Duration of pauses[a]	7.9	7.3	7.2	7.2	7.1	6.7	6.1	7.9	8.1
Selection 2 (silent)									
Fixations	11.1	9.1	8.7	8.8	8.2	7.6	—[b]	—	9.3
Regressive movements[a]	2.3	1.7	1.7	1.8	1.6	1.5	—	—	2.1
Duration of pauses[a]	8.2	7.9	7.7	7.5	7.6	7.3	—	—	8.9
Selection 3 (silent)									
Fixations	9.9	8.9	8.7	8.6	8.1	7.3	—	—	—
Regressive movements[a]	1.9	1.6	1.5	1.6	1.5	1.2	—	—	—
Duration of pauses[a]	8.2	8.1	7.9	7.8	7.7	7.6	—	—	—
Selection 6 (oral)									
Fixations	13.2	10.6	10.3	10.0	9.6	8.8	—	—	—
Regressive movements[a]	2.7	2.0	2.0	1.9	1.8	1.5	—	—	—
Duration of pauses[a]	9.1	8.4	8.3	8.1	8.3	8.2	—	—	—

[a] In thirtieths of a second.
[b] Not tested.

mover directs the eyes' movements. Model III contains two feedback loops, one from the looker to the mover, and the second from the understander to the mover. The one from looker to mover is concerned with distortions in the pattern analysis (P.A. override), such as are illustrated in Fig. 10a, whereas the second feedback loop or override is concerned with distortions of comprehension. This third model, derived from Buswell, would be amplified as follows.

Suppose that the eye were driven by two impulses and possessed a gain control. One vector is lateral, the other is downward. The eyes' movement along a line of print is created by a "kicker" that bumps the eye along with a near-constant force on each kick. The distance each impulse drives the eye depends upon the setting of the gain control. That setting is established by cognitive factors related to difficulty of the text, vocabulary, familiarity of the subject matter, and the like. The easier the reader finds the text, the higher the gain setting, that is, the larger the distance moved for each "kick." In other words, the eyes' successive fixations on a line of print, or on a picture, are not determined movement by movement, as the semantic theories imply. Rather, a semiautomatic process drives the eye about the material in jumps that accord with the reader's processing ability.

Just such a model seems to be implicated by close examination of some of Buswell's results. The figures already displayed eliminate from consideration the idea of rigidly preprogrammed movements. The movements differ among people, and differ also for the same person on different parts of a passage. A simple semantic system is far too slow; moreover, we know from the eye–voice span that the eye is not looking at what the mouth is saying or the mind entertaining. For other reasons, a bifunctional model based on terrain assessment by the periphery and semantic analysis by the center may not be correct (Kolers & Lewis, 1972).

Consider the quasi-random model in light of the eyes' movements around a picture. Figures 12–15 are from Buswell (1935): Fig. 12 is a black and white version of the colored print that was examined; Fig. 13 shows all the fixations made by 42 subjects in a few seconds of viewing; Fig. 14 shows the first three fixations made by each of 40 subjects—notice the wide variation in sequence followed by different subjects; Fig. 15 shows the last three fixations. Again, wide individual differences in sequence of fixations can be seen.

A model that supposes that the grammatical regularity of a sentence or the semantic regularity of a picture must be preserved as the input to the visual system assumes that the perception of language, like the production of language, has to follow grammatical rules; that is to say, the assumption would be that the input into the eye must preserve the grammatical regularity of the sentence printed on the page. On this model, the eye would then look for the syntactic, semantic, and related regularities of the sentence; thus it would look at a sentence and present it to the mind in a way that preserved its linguistic sequence on the page. Similarly, in looking at a picture such a model would

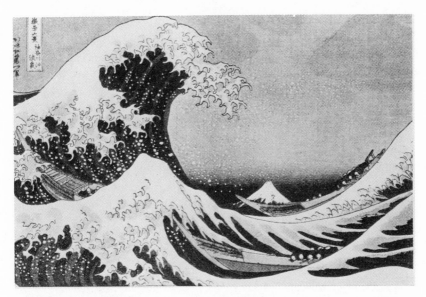

FIG. 12.   Black and white copy of Hokusai's "The Wave." (After Buswell, 1935.)

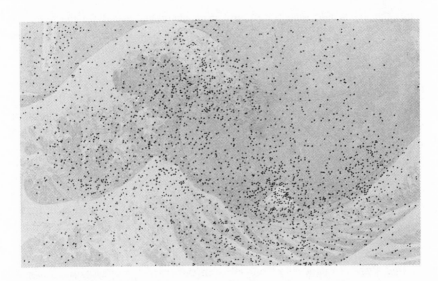

FIG. 13.   The black dots show the fixations made by 42 subjects looking at the print of Fig. 12. (After Buswell, 1935.)

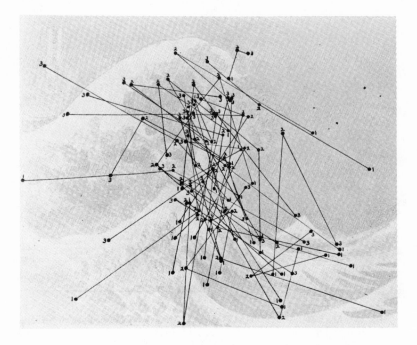

FIG. 14. The first three fixations by 40 subjects on the print of Fig. 12. (After Buswell, 1935.)

hold, the eye would scan the picture in a way that created for the mind the thematic or semantic message of the picture. The data, however, simply do not square with such models, and the assumptions underlying such models may be wrong.

Rather than supporting a grammarian's view, the enormous variation in sequence of looks says two other things. One is that different lookers take away substantially different messages from their encounters with the same sentences and pictures. They do not look in the same sequence; therefore, this assertion would be, they have not read the same sentence or seen the same picture. And yet, if we were to ask a dozen people, each of whom examined a sentence in his own way, what the content, message, or meaning of the sentence was, we would, I am sure, obtain a fair measure of agreement. Hence, a considerable degree of cognitive similarity would be obtained despite considerable difference in input. The second point the finding of irregularity makes is related to this: The input sequence has a wide range of tolerable variation, and cognitive processes act to regularize or "normalize" the input from radically different sequences of looks.

I find Buswell's data quite compelling in this respect, emphasizing the cognitive reordering of inputs made irregular by sampling eye movements rather than insisting on a regularized order of inputs. With such a model the control processes of eye movements are reduced to fairly simple form, as is appropriate to so peripheral an activity. Two vectors and a gain control seem sufficient for text and pictures, the gain control under continual adjustment by feedback from interpretative processes. Most movements are forward, but an override can interrupt the usual processing to search, to check out, or to recover something dropped. In other words, it is not necessary, on this model, that the content of each fixation be used to calculate the position of the next or the next-but-one fixation. The actual sequence can take on a near-random variation in amplitude and position, and the regularizing or ordering of inputs be carried out cognitively.

An illustration of such processes can be made with speech. A sentence spoken aloud, such as, "Floor dirty cleaned the she," is readily understood by people. In informal experiments I have found that simple declarative sentences up to about eight or nine words in length can be scrambled in many ways, and still be understood. When they are written down, even longer ones can be worked out, of course.

Cognitive Reordering

The principal thrust of this notion is that the brain can cope with irregular inputs because it has the power to localize them in respect to a sentence frame. The brain does not require that the inputs preserve the printed grammar. The point is made clearly with respect to the picture by Hokusai (Fig. 12). One's

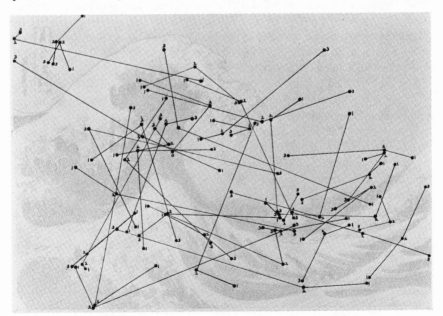

FIG. 15. The last three fixations by 40 subjects on the print of Fig. 12, with 3 representing the final one. (After Buswell, 1935.)

visual experience is that one is seeing the whole print all at once; but records of the eyes' movements tell us that a person samples the print, and knowledge of the anatomy of the eye tells us that the sampling is carried out best through segments extending only about 1° or 2° in diameter. As the eye moves about the print, the perceiver does not get a faulty impression about the location of parts of the picture. The location looked at second is not assigned erroneously to a location next to that sampled immediately previously; the temporal order of samples, that is to say, does not govern the spatial location assigned to them in the mind. The visual system must keep track of the spatial frame of reference within which it is sampling contents, and keep track of the location within that frame that each sample is derived from. Analogously, in reading sentences, the visual system samples different parts of sentences at different times, but the perceiver does not necessarily run the sentence parts together in the mind in correspondence to the order in which they are sampled. Rather, he manages to keep track of where in the sentence the different samples come from. To do so, his brain must tag samples with respect to their location, both in pictures and in sentences, mapping temporal order onto structural locations. Hence, neither the perception nor the memory of what is perceived can be the result of a straightforward listing or recording of samples.

Buswell never formalized this theory but he implied it. And the consequences of believing in an alternative theory are beautifully illustrated by him and Judd (Judd & Buswell, 1922). For this purpose they assumed that a normal fixation while reading a sentence extended over about 10 letter spaces (about 2° of visual angle). The subject for the test was a high school student studying a passage for paraphrase. Part of one sentence studied is illustrated, along with the sequence and duration of fixations, at the top of Fig. 16. Below that the figure lays out in order what each of the fixations 10 letters long would contain.

What is produced is gibberish. The wave of movement is roughly from left to right along the line of print, but successive lines are individually almost incomprehensible. Of course we don't know what the person was actually seeing; he may have concentrated his gaze upon single words in such a way that displays 10 letters long only caricature the real process. He may have "turned off" cognitively while his eye fixated. We know, after all, that one need not see all that the eye is pointed at; many selective processes intervene in perception, and such selective operations may have come into play here. There are, that is to say, many ways to divide the successive lines of print into words and phrases that make the content of individual fixations more coherent than is shown in Fig. 16. But no matter how one divides them to preserve coherence on a line-by-line basis, the sequence of fixations produces radically disordered messages. Hence, not all discrete inputs are represented discretely in consciousness. Disorder is not usually present in the reader's conscious experience; our experience is of coherent and regular messages. The implication is clear, therefore, that the order and clarity of the messages are properties achieved by some powerful cognitive operations, and are not merely reflections of the message the eye picks up from

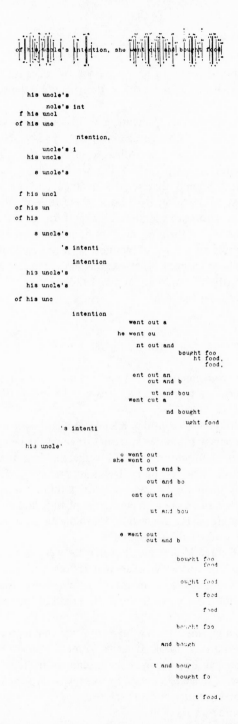

FIG. 16. The content of each of the fixations, 10 letters wide, made on the phrase shown at the top of the figure. (After Judd & Buswell, 1922.)

391

the printed page. More seems to be suppressed by saccades than theories of saccadic suppression allow for, and more is constructed by the mind than theory acknowledges.

The mind orders, arranges, supplements, and fills out the information the eye delivers to it. That is Buswell's message, very clearly. The ability to carry out these reconstructive processes varies with age, linguistic skills, IQ, interest, and many other properties of the perceiver. The work is done, moreover, by distributing attention to stimuli that require detailed analysis. In other words, perceivers learn how to perceive; they learn where to look; they learn how to find what they need. These are acquired skills, performed in service of a person trying to make sense out of the array he finds himself confronted with, whether it is the array of words on a page, of pictures, or of objects in the environment. Perceiving is in terms of meaning. That was Buswell's message. A strange remark to come from a dustbowl empiricist of the 1920's; but perhaps all the more believable, given that time and place.

DISCUSSION

COOPER: Could you comment to some extent on what is known about within-word sequences of fixations, i.e., between letters in the same word, in normal reading.

KOLERS: I don't know of anything reliable. As hard as it is to measure eye movements when a person is looking at flashes singly in the laboratory, it is, say, three or four orders of magnitude as hard to measure eye movements reliably when a person is reading. No reliability figures are presented with Buswell's data and, in light of the apparatus he had available, I think one has to be a little cautious. The data presented are all from frames of film, and one must allow for some variance. You are asking a question directed at a measure of precision in analysis that I think we haven't arrived at yet.

MACKWORTH: George Miller said that maybe psychology should be given back to the people, and one way to do that is for us to give each other new methods. I think that Buswell's approach of eye–voice span measurement suggests a new method, that is, to find out the length of the span at the start of reading a sentence.

In other words, simply measure the time from the moment a person starts to read to the time he starts to speak. It seems to me that point you emphasized, about the eye–voice span being long at the beginning of the sentence, might be shown over a very wide range of subjects by this relatively simple method, rather than getting involved in a series of data analyses.

KOLERS: I am sure you are right.

MACKWORTH: This should be compared to the blanking out method (cutting off the light and measuring how long they continue to speak) because I'd be interested to know if Buswell's method gets at the same things as were found in the Project Literacy studies.

KOLERS: The technique, for those not familiar with the method to which Dr. Mackworth is referring, is another way of studying the eye–voice span. The method is to let a person start reading aloud, then shut off the display and measure the number of words the person continues saying. You can do it just once to the naive subject and then he is forever alerted to what you are doing. I think what Buswell was doing was monitoring this eye–voice span in a continuing way, finding that it varied through the course of the sentence.

NICKERSON: How much of the eye–voice span data can be accounted for by the simple assumption that the subject or reader is always exactly one fixation point ahead of what he is saying?

KOLERS: I am not up on the eye–voice span literature. I do remember that John Geyer, a psychologist at Rutgers, did rather an elaborate study on it a couple of years ago. My recollection is that he found the fixity was not in distance, but in time. That is, the mouth lagged the eye by about a second, which, of course, is more like three or four fixations than one fixation.

HABER: It also varied with difficulty though.

KOLERS: Sure, it varied with difficulty, short-term memory, and so on. I don't think you can necessarily point to a constant. The idea of information being quickly fed back within one fixation doesn't strike me as reliable.

COOPER: Yet by making a conscious effort you can reduce the eye–voice span to zero.

KOLERS: Yes, if you have a subject who has a great deal of practice in controlling fixation patterns of his eyes. You can train him so that he doesn't move his eye until after he's said what he is looking at. But that is not really normal reading.

MACKWORTH: Recently, Wood (1974) has shown that when you are matching letters by matching an audio letter to a visual letter or two audios and two visuals, there is an enormous rapid switch from the visual letter to the audio letter. In other words, in 150 msec the visual presentation is converted into an acoustic image, if you will.

Now, I wondered how you would handle that kind of data. I know that it may not be a necessary channel, but it is an available channel.

KOLERS: How can congenitally deaf people learn to read, as they do?

MACKWORTH: I have examined them on the eye camera, and I have found that they do not in fact read beyond the third-grade level even at Gallaudet College. So the point I would ask you about is, if we have normal people, how can you be so sure that it doesn't go into the acoustic system as well as through the visual system if there is this available processing mechanism?

KOLERS: As I said in my paper, there is a considerable controversy over whether reading requires some kind of translation into auditory representations. For myself, I believe that the auditory translation is not necessary, although it often occurs. I think Dr. Hochberg is going to make the opposite argument, and that strikes me as a good point of transition.

HOCHBERG: Not really the opposite.

KOLERS: Good. I have persuaded you already.

Afterthoughts

After returning from the conference, I sent a copy of my paper to Dr. Buswell to insure that I had not misquoted or misrepresented him. The reply I received pointed out a couple of errors of citation and localization; but more than that, it conveyed a sense of the spirit and concerns that motivated Buswell and his colleagues in their work. I found the letter so evocative of the spirit that I thought others would like to read it as well. It follows in its entirety edited only to reflect the appropriate page numbers.

> 202 Zephyr Circle
> La Crosse, Wisconsin 54601
> August 11, 1974

Dr. Paul A. Kolers
Department of Psychology
University of Toronto
Toronto, Canada

Dear Dr. Kolers:

Thank you for your letter of August 2nd and for the copy of your paper on eye movements. It is both interesting and pleasing to find a renewed activity in a type of research that kept me busy for a good many years. Your treatment of my early work is generous. Describing it as "data-oriented empiricism" is quite correct. In the 1920's our main concern was to break away from the a priori pedagogy of that time and to build up a body of objective data as a base for defensible educational theory. Statistical sophistication had not gone much beyond correlations and the terminology of theoretical models was yet to come. Yet, they were thrilling times for young researchers.

May I suggest two additional items that might be of interest to you. First is a paper (copy enclosed) written in 1946[1] in which I tried to bring together some of the findings of perceptual research and to apply them to the teaching of reading. The second is a monograph on eye movements in reading modern languages which carries a little further the work reported by Judd and myself in 1922. I was the junior contributor to the earlier monograph and major credit for it belongs to Judd rather than me. The later study, entitled "A Laboratory Study of the Reading of Modern Foreign-Languages" (Macmilliam, 1928)[2] is probably in the university library. If not, I have an extra copy that I will send you. You may wish to add these two items to your bibliography.

A few trivia: On page 374, line 29 is the phrase "frame by frame." Since our film ran continuously, rather than by jerks or frames as in moving picture photography, it might be more clear to say "foot by foot". On page 379, line 7 from the bottom and again

---

[1] Dr. Buswell is referring to Buswell (1947).
[2] See Buswell (1928).

in the 24th line on page 386 you use the word "mouth." Although your use is probably more correct, the term "voice" has become customary in the literature, as in eye–voice span rather than eye–mouth span. On page 392, 14th line you use the word "dustbowl" empiricist. Since Chicago was a thousand miles from the dustbowl I would feel more natural to be a "Midwest" empiricist.

I am glad to have this opportunity to make your acquaintance by letter. I hope that you will keep me informed of further work that you do. With best wishes, I am

Sincerely yours,
Guy T. Buswell

VI.2

Toward a Speech-Plan Eye-Movement Model of Reading[1]

Julian Hochberg

Columbia University

Dr. Kolers ended in an emphasis on the importance of cognitive functions in sorting out the scrambled input to the visual system, and on the importance of selective attention. I would like to do the following: discuss briefly a cognitive model of the reading process; take a first stab at just how that sorting out of the scrambled input occurs, and how selective attention works in the course of highly skilled reading; and report a number of experiments that serve to support that model.

If I have to characterize the model that I will discuss, it will be in terms of two features that Kolers indicated he thought were contraindicated. First, this will be a *bifunctional* model, in the sense that it holds parafoveal vision to be extremely important in the skilled reading process. Second, skilled reading will be viewed as being "merely implicit" speech (in his terms), or more specifically, as being mediated by speech programs. As we shall see, implicit speech is a far more complex psychological function than a mouthing of phonemes and I think implicit speech itself is not "merely implicit speech."

The model is outlined in Fig. 1. It was constructed to deal with the data and phenomena of selective attention (Hochberg, 1968; 1970a) and of attentive listening in particular, and was not originally designed with the reading process in mind. But I think that the same implicit speech mechanisms are at work in both skilled reading and attentive listening (Hochberg & Brooks, 1970), and that is my excuse for starting with this model. I will outline it now, and come back to it from time to time.

[1] The research described here was supported by the National Institute of Child Health and Human Development, Grant No. HD-4213-01.

It runs like this. At the top of Fig. 1 are message strings A, B, and C in row I. These are units of utterance. These units are flexible and not rigidly fixed. Basically they are chunks (Simon, 1974). Each unit of utterance has a set of distinctive features in the linguistic sense of the term and as Gibson (1965) uses them. The features are represented by the numerals below the boxes, 1, 2, and 3 on chunk A, 1 and 2 on chunk B, and 1, 2, 3, and 4 on chunk C.

The listener's responses are represented in the next row, II. He produces *speech plans* in response to the message strings, i.e., in response to the auditory stimulus patterns. Now, it is my assumption (and the assumption of at least some other people who have thought about the problem [e.g., Neisser, 1967)] that the picture I am giving you holds for listening in general. It seems quite likely that it holds for selective listening. Whether it does or not, something very much like this must hold for the *shadowing task* with which selective attention is often measured: in this task, the subject's job is to repeat *with as little lag as possible* what it is that the speaker is telling him. The model quite naturally explains why subjects who are asked to shadow a message on one of two competing channels can recall the contents of that channel, but not the contents of the other channel: it is the formulation and testing of speech plans that comprise the act of attentive listening, and with the right selection of information load, the listener will be able to formulate such plans for only one channel (Hochberg, 1970a).

If it is a single channel to which the subject is listening (or which he is shadowing), there is of course no need to invoke *selective attention* in describing his performance. But I believe that the process remains essentially the same whether the subject is listening attentively to one channel or to one of several competing channels: the very nature of listening is a selective activation of sets of speech plans (row II in Fig. 1). Which plans get activated depends both upon what the subject's intentions are (e.g., who it is he is trying to shadow) and upon the constraints imposed by what he has *encoded* up to this point.

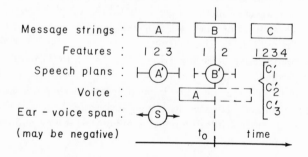

FIG. 1.   A model of speech plans in shadowing spoken messages.

In Fig. 1, the speech plans are inscribed in circles with brackets coming out at each side; the ends of the brackets are drawn so as to be coterminous with the message string to which the speech plan refers. Message string A is in the speaker's past. The present is marked as t_0 at the bottom of that diagram. (The arrow showing the lag between the presentation of the message string and the beginning of the utterance—the *ear–voice span*—is of some magnitude that has not been of particular concern in connection with the problem of listening to speech. But if time permits, we will talk about what that magnitude is in the reading process where it has been of much concern indeed—i.e., where the lag appears as the *eye–voice span.*

At t_0, the listener is shown about to activate speech plan B'. This is fortunate because, in fact, the speaker is then uttering message string B. The listener has started to activate speech plan B' on the basis of one of the features that he has received (feature B_1) and, of course, on the basis of whatever anticipations he has been led to form by the contingencies set by the previous speech plan (A'). He is not yet fully certain that the message string is indeed unit B; he has another feature yet to test (feature B_2), and he is waiting for the confirmation he will receive when that stimulus feature appears.

The speech plan B' is the one that he holds in readiness to utter when he comes to the next string after A', and the one that he will in fact be able to recall later. *What he does not encode in his own speech plan he will not remember* (at least he will not remember it very long). Note that in this interpretation, selective attention follows from the fact that the listener has time and resources to anticipate, test, and encode only one line of discourse. The other channels (if there are other messages competing for his attention) are not rejected by any "filter"—they are simply lost because they far exceed his memory span in their unencoded form. If some compelling signal, like the listener's name, is spoken on one of the competing channels, he will of course hear it and switch attention to that channel. We will see that a similar phenomenon can be generated in reading as well.

Still waiting in the wings are the responses that the listener is ready to make to the next message string, which has not yet been spoken by the speaker and which I have indicated as C_1', C_2', C_3', C_n'. The listener doesn't *know* what the next string is going to be, of course; but the fact that he has heard the previous message strings, and is now entertaining B, usually strongly constrains his choices for C.

Now we have to get to the listener's own utterances. Normally, it is reasonable to assume, I think, that active listening entails some equivalent of the beginning of the utterance, whether or not the listener's vocal apparatus is fully activated (and he therefore speaks aloud—let's call these token speech readinesses "articulatory plans"). In normal listening, the articulatory plans are readied but are not fully activated; in the shadowing experiments the subject is required to activate his articulatory plans as rapidly but as correctly as possible. And so he will, in its turn, utter a message string which has some lag or latency with respect to the speaker's utterance. This lag is indicated by the arrow S, indicating the ear–voice span between the speaker's utterance of the message string and the listener's own corresponding utterance of that phrase.

Now, notice that in Fig. 1, the subject is saying "A" well after A was spoken, while he is engaged in formulating or testing the speech plan for B'. So the ear–voice span in this case has a positive value. But the ear–voice span can have a *negative* value: It is easy to demonstrate a negative ear–voice span by asking your audience to shadow something that is *very* familiar, like the Gettysburg Address, as closely as possible, and then stopping short. In fact, if you merely pause, you will find that your shadow will actually *lead* you–as long, of course, as you are speaking highly redundant material. So the ear–voice span may be negative, which is going to be important later.

Now, it seems most likely that the same processes that go on in attentive listening to message strings occur in skilled reading: that is, that we anticipate what is going to come next (and interpolate what has been said in some part of the text that we have not looked at closely); that these "constructions" are determined by context; and that in fact the processes of shadowing and skilled reading are identical in all respects save two. The two differences are these: (1) in the reading process, when the subject need not speak aloud, he can elide great chunks of the material, skipping entirely the redundant or uninteresting material without anybody's telling him that he's failed in his task; and (2) the reader can use his eyes to select what he will receive (which of course he cannot do while he is listening) and, more important, he can move his eyes so as to pace the input to his own needs.

And consequently, the eye-movement aspect of the looking–"subarticulating"–listening–reading process is our main entry to understanding both active listening and skilled reading: the reader's eye movements are sensitive to the intake and comprehension process simply because they mediate his choice in what he is going to "hear" and when he is going to hear it.

At this point, I think we have to start getting more precise about the control of the eye movements, and about the way the results of those eye movements must be interpreted. We have had pretty good general statements about how eye movements serve the reading process, as Kolers pointed out, for 50 years. I think that Buswell's conclusions (1937) were right, by and large, with some minor elaborations and revisions that I will propose.

First, I would like to distinguish the two different kinds of guidance systems that must move the eyes: we can distinguish *peripheral search guidance* and *cognitive search guidance* as separable functions (Hochberg, 1970b). Let me give you pure examples of each function simply to indicate that there are such different systems, and that they can be called upon when needed. And then we will try to see how they interact.

Examples of peripheral search guidance are provided by the experiments represented in Fig. 2. These are sequences of presentations (sometimes produced tachistoscopically, sometimes produced by motion pictures serving as a multi-field tachistoscope) in which the following generic procedure is used: In Fig. 2a, frame i (shown at the extreme left of the series of presentations) is a fixation point. The subject starts the sequence of views by pressing a button. The next presentation (frame ii) displays a stimulus at some place at some randomly determined distance and direction from the fixation point. In this case (Fig. 2a), the stimulus is a word, "wood," that appears in the upper right-hand corner of the screen for 125 msec (which is not enough time for the subject to move his eye to the word). This is followed by a blank screen (frame iii) for a brief period of time (whose purpose is to decrease the sensory detectability of the change per se, between frames ii and iv, if there is any change on that particular trial). In the last frame (iv), the stimulus appears again, for some variable duration; in the trial shown in Fig. 2a, that duration is 125 msec. By the end of this frame, the subject has indeed gotten his eye from the fixation point (which was at the center of the screen) to the point at which the stimulus appeared. If the reader has obtained any information from his peripheral view of the initial presentation (frame ii), before his eye had a chance to leave the fixation point, he should be able to recognize the stimulus in frame iv with a shorter exposure—i.e., there should be a *saving*—than would be required if he had not seen frame ii. If the stimulus has been changed between frame ii and frame iv, as it was in Fig. 2a, the amount of the savings (which can of course be negative, as well as zero or positive) can tell us whether his peripheral vision can distinguish the features by which the stimuli differ (e.g., "word" in frame iv versus "wood" in frame ii). This procedure was devised by Roger Nelson and myself (Nelson, 1972; Nelson & Hochberg, unpublished data) to measure the functional acuity of the periphery to features like those used in recognizing text. Traditional measures rely on the subject's report of what he sees at some point in the periphery, and such measures could be invalid because it might well be the main function of peripheral vision to constrain the effects of subsequent foveal fixation (and not primarily to permit recognition on the basis of peripheral vision alone). What Nelson found was that this procedure gave gross acuity curves similar to those produced by more traditional measures; that specific letter information was not picked up much into the periphery; and in fact that any word (regardless of the letters of which it was composed) would produce some savings when compared to a line of equal size (Nelson, 1972). This procedure is a promising one, and does give us a measure of the functional acuity of the periphery. But it does not permit us to measure the *functional reading acuity* of the periphery, i.e., to measure what features, at what distances from the fovea, affect the ongoing course of reading. That aspect is being studied elegantly by McConkie and by Haber.

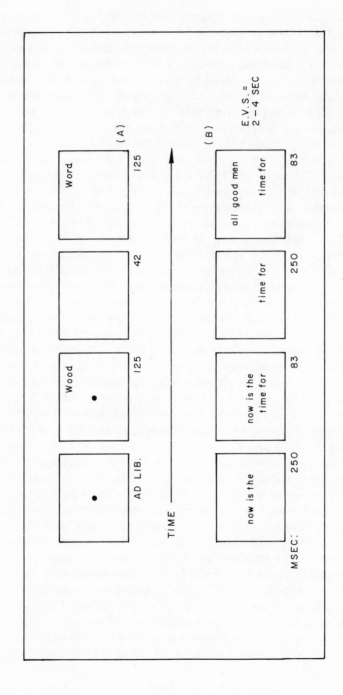

FIG. 2. A demonstration of reading by means of eye movements that are directed by peripheral search guidance alone.

Notice what we do have in this procedure, however: only the peripheral information can guide the eye to the word, and the savings that *are* found show that the eye movements that connect the two views of the words do serve a reading-related function. Moreover, subjects can actually read continuous text, presented in this discontinuous fashion. In a pilot study by Virginia Brooks and myself, sequential presentations were as shown in Fig. 2b. As some thought will show, this procedure requires the subject to move his eye to randomly determined places, for one fixation at a time, to pick up the successive segments of the message.

People differ widely in their ability to perform this task. It is not a comfortable task under any conditions, and eye–voice span rises to 2–4 sec of lag. (This is the equivalent of a fairly large number of fixations for the voice to lag behind the eye, and obviously requires redundant text.) But the point is that the subject's eye movements, by means of which he reads, are clearly being guided solely by peripheral indications of where he should look next. And that is a pure example of peripheral search guidance.

We don't know how much the peripheral guidance system contributes to normal reading ability because peripheral acuity is too poor to provide more than the grossest sort of information about the text. Various attempts that we have made to modify the individuals' use of peripheral search guidance in reading, by means of training sessions, have had only small effects. Although this may in part be attributable to the relatively short training periods that could be provided in the experimental sessions at our disposal, we shall see that there are other reasons to consider peripheral guidance to be less important in determining reading ability than the cognitive guidance system, which we will consider next.

Cognitive search guidance is somewhat more difficult to demonstrate in a pure case. I think it has been done in one or both of the following two experiments.

In Fig. 3 is an example from some work by Fisher (1973) in which the subject has to search out a word that is embedded in a paragraph, and the time required for him to find the word is measured. The paragraph is subjected to various kinds of mutilation. What is important to us in that particular experiment is that the subject may be searching exactly the same paragraph, for exactly the same word spelled in the same way, but with two different meanings. One of the meanings would lead the subject to expect the word in a particular part of that sentence, the other meaning would not. The subject is given one of the two different meanings by means of a defining phrase, as shown in the right-hand part of Fig. 3. His search time is affected by the meaning with which he searches the paragraph. This implies strongly, but not unequivocally, that the subject knew where to move his eye because of the grammatical constraints on the word for which he was searching. The reason I say "not unequivocally" is because something else must also be happening (an hypothesis that I think Fisher also raises). The subject may not be recognizing merely the word itself—he may be recognizing an entire phrase or even a clause in which that word is embedded, in

404   JULIAN HOCHBERG

Stimulus phrase	msec / word	Use in paragraph
a royal <u>subject</u>	146	rights of the subject
to <u>sub</u>ject oneself	186	(D. Fisher)

FIG. 3. A demonstration that cognitive factors affect search time: knowing the meaning of a homonym decreases the time required to find it. After Fisher (1973).

which case he's got a wider target than a word to aim at. That is, his eye may not actually have reached the target word at the time he reported its presence. But even if that target-size factor contributes to Fisher's results (and to all of skilled reading), I think one can demonstrate that in fact eye movement is guided by knowledge of where to look.

Figure 4 illustrates an experiment by Brooks and me (unpublished data) in which a subject is shown a nursery rhyme (which he knows). A word is given to him, and hs is supposed to tell us whether it is correctly spelled or misspelled, and we record his eye movements as he searches. As soon as he sees the word, he is told to freeze on it—not to look further—and then to report on whether the word is correct or not. In this case (Fig. 4a) the word is "fetch," and it is spelled wrong. The reader will reach that word in an average of 1.5 fixations.

The control paragraphs are matched in various ways. The one shown in Fig. 4b is matched for word length and for some other features. The word for which the subject must search (which would also be one of the words used in the Jack and Jill selection) would be "crown." When it is in the same location that "fetch" was shown in, it takes the reader's eye about three or four saccades to get there.

The fact is, then, that his eye's movement is guided to some degree by what the reader knows about the terrain. That is, if he knows where information is

Jack and Jill went up the hill to tetch a pail of water Jack fell down and . . . (a)	Tom and Bill goes in and rill Up crown a file to bacon Like mall loud . . . (b)

FIG. 4. A second demonstration of cognitive search guidance: it requires fewer eye movements to detect (a) whether or not "fetch" is misspelled, than (b) whether or not "crown" is misspelled.

likely to appear, the reader can move his eye there. And we now know with reasonable assurance that the subjects had no way of knowing that the word was there by picking it up in peripheral vision: as McConkie has shown us, the readers can't recognize words that far out from the fovea. These experiments provide examples of cognitive guidance: they show that the eye can be directed to where the reader knows information should be found. But they do so in the context of search instructions, and I know of no experiments directly to this point in the context of skilled reading. Perhaps the large regressive movement back to a word that the reader makes when he discovers later on that he must have misread the word (Geyer, 1966) is the closest we have come to a direct record of cognitive guidance in the course of reading.

Now, this raises another point: as Buswell says, the good reader is a flexible reader. That could be a scary statement. If flexible means that his eye movements are unpredictable, then the model that we are going to end up with can only be a qualitative and descriptive one. But I think we can fill in the model that I have been outlining so that it can make a start at being reasonably specific about the changes in behavior that comprise "flexibility" of eye movements in skilled reading.

There have been various ways devised to study peripheral search guidance and cognitive search guidance. Until recently, filling in the text (or mutilating it in some other fashion) was the main method: e.g., if the space between words has been filled in, as in Fig. 5e, reading rate decreases very considerably. It was originally proposed (Hochberg, 1970b) that the filling in of the interword spaces interferes with peripheral search guidance, in that the eye doesn't have any indications of where to fixate next because word boundaries (and hence word length and punctuation cues) are obscured by this method. Research of this sort has continued, but we should note that the method also introduces additional sources of confusion and possibly masking effects (Woodworth, 1938, p. 720), and it is clearly subject to very strong limitations. The most direct method for studying peripheral and cognitive guidance in the reading process, a method that various people have been tooling up for quite a while, is to change what the subject is reading or looking at, at various distances from his fixation point, before he has moved his eye to that point; in other words, to give the reader a "window" of some size that moves as his eyes move. Outside of that window, we can alter the text in various ways, and see how those alterations *which always remain in the reader's peripheral vision,* affect his reading behavior. For example, in our laboratory, we have tried to shape reading behavior (and investigate form-scanning behavior) by using motion pictures to simulate the sequence of retinal images that the viewer would receive if his eye movements followed some particular sequence of fixations. In general the procedures were as follows: The window of clear vision exposed the text by being moved (with or without some signal as to where it would be moved to) from one place to the next at from 2–4 times per sec; outside of the window, the text was degraded (e.g., blurred), so as

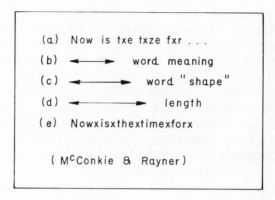

FIG. 5. Methods for studying the distances from the fovea over which different kinds of information are picked up, and some schematized findings. After McConkie and Raynor (1973).

to be illegible. In order to read the text, therefore, the viewer had to move his eyes so as to keep the window fixated. Although this set of experiments was concerned primarily with simulating and modifying eye movements, the distance into the periphery that letter information is used could be estimated by determining the effect of window size on reading performance. (The estimate was about eight letter spaces.) But the procedure obviously has major disadvantages as compared to the most desirable method, in which the window is made to coincide with the viewer's fixation point by having eye position measures control an on-line computer display.

The most complete and successful use of this method appears to have been accomplished in McConkie's laboratory. McConkie and Rayner (1975) have done some really beautiful work on this problem, and I want to talk about just one point of their conclusions because I want to build on that point.

Figure 5a is like one of their conditions. The window is around "now is." The words that are in the text that is outside of the window have the same terminal and initial letters that they normally possess, but their internal letters are changed, so the "h" has been taken out of "the," the "im" is out of "time," etc., and the deleted letters are replaced by meaningless filler. Or "the" might be replaced by "tie," when it is outside of the window, so that the word has been altered but remains meaningful. If the reader detects that a change has occurred when his fovea (and the window) reach the word that has been altered (e.g., from "tie" to "the"), his fixation duration is found to increase, and that finding tells us that the window was not large enough to include all of the peripheral retina that the subject used to detect those features that are being manipulated.

Now, what McConkie and Rayner find is that within about four letter spaces to the right of the fixation point the actual letter-by-letter word meaning is picked up (i.e., the subject can tell the difference between a meaningless string of letters and a meaningful string of letters within that distance). Beyond that out to about 10 letter spaces, the shape of the words (in the sense that word shapes are preserved in Fig. 5a) is important. Out to something like 13 or 14, the interword spaces (i.e., the cues to word length) remain important. Past 13 or 14, word-length cues are no longer important.

In general, then, we have strong indications that out to about 13 or 14 letter units, the reading system does use word-length cues (and it avoids functors), which is the main function that it originally seemed plausible to me to attribute to peripheral search guidance (Hochberg, 1970b); but more, it also uses word shape in the sense of the initial and terminal letters' being important out to about 10 spaces.

Now, this finding is at first glance very surprising, because according to the model in Fig. 1 we should be able to process only one unit at a time. That was a central feature of the listening-speaking-reading model, a feature that automatically accounts for selective attention, and I'm naturally reluctant to discard my entire model. Also, Kolers and Lewis (1972) have in fact shown that you cannot recognize two words that are simultaneously presented (this is a simplification of their findings, but is a reasonable one).

So the question I have to answer is this: *Why is peripheral search guidance so good,* i.e., how come word shape is used that far out in the periphery?

In order to answer this question, we will have to return to what the implicit speech units are that I invoked in Fig. 1. In Fig. 1, strings A', B', and C' are not necessarily syllables or words. They may be entire phrases. It depends upon how strong the internal constraints are within the word strings that are being shadowed; that is, the size of a listening-speaking-reading unit is highly variable, and a unit may be many letters long. What evidence is there for the existence of such units, and how might they be measured?

First, of course, is the old finding, dating back to R. B. Cattell, that although only a few unrelated letters can be identified in a single brief glance, a familiar word or phrase, many letters long, can be recognized in the same time (cf. Miller, 1956). Second, indirect evidence suggests that these perceptual differences between familiar and unfamiliar words are due largely to encoding or memory differences, not primarily to changes in sensory reception. Most directly, a series of experiments by Glanzer and his colleagues has shown that learning is almost identical for phrases and for nonsense syllables (cf. Glanzer & Razel, 1974), and Simon (1974) has demonstrated a very similar phenomenon, that is, the time it takes a subject to fix a phrase in memory is just about the same as the time it takes him to fix a single digit. In fact, Glanzer and Razel found that the serial position effect (which appears to be a measure of the number of units being loaded into memory), as measured in free-recall learning, is essentially the same for entire proverbs (independent of length) as it is for nonsense syllables. What makes a sequence of sounds into a unit of listening–speaking–reading behavior is, it seems clear, the fact that the subject can generate the sequence himself once he is given the label (or some characteristic features) by which to identify it. [In the literature on speech sound recognition, a directly analogous theory is called *analysis by synthesis* (cf. Neisser, 1967); at the level that we are discussing, the term that Neisser uses is "constructionist."] But to return to why the McConkie and Rayner data seem to show that we process peripherally and foveally recognized words simultaneously: I think that we aren't really doing that at all, and that the data reflect a quite different process.

What I am proposing is that one of the things that the peripheral word shape does for the skilled reader is that it helps him to identify message strings up to 12 to 14 characters long as units—*if* they are indeed speech units, and are highly redundant ones. For example, in Fig. 5a, suppose you were fixated on the "N" in now, and you have "the time for" out in peripheral vision. You could probably recognize the terminal and initial letters of "time" and the initial letter of "for." The four letters that are discerned foveally, plus what is seen peripherally, comprise the *distinctive features* by which you can recognize the string as a single unit. And, of course, the previous context may so constrain your anticipations that fewer features will be sufficient to enable you to recognize what the group of words must be—perhaps word length alone will suffice for recognition of the string much of the time (as rhythm or inflection will often suffice in listening). (And the fact that you do not actually have to discern the letters within each of those strings out in the periphery is something we know is true, anyway, from the kind of "proof readers' errors" that normally occur in reading.)

So the first thing that the peripheral vision does in reading is to provide us with extended views of strings that help us to identify them as strings. Next, it gives the eye a definite place in the field to go when it is time to move. That is still another reason why the filling in Fig. 5e is important and interferes with reading. (Another reason, as we saw, is that it masks both word-length and punctuation cues, and the terminal letters.) A third thing that the periphery contributes to reading is that it gives you a second view of the other end of the string when you have moved your eye to the new position, thus providing an additional view of the speech hypothesis that is being tested.

The processes that I have described should generate at least four different kinds of reading. We would expect the skilled reader to be able to produce these different kinds of reading as they are as needed. And we should be able to make some sort of a stab at specifying the characteristics of those four kinds of components of normal reading.

Type I reading (word decoding by analysis of the word) requires the viewer to determine each letter's location in the word relative to the other letters. Because a skilled reader knows what the "shape" of syllable-length or word-length letter strings is, he has to do Type I reading only infrequently. With a totally new word (or with a random collection of letters), however, even the skilled reader should have to move his eye back and forth within a word; unskilled readers (and this includes those who are unfamiliar with the vocabulary or with the internal syntactic and semantic constraints of the text in question) should have to do this more frequently. We can't state this kind of reading speed in words per minute, because we don't know its frequency of occurrence and because the speed of recognition will depend on the word (e.g., on the amount of internal masking, on how familiar the reader is with the word, on how much it is constrained by context), and because the process of word recognition is itself complex and not well understood. So Type I reading introduces an indeterminate factor into overall reading rate, but its occurrence should be at least statistically predictable (given measurable characteristics of reader and text), and it has identifiable characteristics (e.g., we should expect out-of-order fixations on such words, like letter 1, 4, 3, 2, etc.). We can therefore attempt to partial out Type I reading in order to examine the other components.

In *Type II reading*, the skilled reader can pick up words out to about four to six letter spaces per fixation. He does this when the material is not highly familiar (which will be true with most text, for many readers), and/or when the task is to read "well" or carefully. If we figure about four eye movements per second, 4 to 6 letters per fixation, and approximately 5 letters per word, that gives us a reading rate of 4 X 60 X 5/5 = 240 words per min. This is illustrated in Fig. 6.

In *Type III reading*, the reader is using features like word length, from as far out as 12 to 14 letters, to the right of the fixation point, which should give approximately 4 X 60 X 12/5 = 580–680 words per min. This is usually the upper limit of what we are willing to call reading—that is, performance in which the reader has *some* information, even if it is only word length, for *each* word in

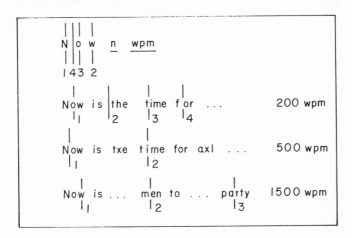

FIG. 6. How reliance on the different kinds of information generates different reading rates.

the speech plan that he is fitting to the text. At this speed he is using letter strings for all they are worth, and he can only do it with material that is heavily redundant to him: i.e., this rate should be possible only with strings that are three or so words long, strings that he is able to recognize when he is given one clear word, plus the initial letter and word shape of another word, plus the word length of the last word. With such strings, Type III reading rates should be possible.

It is interesting with regard to Type III reading to consider how pictures are looked at. We know that eye movements are directed to those parts of the display that viewers rate as being informative (Antes, 1974; Brooks, 1961; Hochberg & Brooks, 1962; Mackworth & Morandi, 1967; Pollack & Spence, 1968), which implies that the periphery has guided the eye to the informative regions. Antes finds that the first eye movements made on viewing a picture are large in extent and that the pauses between eye movements are of short duration; subsequently, fixations are longer and saccades smaller: the eye first surveys the field, then examines the details (see Fig. 7). I think Antes' data are of general importance and will repay close examination. But they are suggestive here for the following two reasons: first, we should note that the saccades are directed to definite places in peripheral vision, and are not merely sent off for some excursion whose extent is determined by internal factors, regardless of what awaits the eye at the end of the saccade; second, the first few saccades are about 4.5° in extent, which is about 9 letter spaces in McConkie's setup, and the first few fixations are 200 msec in duration, so that the looking behavior in the rapid initial survey is roughly equivalent to reading rates of about 500 words per min. Admittedly, Antes' tasks did not demand cognitive search guidance, nor directed skimming; furthermore we don't know how illiterates would perform

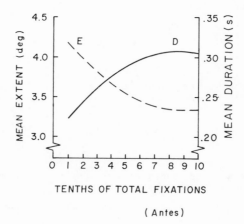

(Antes)

FIG. 7. In looking at pictures, fixations become progressively longer in duration and closer in space. (After data by Antes, 1974.)

with his pictures, so that we can't say whether fast reading performance taps the same eye movements that we normally use to scan scenes and pictures, as has been suggested (Hochberg, 1970b, 1972); whether Antes' data reflect reading habits transferred to pictorial inspection; or whether the rough similarity of the numbers is mere coincidence. But it does seem worthwhile to explore reading and picture-looking in tandem in the hope, not without some basis, that the two will illuminate each other.

The same number appears in another context: if the redundancy of text is decreased (by compressing it), then silent reading proceeds at what looks like the same number of ideas per minute (cf. Keen, 1973), meaning of course that the number of words per minute goes up as the speech is compressed. But word length increases in the process, so translating the reading rate back into letter units brings it to about 7 letters per fixation.

Considering that we don't know the mix of Types II and III reading that went into these experiments, the numbers seem nicely poised between the 4–6 and 10–14 magic numbers that McConkie and Rayner have given us.

Type IV reading, a fourth kind of skilled reading, like the first is too variable to assign an inherent number. Unlike Type III, it doesn't require the reader to look at, or get any information at all about, each and every word: in Type IV "reading"–or skimming–the subject doesn't have to pick up information except maybe once every 8, 10, or 15 words if the text is really redundant: if the text is the Gettysburg Address, I just have to sample it every couple of sentences to see whether it is still the Gettysburg Address. And since I know the material so well, it is not even very important that I look at it in some particular place or order. As Kolers' example showed, we are perfectly capable of supplying the canonical order of a disordered presentation like: "the floor dirty clean up she will," or whatever, as long as we know that it's a sentence.

KOLERS: That's the wrong order.

HOCHBERG: Strange, it sounded right to me.

We really have a lot of knowledge about what some message is likely to be, given pieces of it. The ability to "reconstruct" distal objects from fragmentary views is central to the perceptual process in general, and we should not be surprised to find that ability exploited in highly skilled reading. But more of that later. In Fig. 6d, I have given an example that will generate a rate of 1,500 words per min: if you know the phrase, "now is the time for all good men to come to the aid of their party," you can certainly check whether a given string of letters really is the phrase merely by looking at *now, is, men, party,* and thereby read the text at the 1,500 words a min. (We don't know, at present, whether such widely separated fixations are directed toward where information is likely to be found—which is what cognitive search guidance would do, and which we know is possible, from the experiments represented in Fig. 4—or whether where the large saccades land is determined by more mechanical factors, and the reader interpolates between whatever features these saccades furnish him.) We have some shaky and indirect evidence that subjects can learn to adjust their eye movements to the "padded" material shown in Fig. 8, which suggests that those movements are at least partially under cognitive guidance, but more reliable and direct data are needed on this point. We do know that the subject can use his knowledge of where information should be found in order to speed his search (e.g., Fig. 4), but we do not know whether this ability is normally used in reading. Instead of casting his eye ahead to seek some specific piece of information, the subject, when skimming, may merely look ahead, beyond what he has just fixated, and either fit what he finds there into the speech plan he has anticipated, or interpolate a plausible connective between what follows and what preceded. I shall return to this question shortly. Let me summarize up to this point.

Of the four components of reading performance that I have described, Types I and IV are indeterminate as to extent of saccade and duration of fixation, making reading rate correspondingly indeterminate. But Type I fixations can be partialled out post facto (and perhaps predicted in advance by some combination of vocabulary and Cloze tests). And when we do remove Type I fixations, the eye-movement records of three good and three poor readers, reading the same copy (Buswell, 1920), show us the good readers to be averaging 8.8, 9.1, and 10.4 letters per fixation, and the poor readers averaging 5.1, 4.5, and 4.8—just about what we would expect from Type II and Type III reading, respectively (see Fig. 6). (Interestingly enough, the two poor readers who made substantial numbers of regressive movements averaged 12.8 and 7.8 in their subsequent fixations of fresh text—presumably because those movements traversed old territory. Type IV, which is skimming or speed reading, doesn't occur much in most laboratory reading studies, but it probably does occur a great deal

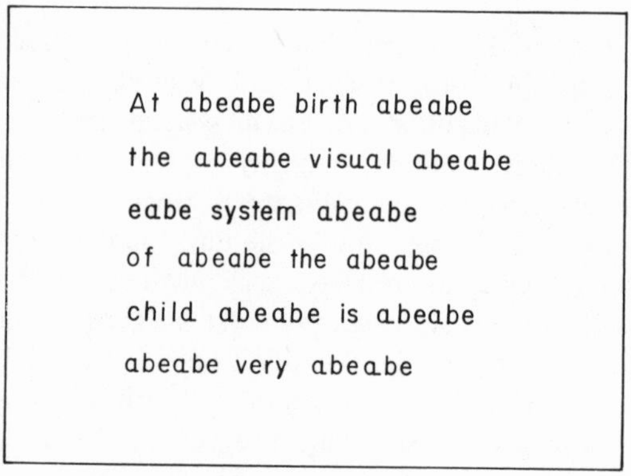

At abeabe birth abeabe
the abeabe visual abeabe
eabe system abeabe
of abeabe the abeabe
child abeabe is abeabe
abeabe very abeabe

FIG. 8. An attempt to shape fixations to avoid uninformative letter strings.

in natural settings and deserves study. It may be possible to predict the characteristics of Type IV reading, in any case, from the parameters of the individual's ability to shadow the text in question, or from his ability to reconstruct the message from randomly selected fragments.

In this model, then, the general parameters of reading follow from the length of letter-and-space strings that the subject has anticipated and tested in each glance, and from the acuity limits that are imposed on each fixation. I would like then to address a question that McConkie has raised, which is, "why talk about anticipation?" I guess you could ask why all the elaborate anticipatory speech-plan structure of the model in Fig. 1 is needed when you might simply say instead that the reader uses whatever prior information he has to help him pick up the information about what the presently viewed text is, and then goes on to the next section of text.

I cannot make a really powerful case against this simple formulation, except that it overlooks a lot of coincidences and a lot of marginal information that seem to fit the model in Fig. 1. I think we will need a lot of research before we can separate these formulations. Let me show some of what would have to be overlooked if we were to discard the anticipatory speech-plan model:

1. There is a great deal of similarity between the characteristics of active listening, or shadowing, on the one hand—which demonstrably involves anticipation, as I indicated at the beginning of the talk—and reading on the other.

2. Eye–voice span and silent reading are correlated (which Kolers referred to and interpreted in a different way). And specifically, to the same point, there is the following demonstration by Buswell: the better the reader (that is, the more rapidly he reads and the closer his fixations approach the Type III limit of 14 letter spaces per fixation), the more his silent reading is interfered with by a "tongue twister" in the text (this is graphed in Fig. 9).

Now, that to me is a dead giveaway that the reader has been formulating speech programs. Why should a tongue twister be a tongue twister to him otherwise, considering the fact that he is not reading aloud? (By the one piece of Buswell's logic that I fail to follow—and my admiration for the man is as strong as Kolers' is—he takes this finding as evidence that the good silent reader is *not* using implicit or silent speech. I think that he may have done this because the grand idea of plans had not occurred back then, and implicit speech would probably have meant to Buswell actual and real-time movements of lips and tongue and larynx.)

3. By the Stroop test (1935), if I show you a printed word, the odds are very good that you will say that word, especially if I potentiate it, i.e., if I force you to utter *some* sound.

In the usual demonstration, the word might be "green," printed in red ink, and the subject required to name the color of the ink. He either says "green," or displays an unusually long latency before saying "red." The paradigm can be used to study how words constrain each other (Warren, 1972) which should

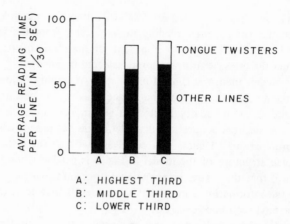

FIG. 9. How tongue twisters affect silent reading by readers of three levels of ability (after data by Buswell, 1937).

make it of considerable use in predicting the occurrence of Type III and IV reading, but the point here is that there are very close links (undoubtedly strongly learned links) between the printed word on the one hand and potential speech on the other.

4. If it is true, as I argue, that the printed word normally (or frequently) serves as the set of visual features by which to test an anticipatory speech plan, we should be able to use that fact to teach children to recognize printed words. Now, we had previously tried a variety of "interventions" designed to help people learn to make shorter fixation pauses and longer saccades. Believing from the model in Fig. 1 that the eye movements serve the active speech-plan-testing process and not vice versa, it seems plausible that no amount of training of the eye-movement process as such is going to have any effect (and in fact, we have tried a variety of training procedures that have recapitulated old data to that point). If, however, we use the following procedure, derived from the model in Fig. 1, we find that we can apparently teach a subject to read words which otherwise are not within his reading vocabulary (Hochberg, Brief, & Glanzer, unpublished data; Brief, unpublished data).

Consider Fig. 10, the top row: "opened the door of the apartment. . ." is shown to the reader (a child) on a rear-projection movie screen. A ball (for which Sam Gibbon is partly to blame) bounces from word to word or from syllable to syllable over the text. The filled circle in Fig. 10 signifies that the ball is now over the final syllable of "apartment"; the other unfilled circles show where the fixation points were previously. At the same time as he watches the ball bouncing along, the child hears a voice reading part or all of the sentence (in language reasonably congenial to his normal dialect). In the experimental condition, unlike the control condition, a word of text is left out—is not spoken aloud—by the voice.

The child's task is to shadow the speech, i.e., to repeat what the voice says as closely as possible. Since he is under pressure, he should use whatever his eye can do to help him. Let's say that the word "apartment" is one that is within his speaking vocabulary, but is not within his reading vocabulary, and is the word that is omitted from the spoken channel in the experimental group: that is, the child, shadowing the voice, says, "opened the door of the." When the voice that he is shadowing "goes blank," he's got to say something, and he has only the text word there before him, with all of the context of the previous message to constrain his response alternatives to the printed word. So he says "opened the door of the apartment," and goes on shadowing the voice, which has resumed. If we test his reading vocabulary again after such a performance, we find that those words which were both constrained by the sentences (as measured by Cloze test), and are outside of his reading vocabulary but within his speaking vocabulary, *and* which were left out of the sound track, he now can read. There are certain controls needed (for possible differential emphasis of the omitted words, by virtue of their omission) before we can be sure that we have an interesting and painless way to increase reading vocabulary at a practical level. More to the present point is the fact that the subject's speech plans, on which he bases his shadowing of the voice, can provide him with the correct response to make when next he sees the word, which was previously beyond his ability to read without context, in a list of other words.

This experiment comes close to (but falls short of) being a real demonstration that reading may proceed by the formulation of speech plans. One of the main things it lacks by way of being such a demonstration is that the reader is, after

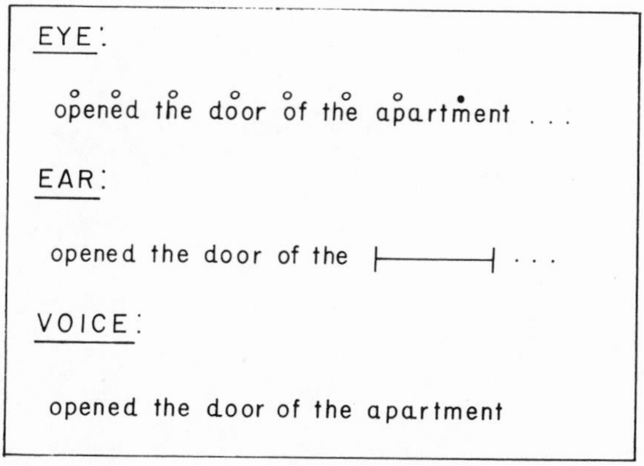

FIG. 10. A shadowing experiment, using the model of Fig. 1 to lead the reader to guess (correctly) at a word that is not yet in his reading vocabulary.

all, shadowing aloud. And he may not do anything of the sort when he reads silently. We have to do the experiment over again, bouncing ball and all, and see if we can get the same results when the subject doesn't ever actually say the words. If that happens, I think the burden of proof will then rest upon the proposal that the subject is merely "picking up information."

All of this is not to say that we *must* use anticipatory speech plans in order to integrate successive glances, or even that this is the only way to read. It is quite clear that we do have the ability to store structure, and test structure, and anticipate structure in ways that have nothing to do with words, and that requires a different line of research than I am going to be able to discuss.

But in any case, I believe that any "information-retrieval" model of skilled reading (Type III and better) will have to have the following characteristics: it will need a buffer store; a provision for selective attention (or selective testing and retention); a capacity for dealing with chunks of verbal material (*and once we allow chunking, we automatically provide the capacity for anticipation and interpolation*); and a set of susceptibilities to influence by the factors that influence speech and speech plans that I have noted here. I don't see how that account can differ much in its general features from the model presented here.

VI.3

Spatial Factors in Reading and Search: The Case for Space

Dennis F. Fisher

U.S. Army Human Engineering Laboratory

Many of the previous papers have emphasized hypotheses about changes in visual processing from peripheral and foveal retinal involvement to foveal processing alone or what I will call the shrinking functional visual field. I am going to describe data which I feel lend support to the assumption that the two processes described by Hochberg (1970b), i.e., peripheral search guidance and cognitive search guidance, are active. Basically, these are locating and identifying processes. Peripheral search guidance was hypothesized to be a process that is activated during eye movements and tuned to pick up contours (physical cues and features) in the periphery. Information about important cues and features is sent to a higher order processing unit, cognitive search guidance, for integration and meaning extraction. As meaning increases, the peripheral search guidance process interrogates larger areas of the text. The primary concern in the experiments was to examine the effects of manipulating two spatial features, namely, word shape and word boundary on reading and on search. These features are considered particularly relevant cues for the visual periphery during reading.

I am going to separate the experiments into two distinct phases representing very basic examinations of word-shape and word-boundary information processing. In the first phase I will describe adult data to provide estimates of skilled reader performance. In the second phase I will describe developmental data to show progressions in performance efficiency resulting from experience with the various cues and features in printed text. The data for both phases were collected with and without eye-movement recordings while subjects read and searched paragraphs of normal and spatially transformed text.

The nine typographical variations that were used in these experiments (Fisher 1973, 1975; Fisher & Lefton, 1976; Spragins, Lefton, & Fisher, 1976) are

417

shown in Table 1. Number 1 shows the *normal-type* (case)–*normal-space* condition. Numbers 4 and 7 show normal type with the spaces filled and absent altogether: three spacing manipulations were used in an attempt to eliminate word-boundary information in successive steps. Numbers 2, 5, and 8 show the three spacing conditions combined with capital letters: the spaces between the words were filled with larger symbols corresponding to the size of the capitals. Numbers 3, 6, and 9 show the three spacing manipulations combined with alternating capitals and lower case letters.

Reading and search measures for all these variations will be presented; however, for simplicity I will concentrate on the most extreme cases, i.e., numbers 1 and 9. The sizes of the displays were approximately 18–20° of visual angle and a typical five-letter word subtended and angle of approximately 2°.

Figure 1 shows adult reading speeds for the nine stimulus variations. The subject was asked simply to read nine 200-word paragraphs, one in each of the nine variations. The numbers in the data points correspond to the number of the variations in Table 1. As an inducement to read for comprehension, subjects were asked multiple-choice questions after each paragraph. It can be seen that there was about a 3:1 decrement in reading speed moving from the control, or normal-type–normal-space condition to the *alternating-type–space-absent* condition.

Knowing that these manipulations slow down reading, how do they affect high-speed visual search through paragraphs? More importantly, can we draw an analogy between reading and search processes if the data for each task are affected similarly by these manipulations? To examine these questions, the same nine typographical manipulations were shown to another group of subjects, whose task was to find a target word embedded in the paragraph. Once the paragraph was presented, the subjects had to respond as quickly as they could by pushing a reaction-time button and identifying the location of the target word. The search data are shown in Fig. 2.

It can be seen that these curves are very similar to those shown in Fig. 1. Again there was a 3:1 slowdown in search time with the most extreme spatial manipulations. Unlike the data from the reading task, however, no differences were found during search between the filled and space-absent conditions. However, the over-all features of the text affected both reading speed and search speed similarly.

It can be seen that there was a 3:1 speed reduction from condition 1 to 9, and also a 3:1 decrease in speed from reading to search. Search was three times as fast as reading, and both reading and search speed were greatly reduced when the word-boundary and word-shape information were disturbed. What are the effects of these task and spatial manipulations on eye movements?

Figure 3 shows eye-movement records for the normal-type–normal-spacing condition. These were recorded on the EG&G/HEL Oculometer developed by EG&G Inc., Las Vegas for the U.S. Army Human Engineering Laboratory that was

TABLE 1
Space and Type Combinations

1

The government of Henry the Seventh, of his son, and
of his grandchildren was, on the whole, more arbitrary
than that of the Plantagenets. Personal character may

4

The+government+of+Henry+the+Seventh,+of+his+son,+and++++
of+his+grandchildren+was,+on+the+whole,+more+arbitrary++
than+that+of+the+Plantagenets.++Personal+character+may++

7

ThegovernmentofHenrytheSeventh,ofhisson,andofhis
grandchildrenwas,onthewhole,morearbitrarythanthat
ofthePlantagenets.Personalcharactermayinsomedegree

2

THE GOVERNMENT OF HENRY THE SEVENTH, OF HIS SON, AND
OF HIS GRANDCHILDREN WAS, ON THE WHOLE, MORE ARBITRARY
THAN THAT OF THE PLANTAGENETS. PERSONAL CHARACTER MAY

5

THE@GOVERNMENT@OF@HENRY@THE@SEVENTH,@OF@HIS@SON,@AND@@@@
OF@HIS@GRANDCHILDREN@WAS,@ON@THE@WHOLE,@MORE@ARBITRARY@@
THAN@THAT@OF@THE@PLANTAGENETS.@@PERSONAL@CHARACTER@MAY@@

8

THEGOVERNMENTOFHENRYTHESEVENTH,OFHISSON,ANDOFHIS
GRANDCHILDRENWAS,ONTHEWHOLE,MOREARBITRARYTHANTHAT
OFTHEPLANTAGENETS.PERSONALCHARACTERMAYINSOMEDEGREE

3

ThE GoVeRnMeNt oF HeNrY ThE SeVeNtH, oF HiS SoN, aNd
Of hIs gRaNdChIlDrEn wAs, On tHe wHoLe, MoRe aRbItRaRy
ThAn tHaT Of tHe pLaNtAgEnEtS. PeRsOnAl cHaRaCtEr mAy

6

ThE@GoVeRnMeNt@oF@HeNrY@ThE@SeVeNtH,@oF@HiS@SoN,@aNd@@@@
Of@hIs@gRaNdChIlDrEn@wAs,@On@tHe@wHoLe,@MoRe@aRbItRaRy@@
ThAn@tHaT@Of@tHe@pLaNtAgEnEtS.@@PeRsOnAl@cHaRaCtEr@mAy@@

9

ThEgOvErNmEnToFhEnRyThEsEvEnTh,oFhIsSoN,AnDoFhIs
GrAnDcHiLdReNwAs,oNtHeWhOlE,MoReArBiTrArYtHaNtHaT
oFtHePlAnTaGeNeTs.pErSoNaLcHaRaCtErMaYiNsOmEdEgReE

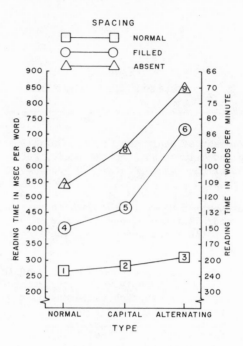

FIG. 1.   Reading times for the nine space–type combinations.

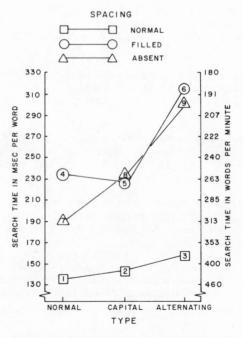

FIG. 2.   Search times for the nine space–type combinations.

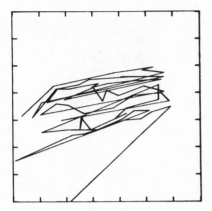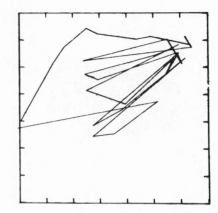

FIG. 3. Scan-path records of reading (left) and searching (right) through text of normal type–normal spacing.

previously described by Lambert. The left side of the figure shows the reading record and the right side shows the search record using the same paragraph. The subject indicated he was finished by moving his eyes off the screen. Scan path-discontinuities within the records indicate fixations, while those at the end of the records indicate that the end of the passage was reached or that the target was found. Subjects read and searched through approximately 50 to 100 words. The results are summarized in Table 2. It can be seen that with normal text, reading speed was slower and perceptual span (words and spaces per fixation) smaller than when engaged in search. Fixation duration, however, was the same for both tasks.

TABLE 2
Reading and Search Efficiency Measures
for Scan-Path Records in Figs. 3 and 4

Measure	Normal case–Normal space		Alternating case–No space	
	Reading	Search	Reading	Search
Rate (words/min)	180	256	36	148
Fixation duration (msec)	266	260	417	310
Words (read or searched	66	47	116	59
Words per fixation	1.05	1.9	.27	1.00
Spaces (read or searched)	351	270	511	260
Spaces per fixation	5.6	11.8	1.2	4.4

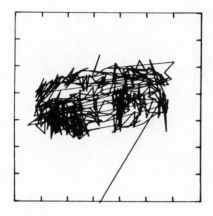 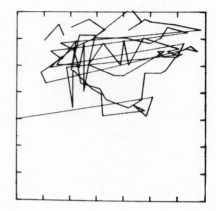

FIG. 4. Scan-path records of reading (left) and searching (right) through text of alternating type–absent spacing.

Figure 4 shows the eye-movement records of reading and search for the alternating-type–space-absent condition. Once again the reading record is on the left and the search record is on the right. A summary of these data is also found in Table 2. In this condition, search progressed more than four times as fast as reading, fixation duration was two-thirds as long, and perceptual span was about four times as large as in reading.

In general, for both search conditions (normal-type–normal-spacing and alternating-type–space-absent), there were fewer fixations while fixation durations remained about the same. Not so for reading: reading speed decreased to about one-third normal rate and the number of fixations increased with increasing spatial complexity. Perceptual span (character spaces per fixation) was smaller for reading than for search and decreased further in both tasks when spatial cues were perturbed.

What causes the differences between reading and search? One factor is most likely the comprehension demands of the tasks. Reading requires the extraction and retention of meaningful information, whereas search simply requires locating a specific target. Another difference was reflected by the lack of space–case interdependence in search that was found in reading. The differential priorities to comprehension and spatial feature demands between the two tasks are probably reflected in the eye-movement data. In short, these data generally show that both comprehension and spatial factors can reduce the functional visual field of view.

One of the other interesting and potentially important aspects of the reading record in Fig. 4 is the large number of vertical eye movements. They are essentially nonexistent during search when the same stimulus materials are used. They are not typical regressions; they are practically vertical. The movements are intriguing and we are going to continue to investigate them. In addition, the angular extent of the saccadic movements, between the two records, is dramatically different.

Table 3 (from Taylor, 1965), shows the developmental progression of a number of eye-movement parameters. There seems to be a developmental progression in reading efficiency (perceptual or recognition span), reading rate, fixation duration, and number of regressions. Generally, the average perceptual span increased from .45 words at first grade up to 1.11 words per fixation for college students. Average duration of fixations also decreased slightly (about 40 msec) over an 11-year span.

Figure 5 shows developmental data that were collected at the University of South Carolina (Fisher & Lefton, 1976) using the same typographical manipulations described above. The paragraphs were standardized for difficulty within but not between grade levels. All of the data are represented here, but comparing the most extreme age groups (third grade and adult) and the most extreme typographical conditions (numbers 1 and 9) will best serve the purpose of the remainder of the discussion. There is a very definite developmental progression with normal spacing. That is, reading speed increased dramatically with age. When we perturbed the text, the youngest children showed only minor changes in reading speed. The older children and adults, however, showed large decrements in speed between normal and perturbed conditions. Essentially, all groups were reduced to the word-by-word reading technique used by the youngest children. The basic reading speed of the third graders stayed fairly constant even

TABLE 3

Averages for Measurable Components of the Fundamental
Reading Skill

| Measure | \multicolumn{13}{c}{Grade level[a]} |
	1	2	3	4	5	6	7	8	9	10	11	12	Col.
Fixations (per 100 words)	224	174	155	139	129	120	114	109	105	101	96	94	90
Regressions (per 100 words)	52	40	35	31	28	25	23	21	20	19	18	17	15
Average span of recognition (words)	.45	.57	.65	.72	.78	.83	.88	.92	.95	.99	1.04	1.06	1.11
Average duration of fixation (sec)	.33	.30	.28	.27	.27	.27	.27	.27	.27	.26	.26	.25	.24
Rate with comprehension (words/min)	80	115	138	158	173	185	195	204	214	224	237	250	280

[a]First-grade averages are those of pupils capable of reading silently material of 1.8 difficulty with at least 70% comprenhension. Above grade 1, averages are those of students at midyear, reading silently material of midyear difficulty with at least 70% comprehension. (From Taylor, 1965, Table 2, p. 193. Reproduced with permission of the American Educational Research Association.)

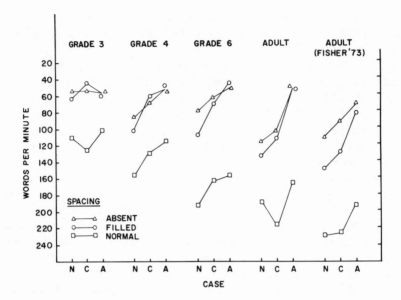

FIG. 5. Reading times for the nine space–case combinations for each of four developmental levels.

under the most perturbed conditions and, in fact, turned out to be the basic reading level for all groups in the most perturbed conditions.

From these data it was hypothesized that constraining the number of available peripheral cues causes a constriction in the field of view. This constriction results in a functional "tunnel-vision reading" situation. Everyone gets down to that very basic word-by-word reading rate when the periphery is rendered nonfunctional. The third grader has probably not yet learned to use peripheral cues; therefore, he remains relatively unaffected by the typographical changes. The detrimental effects of these manipulations increase with age as the reader relies more heavily on the peripheral cues. In effect, an increased reliance on peripheral cues leads to faster reading of normal type, but when the cues are perturbed in the alternating-case–absent-space condition, the differences in reading speed between the conditions increased with age. Similar trends are also apparent during search (Fisher & Lefton, 1976).

The next step was to examine the developmental trends as shown by the eye-movement recordings (Spragins, 1974). These data are summarized in Table 4. In the table, reading and search data are contrasted for third graders and adults on a number of measures.

There was a dramatic, almost 2:1, increase in speed for adults between reading and search in the normal-case–normal-space conditions. This was not the case for the young children. In the alternating-type–space-absent condition there was an

TABLE 4
Reading and Search Efficiency Measures

Measure	Reading				Search			
	Normal case—normal space		Alt. case—no space		Normal case—normal space		Alt. case—no space	
	3rd grade	Adult	3rd grade	Adult	3rd grade	Adult	3rd grade	Adult
Rate (words/min)	130	260	50	60	162	440	110	190
Words per fixation	.71 .65[a]	1.24 1.11[a]	.33	.35	1.0	2.2	.60	.85
Spaces per fixation	3.3	5.5	1.3	2.5	4.0	10.0	2.5	4.0
Fixations per minute	184	209	181	172	204	205	160	194
Fixation duration (msec)	400	235	393	365	274	242	348	290

[a]From Taylor (1965).

almost 3:1 change for the adults but only a 2:1 change for the children. Again this reflects the bottoming out situation that we noticed in the previous figure.

A measure previously pointed out in Taylor's (1965) data is perceptual span or the average amount of information in words or character spaces available during a single fixation. The span increased on the average from 1.24 to 2.2 words per fixation for normal text and from .35 to .85 words per fixation for perturbed text during reading and search, respectively.

Characters per fixation may, in fact, be a more sensitive measure and more relevant to an examination and explanation of the shrinking visual field since some of the typography has no spaces. When normal text was read, the average number of character spaces per fixation was 5.5. When we perturbed the typography it dropped to 2.25, a 2:1 shrinkage. The adults' field of view was greatly enlarged, almost 2:1 during search as compared with reading. For the children, whether reading or searching, there was not much difference between perceptual spans. Again this seems to reflect a lack of childrens' ability to use peripheral cues effectively.

The number of fixations per minute was also examined. Adults engaged in reading and search averaged 209 and 205 fixations per min, respectively. In fact, these data did not change dramatically when in the totally perturbed situation. Moreover, regressive eye movements were not affected by case, space, or grade level in either reading or search.

The manipulations of word shape and word boundary generally led to a reduction in the number of fixations per minute and to slower reading rates. Subjects not only looked at fewer character spaces per fixation, but they generally spent more time on each fixation, thus the reading rate was reduced.

Differences between search and reading may reflect a gross measure of comprehension, e.g., reading equals search plus comprehension. It is suggested that when the spatial features are perturbed, the subject is no longer capable of extracting meaningful information, namely word shape and word boundary, from the periphery. This leads to a shrinking of the functional visual field and of the perceptual span. The data presented indicate that contextual as well as physical features affect the size of the functional visual field.

In summary, developmental and adult data have been presented showing the effects of two types of spatial manipulations on reading and search speed as well as a number of eye-movement measures. These data are interpreted as providing support for Hochberg's (1970b) two-stage peripheral-to-central visual-processing model. With increasing development and experience with printed text, readers and searchers tend to rely more heavily on peripheral cues to enhance reading and search efficiency. Data were presented that indicate that contextual as well as physical features affect the size of the functional visual field of view. The most potent of the variables of type (case) and space appears to have been space. Case change does not cause a great decrease in reading or search speed until combined with the additional feature of perturbed word boundary, or what we call a case for space.

DISCUSSION

MACKWORTH: Do you think that the difference you got on the first pair of scan paths, where in contrast to reading, the search record showed a failure to return to the left-hand side of the page, could be an indication of what you might call the right–left processing advantage? As is well known, the right field is better at processing words than the left field and it might be that that advantage is increased in reading as opposed to peripheral search. In other words, the difference between search and reading may be due to the fact that you can search with both halves of the field of view, but when reading you have to use more of the right half. The reason I make that point is that neurophysiologists, such as Marshall (1973), tend to find that the right field is especially good when you are processing verbs. What the question boils down to is, are the noted differences between reading and search really due to the fact that when you are reading English you have to use the right field, but when you search you can use both?

FISHER: I really don't have a definitive answer to your question. To speculate, I think one reason the scan paths show up that way involves a difference in the general level of contextual awareness between the two tasks.

If we can say that the periphery picks up physical-feature information, but not semantic information, it may be able to pick up enough gross features to preclude having to return fully to the left side of the next line. Recent data (Fisher, 1973) suggest that during search, right-side perturbations slow down search more than left-side perturbations when targets are on the corresponding sides. In reading, there is an extra demand of comprehension. We probably become more conservative guessers and must make additionally sure of what is coming next, so we go all the way back to the beginning of the next line.

VI.4

The Use of Eye-Movement Data in Determining the Perceptual Span in Reading [1]

George W. McConkie

Cornell University

I appreciated Leonard Matin's comments earlier in which he recognized the fact that there were some people at the meeting whose basic interest is not really in eye movements. I have to admit to being one of those. I am interested in the nature of reading and hope that the study of eye behavior will lead me to better understand that important activity.

Much of what has been said thus far has been quite interesting and informative to me, although I find that there is much additional complexity when I start trying to consider the nature of eye-movement behavior in reading.

I could spend time trying to respond to some of Hochberg's concerns, but I think the group that is here will probably be more interested in other issues. Hochberg and I can have our discussion in private later. What I want to do now is to deal with the problem of the size of the perceptual span in reading.

When I consider the direction which should be taken in constructing an adequate model of the reading process, one of the first questions I encounter concerns the size of the perceptual span. The rest of the model will look quite different, it seems to me, if I assume a very narrow span that views only a single word or two than if I assume a very broad perceptual span that takes in much visual complexity over a very wide area.

To investigate this question, a graduate student, Keith Rayner, who is presently on the faculty at the University of Rochester, and I spent a year at the

[1] The research described here was funded through a grant under the U.S. Office of Education Basic Research in Education program, and a National Institute of Mental Health Special Fellowship awarded to the author. It was carried out at the Artificial Intelligence Laboratory at the Massachusetts Institute of Technology.

Artificial Intelligence Laboratory at M.I.T. developing the kind of computer-based eye-position-controlled display system which Gould and Senders were suggesting earlier. Let me stress at the outset that I view this as a first try on our part to see if such a system could be developed and to see if meaningful data could be produced with it.

I worked with the basic fear that such strange visual displays, with the stimulus changing on each fixation, might do nothing except produce emotional break-downs in our subjects. But in general the results met our highest hopes. At the end of the year we had to return to real life at Cornell University, much to our regret, and leave our baby behind. However, this month we anticipate delivery of a computer graphics system with which this research can be continued at Cornell. With our previous experience we were able to select a computer system that is much more adequate for the research and we will design our programs differently to produce a more optimal research environment for these types of studies. Hopefully in a year or two we will be able to report more data from this type of research.

Here I will describe two experiments carried out with the M.I.T. equipment. The first I will refer to as the *window study* and the second experiment as the *boundary study*. First the window study.

The goal of the window study was to track the eye during reading and on each fixation to place a range of normal text right at the point of fixation, but to mutilate the visual image of the text in the periphery in some specified manner. To do this we selected passages of about 500 words each from a high school psychology text and then produced mutilated versions of each of the passages in the following manner. For one version, each letter was replaced by a letter visually confusable with it, with ascending letters replacing other ascending letters, descenders replacing descenders, and so on. This produced text which was totally unreadable, but which preserved some of the visual characteristics of the original text, namely gross word shape, certain additional featural details of the words themselves, and the word length patterns of the original text. This version I will call the confusable (C) version since letters were replaced by letters visually confusable with them.

A second form of mutilation was to replace each character with a letter of a different visual shape, including replacing ascenders and descenders with other letters and other letters with ascenders and descenders. Here the word length patterns were preserved, but the word shape was mutilated. This was called the nonconfusable (NC) condition.

For the third form of mutilation, each letter of the original was replaced by an X, again preserving word-length patterns, while giving a constant pattern so far as word shape was concerned. This is called the X version.

And finally, an additional form of each of these versions was produced by replacing spaces and punctuation marks with appropriate letters, X's in the X condition, other letters in the other conditions. This destroyed all word-length information, producing a new form of each version called the filled (F) form. The versions with spaces remaining were called the spaces (S) form. Thus there were six types of text mutilation used, C-S, C-F, NC-S, NC-F, X-S, and X-F.

Now, to conduct an experiment, the original page of text and one mutilated version of it were stored in the computer's core memory. The computer displayed the mutilated version on a cathode-ray tube (CRT), producing a nonreadable stimulus. However, the computer was also receiving input from a Biometric eye-movement monitoring unit and sampling the eye position 60 times a sec. When it detected the person fixating the first line of text, the computer immediately replaced the characters on the CRT with corresponding characters from the normal text within a certain region on that line around the point of fixation. Thus, a window was created around the fixation point within which normal text was seen. Beyond the window the mutilated text remained, presenting a pattern to peripheral vision which preserved certain visual characteristics of the original text, but destroyed others.

When the reader made a saccade, the letters in the window returned to the mutilated form and the letters in the new window area around the new fixation were transformed to normal text. Thus the subject could read quite normally, for wherever he looked he saw normal text in his central vision. However, the experimenter could modify the size of that window and could determine the type of visual pattern which was presented to the periphery.

Figure 1 illustrates this process. The top line of the figure shows the original text, actually a shortened line from one of the passages. The second line shows the X version of the passage with the spaces retained (X-S). The dots under the first line show the location of four fixations on that line, and then the bottom four lines show what that line looked like during each of those four fixations. You see the window moving across the line.

In the experiment we had six subjects, all juniors and seniors in high school, who were identified as being superior readers. We used eight window sizes

```
  I.  distributed.  It appears that pitch-naming ability can be improved,
                        o          o             o
 II.  xxxxxxxxxxxx.  Xx xxxxxxxx xxxx xxxxx-xxxxxx xxxxxxx xxx xx xxxxxxxxx,

III.  xxxxxxxxxxxx.  It appears xxxx xxxxx-xxxxxx xxxxxxx xxx xx xxxxxxxxx,
                        o
 IV.  xxxxxxxxxxxx.  Xx xxxxxxx that pitxx-xxxxxx xxxxxxx xxx xx xxxxxxxxx,
                                         o
  V.  xxxxxxxxxxxx.  Xx xxxxxxx that pitch-naxxxx xxxxxxx xxx xx xxxxxxxxx,
                                              o
 VI.  xxxxxxxxxxxx.  Xx xxxxxxx xxxx xxxxh-naming abilxxx xxx xx xxxxxxxxx,
                                             o
```

FIG. 1. An example of reading with a window 13 characters wide. Line I shows the original text, and line II shows the X-S version. Dots under line I indicate the locations of four successive fixations, and lines III–VI show the appearance of that line of text during each of these fixations. The dot was not present on the CRT display.

ranging from 13 to 100 characters. A 13-character window presented normal text at the letter fixated and six character positions to either side. Incidentally, I will talk about distance in number of character positions. The display was such that there were about four character positions per degree of visual angle, so you can make the translation if you wish.

The window sizes were 13, 17, 21, 25, each enlarging the window by extending it two character positions at both ends, as compared to the next smaller size. Then 31, 37, 41, and 100 for larger size increases. Since the text lines had about 70 characters, a window size of 100 actually produced a complete line of normal text unless the reader was within 20 character positions of either end of the line.

Six text mutilation procedures and eight window sizes resulted in 48 experimental conditions. Each subject read 96 pages of text, being tested in all conditions twice, and a complete record of his eye-movement behavior was recorded and summarized for each of the pages.

They were also tested for retention of information after each six-page passage and paid according to their performance on those tests. We were trying to induce them to concentrate on learning what they were reading.

The assumption we were making was that if at a certain window size one form of text mutilation provides visual information outside the window area which the reader actually acquires and uses in reading, whereas another mutilated form removes that information, a difference will be produced in reading which should have an effect on the eye-movement pattern. Thus, if useful visual information is present in certain areas of peripheral vision with one type of text pattern, and is removed with the other type, removal of the information should have an effect on the reading pattern.

I will now describe some aspects of the data.

The variables seemed to have little or no effect on test-question performance. In another study we reduced the size of the window to nine character positions, essentially turning good readers into word-by-word readers visually. Their test performance, even under these extreme conditions, did not drop significantly. Reading time increased, but understanding failed to go down. Thus it appears to me that failure to understand during reading is not the result of simply perceiving one word at a time rather than perceiving larger word groups, as has frequently been suggested.

Figure 2 shows the effect of the variables on saccade length. Length of saccades was influenced only by the presence or absence of spaces, not by the type of letter substitution made. Here you see plots of the first, second, and third quartiles of the distribution of saccade length under filled versus space conditions. Filling the spaces produced shortened saccades. The effect was greatest on the longer saccades represented by the third-quartile data. It appears that the word-length patterns are probably used in guiding the eye and are acquired at least 12 to 13 character positions from central vision and perhaps

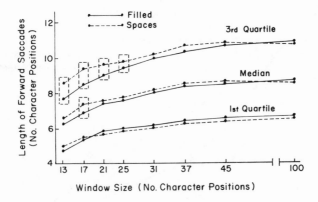

FIG. 2. The length of forward saccades as a function of window size and of the presence or absence of word-length information in the region outside the window. Boxed points were significantly different at the .06 level.

even further than that. It is hard to say just where the two curves come together, particularly on the third-quartile data.

The duration of fixations was significantly affected by the type of letter substitution used and not by the presence or absence of spaces. These data are shown in Fig. 3. Comparing the two top curves on the left, the C and the NC conditions where correct versus incorrect word-shape patterns were presented to peripheral vision, it can be seen that correct visual shape produced shorter fixations at the two smallest window sizes. However, by window size 21 that difference disappeared. Thus, the presence of correct versus incorrect word-shape information in the periphery made no difference more than about nine or ten character positions from central vision.

However, reading at all of these window sizes was facilitated most by having X's in the periphery. I believe that the reason for this is that the homogenous pattern provided by the X's made it very clear just where the window ended. In the other conditions with the small window it was not unusual for the reader, at least in my experience, to pick up letters outside the window and make misinterpretations of the words on that basis. This did not happen so much with the X's because the boundary of the window was clearly defined.

Thus, X's in the periphery eliminated one source of confusion to the subjects. Now, notice that the difference between the X's and the other stimulus patterns in the peripheral areas disappears at window size 25. At that point apparently the subjects were no longer acquiring this sort of letter information from outside of the window.

Now, if these speculations are correct, the data indicate that the reader may have been picking up visual letter information as far as 10 or 11 character

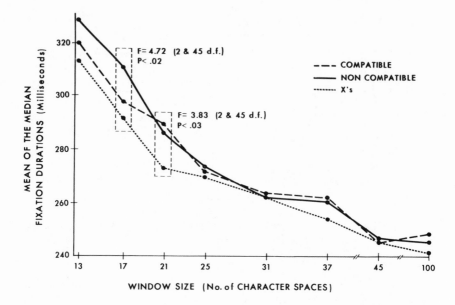

FIG. 3. The duration of fixations following forward saccades as a function of window size and of the type of word-shape information in the region outside the window.

positions from the point of fixation, or about 3° of visual angle. There is no evidence here that they were detecting and using word-shape information further into the periphery than they were picking up specific letter information.

Let me comment on one final aspect of the data shown here. Notice that the curves do not asymptote until a window size of about 45 character positions or so. At first I thought this was evidence for the pickup of useful information far into the periphery. I have since changed my mind and am concluding that this is a result of some artifact produced by the presence of the stimulus changes taking place in the periphery. My reason for this is twofold. First, if in these further areas the readers are not acquiring features of specified letters or gross word-shape or word-length patterns, I can't imagine what information they are picking up that is facilitating their reading; and second, another set of studies has produced earlier asymptotes. Steven Reder, a student at Rockefeller University, has conducted similar experiments, but he was able to produce faster display changes than we were making. In most regards, our data agree quite well, but his curves asymptote much sooner than ours do. This leads me to suspect then the slowness of the display change in our studies may have been producing some sort of artifact that was interfering with reading.

To summarize the results, we found no evidence of the acquisition and use of specific letter features or word-shape information further than 10 or 11 character positions from the fixation point, although word-length patterns may be acquired further into the periphery and may be used for eye guidance.

There were aspects of this experiment that worried me. The massive display changes, the gross response measures, and the evidence of the presence of artifacts all led me to seek a more precise way to investigate the same question. The experiment that I am now going to describe was a thesis study (Rayner, 1974) done by the student who accompanied me to M.I.T., Keith Rayner.

Assume that the reader integrates the visual information that he acquires from various areas of his visual field over fixations. On fixation N he may pick up information about the length of a particular word in his periphery. On fixation $N + 1$, the eye is closer to that word and he may add to the prior information more detail about the specific characters, word shapes, and so on.

If the word were changed between fixation N and $N + 1$, however, what effect would that have on his processing? Well, that depends on the type of change that was made. If the change were only of aspects of the word which he did not acquire on fixation N, then the information he previously acquired would not conflict with the new information, the integration process would proceed smoothly, and the change would have no effect. If the change, however, were of aspects of the word which he did acquire on fixation N, there should be some conflict in this integration process which would require added processing of the visual stimulus, probably, we thought, leading to longer fixations.

Our strategy, then, was to select a word position in a paragraph and for different groups of people display different stimuli in that position initially, stimuli which would have certain similarities to and differences from the word which would eventually occupy that position in the passage, called the *base word*. Then while the subject was reading the passage at some specified point, while the eye was in motion, we would change the initial stimulus in that word position to the base word, the word which should normally be there. We could then examine the eye-movement data to see if an abnormality was produced which would indicate that the subjects noted the change. We could see what types of changes then were noted at different distances from the fixation point and in that way tell how far into the periphery certain visual information was acquired. This had the advantage of not requiring massive display changes and it allowed us to look precisely at a specific aspect of the data.

For stimulus materials, Rayner produced 225 three-sentence paragraphs, each containing one sentence which had one word position selected as the critical word location where the change was to take place. Figure 4 shows an example of one of these sentences containing a critical word location.

There were five types of initially displayed alternatives used. There was the base word *palace,* which is referred to as the *W-ident* alternative, because it was a word (W) and was identical to the base word. There was another word, *police,* indicated as W-SL, where W indicates that it was a word, S indicates that it maintained the gross word shape characteristics, and L indicates that it started and ended with the same letters as the original word. And then there were three nonword (N) alternatives which were constructed: *N-SL,* a letter string which preserved the shape of the word and the first and last letters; *N-S,* a letter string which preserved the word shape but which changed the first and last letters; and *N-L,* a letter string which had the same first and last letters, but changed the external word shape.

If the W-Ident alternative were initially displayed, there would be no stimulus change that took place during the reading. On the others, however, there was a change in some of the letters. The N-L condition produced a change in word shape. The N-S condition produced a change in first and last letters. There was also a difference in whether the initial alternative was a word or not, contrasting the W-SL and N-SL, both of which had fairly similar word shapes and characteristics, but one of which had a semantic rendering and the other did not.

The technique used was to display the passage with one of the alternatives initially in the critical word location and have the subject begin reading the passage. We set a boundary in the computer for each passage. This was not visible, but it is indicated in Fig. 4 by a B underneath the top line. When the eye crossed that boundary position on the line containing the critical word location, if the eye were traveling above a certain speed, the stimulus change would be made. The initial alternative was changed to the base word. In Fig. 4 the number 1 on the top line indicates where the first fixation was prior to crossing the boundary. Number 2 on the second line indicates where the next fixation was, and you can see that the word in the critical word location has been changed between those two fixations.

A complete record was made of the eye movements. Paragraphs were presented one at a time. As in the prior study, the subject could bring the next paragraph onto the screen by pressing a button. After the subject read 15 paragraphs, he came off the equipment and took a test. There were 10 subjects, all M.I.T. undergraduates, and each read 225 paragraphs, 15 blocks of 15 paragraphs each.

```
I.   The robbers guarded the pcluce with their guns.
             1    B

II.  The robbers guarded the palace with their guns.
                  B        2
```

FIG. 4. An example of the display change which occurred in the boundary experiment. The B marks the location of the boundary; the numeral 1 indicates the location of the last fixation prior to crossing the boundary, and line I shows the appearance of the line during that fixation; the numeral 2 indicates the location of the first fixation after crossing the boundary, and line II shows the appearance of the line during that fixation.

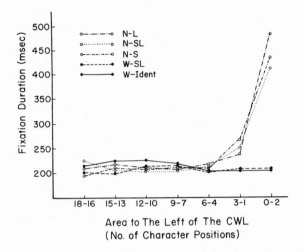

FIG. 5. Mean duration of the last fixation prior to crossing the boundary as a function of its location and of the nature of the stimulus pattern in the critical word location.

Five boundary conditions were used, nine, six, or three character positions prior to the critical word location, and the first and fourth letter of the critical word location itself. The sentences containing the critical word location were all of the same grammatical type, with the base word being subject, verb, or object, and was either five, six, or seven letters long. The variables were counterbalanced as far as possible.

I will now summarize some of the data from this experiment. Some of the stimuli were nonwords. Presumably, if a reader encounters a nonword, this should produce processing difficulty reflected in a longer fixation duration. The first question then is how far to the left of the critical word location one finds lengthened fixation durations for fixations prior to crossing the boundary, when a nonword letter string is present in the text. That is, how far away can we find evidence that the subjects were attempting to make a semantic interpretation of a nonword letter string.

Figure 5 shows results that bear on this question. This shows the mean fixation duration for the different alternatives for fixations located at different distances to the left of the critical word location. These data essentially form two curves, one for the W conditions and one for the N conditions. First, there is clear evidence that the presence of a nonword does affect the fixation duration, not surprisingly. Second, there is no evidence that the subjects were distinguishing between words and nonwords for stimuli beginning more than about four character positions from the fixation point. However, this is weak evidence in view of the possibility of a delayed effect occurring on later fixations.

The next analysis was concerned with the effect of the stimulus change. For data we will consider the duration of only the first fixation made after the change occurred and then only if it fell on the critical word location. Thus, the subject had previously fixated some distance to the left of the critical word location and some stimulus alternative was in that location. Then during the saccade the boundary was crossed, causing the stimulus to change, and his eye came to rest on the word that had been changed. The question is, is there any evidence of a lengthened fixation duration?

These fixation durations were classified by the type of alternative initially displayed and where the prior fixation was. Thus, we ignored the boundary location in classifying.

The results are shown in Fig. 6. Here the durations of the fixations on the critical word location are plotted according to the location of the prior fixation. The different curves present data for different initial stimulus alternatives. The W-Ident condition provides a baseline from which to judge the others and it can be seen that the variables did affect the fixation duration.

There was no difference between fixation durations when the prior fixation was more than 12 fixations to the left of the critical word location. Thus, there is no evidence that the subjects picked up word shape or specific letter information from words beginning more than 12 character positions to the right of the fixation point. There were differences, however, when the prior fixation was 10 to 12 character positions to the right of the critical word location. Here N-S and

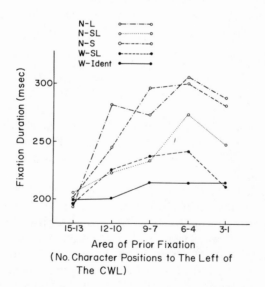

FIG. 6. Mean durations of fixations falling on the CWL immediately after crossing the boundary as a function of the location of the prior fixation and of the initially displayed stimulus pattern in the critical word location.

N-L curves are elevated above the others. The others do not differ significantly. Thus, there seems to be the pickup of both extreme letter information and word-shape information in that region.

The N-SL and W-SL curves rise slightly, but not significantly, above the W-Ident curve when the prior fixation was 7 to 12 character positions from the critical word location. This difference becomes significant for prior fixations in the four- to six-character position region. Apparently when the fixation point was within 6 character positions of the critical word location, the subjects registered the visual features in that location which distinguished the specific internal letters of the word.

When the center of vision was more than 6 character positions from the critical word location, it seemed to make no difference whether that location was occupied by a word or by a nonword letter string; that is, the N–SL and W–SL curves are very close together. However, these two curves suddenly separate when the prior fixation is 6 or fewer character positions from the critical word position. At that point, the subjects appear to have been doing more than simply identifying letter features, but were now sensitive to whether the letter string had a semantic interpretation. Thus, it appears that the semantic interpretation of a letter string was being made for words only if they began no more than six character positions to the right of the fixation point. This generally agrees with the data previously mentioned, where the subjects failed to detect the presence of nonwords which occurred more than about four character positions from the point of fixation.

Although there are many other aspects of this study unexplored, and important questions still unanswered, I will at this time state our present conclusions.

1. There is a fairly narrow region in central vision within which the skilled reader actually makes a semantic interpretation of the word stimuli. We found no evidence for such interpretations for words starting more than about four to six character positions to the right of the fixation point.

2. Certain visual characteristics of the text are acquired further into the periphery than that, however. Features of specific letters may be identified for words beginning as far as 10 to 12 character positions to the right of the fixation. This is slightly larger than the estimate of 10 or 11 characters of the first study but still within the same range.

3. There was consistently no evidence that the general exterior word shape is acquired further into the periphery than specific featural detail about letters themselves.

4. Word-length patterns were acquired still further into the periphery and were used primarily for eye guidance. Although the average saccade for our readers was about $8^{1}/_{2}$ character positions in length, a quarter of the saccades made were more than 11 character positions in length.

5. The techniques that we have used, with the production of precise stimulus changes and analysis of the effects that these changes produce on eye move-

ments, do seem to be useful techniques in studying the nature of the effective stimulation during the fixation while the person is engaged in the normal reading act. We believe these techniques can be used to investigate a number of other very interesting questions about reading as well.

DISCUSSION

KOLERS: I had no idea what Dr. McConkie was going to talk about and I can't decide whether I am pleased or displeased by it, but I think for the most part very pleased. It was interesting to see an old theory confirmed with such new methods. We can have some questions.

LOFTUS: In the W–SL condition of Fig. 5 the data point was right down at the baseline with one to three character spaces. It seems to me if you are really picking up semantic information within one to three character spaces, you should have picked up the fact that the word was going to be different.

It seems a little surprising that when the subject gets there and discovers, lo and behold! the word is changed, he doesn't spend any longer than he would if the word hadn't changed. Would you like to comment on that?

McCONKIE: Yes. I have, of course, found that particular datum point very interesting, too. And the thing that I wonder is whether the person on the prior fixation has in fact rendered a semantic interpretation of that word and, although he fixates it on the next fixation, maybe he ignores it.

We are quite anxious, when we get our computer system, to have people read a passage and find instances where that happens. Then after they will have read the passage, we will ask them to tell us about the passage, and see if we can find out which interpretation they give to that particular word. It may be that the subjects are not processing the thing that is being directly fixated.

GOULD: How fast did your display change?

McCONKIE: I have a hard time answering that question directly because since we did the study I have been learning about delays in the Biometric equipment that I was not aware of at the time. I thought that I was changing the stimulus extremely rapidly.

The actual time necessary to produce a change so far as the computer is concerned is divided into two parts. First, there is the time necessary to change the display list in the core memory, and second, there is the time necessary to wait until the change is realized on the scope. The change in core memory was made in 500 μsec. We were refreshing the image on the CRT something above 60 times per sec since we were just going end to end and not taking off from a timing pulse. I don't know at this point exactly how fast we were refreshing. So there you are talking about a delay, depending on where the word to be changed was on the scope, of up to 12 or 13 msec. But the thing that bothers me is that we had a filter in the biometrics unit that was apparently delaying the signal another 25 msec or so.

GOULD: What did it seem like phenomenally? Did you see a flash, see a change?

McCONKIE: In the window studies, no, you didn't see things change. As soon as we detected the eye as being still, we turned off the scope and then we fiddled with the display list and then turned the scope back on. That, for a small window, was a short enough time that you didn't see a flicker. For a larger window, you saw a definite flicker, and for very big windows it became quite severe. You didn't have the perception of seeing one thing and then seeing it change to something else. But you did have the perception that there is something funny going on in the periphery. In the second study, the change was produced faster.

COOPER: You indicated before that semantic information is not picked up outside of a narrow range of characters, not directly at least.

McCONKIE: What I will say is I was not able to provide evidence in this study that that is so.

COOPER: Yet as they read along people are continuously generating semantic interpretations of word strings based on peripheral information.

McCONKIE: I think that statement is not based on data. That is a common assumption.

COOPER: Let me clarify what I mean. What may be happening is that the person views the initial string of letters within a word, i.e., the initial string of characters, and forms some kind of semantic interpretation of the initial letters within a word string. Then based upon expectancies and clues derived from word shape and spacing between words that come following this initial letter sequence, they form semantic interpretations of what is coming next.

What I'd like to know is, have you done any further studies which go into greater detail to find out how people form interpretations of semantic details based upon what comes next, word shape clues, printed clues of the printed page interacting with semantic interpretations in the first few characters, etc.?

McCONKIE: My answer has to be no. It is clear from what you have said that you and I are going to have the same problems that Dr. Hochberg and I had and we are in for some good discussions in the future.

LEFTON: Did you say there was no effect on comprehension when you used a small window?

McCONKIE: That is what I said. In another study we ran the window size down to nine character positions. After each passage the subjects read they were given five, or maybe seven questions, that were of a "fill in the answer" type so there was not much chance of guessing the right answer. These were kids who hadn't taken a psychology class. If they hadn't read the passage, they simply didn't know the answers to the questions and in that situation we found no significant difference in test performance. The nine-character-position condition was slightly depressed, but not very much.

VI.5

Control of Eye Movements during Reading

Ralph Norman Haber[1]

University of Rochester

In the process of reading, the eye moves over text with saccadic movements. This statement is about the only indisputable one that can be made about eye movements during reading. I will suggest and elaborate three different models which describe the processes that determine the direction and distance moved in each saccade. These models are not original with me although I have talked about them before (Haber, 1972), and Rayner (1974) has described them in related terms. However, because they have not been presented at this conference, I feel it will be most useful to describe them in some detail, hopefully as a means to interpret the earlier papers on eye movements in reading and as a guide to badly needed further research.

The three models place the locus of control of eye movements respectively as the result of three different processes. The first I call *random control* in which the magnitude of each movement is primarily the result of processes in the oculomotor system itself without feedback from higher centers. The principal characteristic of this model is that it predicts that successive movements will be correlated neither with other eye movements nor with the content of the text being read. The second model is called *internal control* in which the magnitude of each movement is determined by information-extraction processes performed by the reader based entirely on the sense or meaning he has made out of what he has already read but still without regard to any specific features of the text yet to be seen. The third model I have called *stimulus control* which includes all the

[1] Partial support for the research that has led to these ideas has come from research grants from the U.S. Army Human Engineering Laboratory (DAAD 05-71-Q-1424), from the National Institute of Mental Health (MH10753), and from the National Institute of Education (NE G-00-3-0090).

processes of the internal control model but goes beyond it. Here the magnitude of each movement can also be determined by graphic, syntactic or semantic features of the text being viewed in peripheral vision before they have been fully processed for meaning.

We know that the durations of eye fixations are pretty constant at about 230 msec ±20 msec, for a practiced reader, regardless of his reading skill, difficulty of the text, or the distance moved. We also know that the duration of each saccade takes about 30 msec ±10 msec, again pretty much regardless of the distance moved, skill, or reading level. These numbers tell us that about 3½ eye movements are being made per sec, or about 210 eye movements per min. Since reading speed and words per min vary over at least 1 log unit for a single reader across different texts or for a single text across readers of different skills, the only factor left to account for this large variation across both texts and readers is the number of fixations being made per word of text. The three models differ on how this variation and the number of fixations per word occur. Let me now elaborate on each of the models.

Random control model. I consider this model to be something of a straw man since I find it hard to think that reasonable people will believe it, but let me try to make it as believable as possible as at least a logical alternative. This model assumes that the oculomotor control system has a rough gain setting which both varies from person to person according to their reading skills and for each reader can be roughly adjusted for the difficulty level of the text. Once this gain control is set, the eye moves a fixed distance each time, plus or minus some small variation. Thus, the pattern of eye movements over text can be fully described by frequency distribution of distances, specified only by a mean and standard deviation. It matters not what the eye encounters on its fovea, that is, with the word or words directly fixated, nor what it might encounter out of its peripheral corner before it moves again. What accounts for the variation around the mean is not at all clear; presumably it is also a random process. However, this variation neatly accounts for regressive eye movements. If the distance moved, for example, averages four character spaces to the right with the standard deviation of two character spaces, then by using a table of areas under a normal curve, it can be predicted that roughly 20% of all movements would be negative, that is, leftward. However, if the mean is eight character spaces to the right with the same standard deviation of two, then regressive eye movements would be exceedingly rare. If the random perturbations are small relative to the mean, then the mean alone is a pretty good descriptor of all eye movements. If these perturbations are believed to be large relative to the mean, then both the mean and the standard deviation are needed to describe the resulting distributions of eye movements. In either case, this model says that neither the moment-to-moment features of the text nor the processing of the text being carried out by the reader is relevant to the determination of the direction and distance of the next eye movement.

One major difficulty encountered by this model is how it determines the difficulty level of the text that is then used to adjust the distance moved. Since difficulty is obviously due at least in part to something about the text, the control system has to have some kind of feedback from samplings of the text and use those samplings to adjust the value of this fixed distance. It seems to me that some very ad hoc feedback mechanism would have to be posited to build this in, and the model does not have any very nice way of doing this.

One direct way to disprove this model would be to demonstrate a correlation between fixation choices and any kind of graphic, syntactic, or semantic features of the text being read. Buswell (1922) has shown one example of such a correlation in which technical words in otherwise straightforward prose are likely to draw multiple fixations. Kolers has already commented upon this as it rather dramatically shows that adjustments in the fixation choices are influenced by what the eye has encountered.

Therefore, in spite of the neat parsimony of the random control model I feel it is both internally inconsistent and inconsistent with what is known about eye movements. Thus, it is not tenable as a reasonable explanation for the control of eye movements made during the process of reading.

Internal control model.   This model places the variance not in the oculomotor control system but in the information extraction processes that are constructing the meaning of the text as it is being read. Thus, each fixation makes some information from the text accessible following the operations of whatever strategies are used by the reader to arrive ultimately at the meaning of the text. If the reader is having an easy time, those strategies can program relatively large positive eye movements. If he is having a difficult time, a smaller movement can be programmed, and sometimes even a negative one if necessary. The important point is that the size of the movement is directly related to the internal information processing that occurs as one reads. The stress here is on internal. The next landing place for the eye is determined not by any characteristic of the landing site but only by the amount of new information the reader thinks he will be able to process next.

This model is very explicit about the relationship of difficulty of the text and the average magnitude of the eye movements—the distance moved will continually be adjusted as a function of the ease or difficulty of making sense out of the text. Thus, the internal control model solves this problem in a straightforward fashion whereas the random control model is embarrassed by this effect.

There still needs to be specified, in the information-extraction sequence, when the decision is made about the distance and direction the eye is to be moved. The timing constraints are fairly severe. Substantial evidence now exists (for example, Westheimer, 1954) that saccadic movements need to be programmed from 150 to 200 msec before they occur and that during this time no new visual information will have any influence on the movement being planned. This means that if the typical fixation lasts 230 msec and the latency for making the next fixation is rarely less than 150 msec, then no more than 80 msec would typically be available to extract and register the features of the current fixation, use those to process the additional text for meaning, and use that processing to make a decision about whether to go forward or back and by how much. Latour's evidence (1962) also suggests that some suppression in visual sensitivity both precedes and follows the actual saccade itself. This postmovement suppression would further cut into the total processing time available before a commitment is made about the next movement. While it is reasonable that *some* information can be extracted in 50 msec, it cannot be too much and it is unlikely that much in the way of a decision can be made in that time. The conclusion, therefore, appears inescapable that any decision about the duration and distance over which to move the eye that is based exclusively on the meaning of the story being constructed must have been made during the previous fixations and not during the current one. It is the logic of this argument that has often been used by advocates of the first model to point out that the second (and the third one also) is unreasonable. If the visual system is so slow in extracting information and if the planning of eye movements takes so long, then why demand that each movement be tied to internal processing (or, even worse, to stimulus information in the text, as claimed for the third model).

Several answers have been made against the timing constraints objection. First, even granting the timing constraints, there is nothing in this model that demands that all decisions and actions be carried out fixation by fixation. As with the eye—voice span effect, the eye may be ahead of comprehension by one or two fixations. All that is required is that comprehension and distance moved be related even if there might always be some lag. I will elaborate an even more effective answer to this in the discussion of the third model. Second, the timing constraints may not be as severe as has been implied in the laboratory research. Maybe no separate decision must be made for each fixation. Rather the oculomotor system may be instructed to move a fixed distance ahead for each saccade unless told otherwise. Thus, for most saccades the latency could be much shorter since no new decision is needed and this would provide much more processing time for the text. When comprehension difficulties arose, new decisions would be made and these would have a lag of one or two fixations in their being carried out.

Most of these comments are quite speculative in that little evidence exists to relate the laboratory studies of eye-movement latencies and suppression on the one hand, and the information-extraction processes on the other, to ongoing reading tasks. In any event, as I will try to suggest in the discussion of the third model, I do not see these objections as serious to either the second or the third model or as providing any interesting support for the first model.

As with the first model, the internal control model predicts no correlation between fixation choice and graphic, syntactic, or semantic features *ahead* of the current fixation. In this sense, the Buswell finding, previously mentioned, is not troublesome for this model. If after having looked at a strange word the reader still does not know its meaning or how to spell it or how to pronounce it, the internal control model says that a refixation would be programmed just as Buswell illustrates. But when moving on the reader does not pick the next landing site by anything he saw out of the corner of his eye but rather only picks a distance which reflects what he thinks will represent the amount of new information he can handle. Thus, refixations on already fixated areas of the text clearly are predictable by the model, although the model does not predict anything about the future fixation sites.

There is one sense in which the internal control model could predict a correlation between fixation choices and some syntactic or semantic features of the text. If the reader, in processing the text or meaning, is doing so by generating hypotheses or expectations about what he is reading, those hypotheses could include predictions about what the next word or words might be. If the reader's confidence about such predictions is very high, then he may not need to actually verify the prediction and can skip the next word. This would tend to produce a negative correlation between the predictability of the syntactic or semantic content of the text and the probability of drawing a fixation on that content.

Notice that what is predicted here is a correlation between fixation choices and syntactic and semantic features, not between fixation choices and graphic features. This model still provides no theoretical basis for generating a correlation between the graphic features of the text and fixation choices because the model says that peripheral vision is not being used to guide future fixations. Yet, McConkie in this volume shows clearly that graphic features are more powerful predictors of fixation choices than syntactic or semantic ones. In this sense, his data show that the eye is sensitive to graphic features farther from the center of the current fixation than it is to syntactic or semantic ones. Thus, it seems unlikely that this extension of the second model is very reasonable or internally consistent.

The two models considered so far place little of the variance of the reading process in the behavior of the eyes. In both, the eye moves over the text pretty much independent of what is there. They differ in how much of the control is influenced by what has already been processed, but neither is interested in the content of the text yet to be looked at. To the extent that either of these models provides an adequate story, they would suggest that eye movements in reading would not be very important, either as a way to understand the reading process itself or as a therapeutic concern in cases of poor reading ability. This is in contrast to the third model which places much more weight on eye movements as a vital and interactive part of the reading process.

Stimulus control model. This model includes all the determinants of the previous one, plus information from peripheral vision picked up during each fixation. This information comes from the graphic features of the text, such as word length (given probably by spaces separating each word), word shape (patterns of ascending, descending, and letter shapes), end of line cues defined by white space, and those phrase and sentence boundaries given by punctuation marks. It probably also includes some graphic features of some individual letters, although this requires better acuity, and it is probably not picked up as peripherally as the textual graphic features listed above.

What this model suggests is that the visual system is both sampling the text centered in the current fixation and picking up peripheral information to determine in part where the next fixation should be centered. Thus, this model specifically predicts that some features of the text will be correlated with fixation choices. The correlation may not be limited to the graphic features alone, even if that is all that the peripheral system is sensitive to. It seems quite likely that if the reader is constructing and testing expectations or hypotheses about the meaning of what he is reading, then we might expect that he can specify what the next word has to be, given its shape alone. Here, then, the reader has used a word-shape graphic feature to generate or test a semantic hypothesis. Similarly, the reader, having processed part of a sentence, must surely be able to predict the syntactic structure over the next few words. Given only a few cues as to word shape or word length, he can verify or create syntactic hypotheses even farther from the center of the area of the current fixation.

To the extent that these peripherally perceived features are used to generate or confirm hypotheses about the meaning of the text not yet encountered foveally, there will be a correlation found between the locations of these features and the locations of fixation choices. The stimulus control model is the only one of the three that predicts such a correlation.

What none of these models describes is the size of the effective field of view. It is tacitly (and I think wrongly) assumed that if the average distance between fixations is 8 character spaces, slightly more than 1 word, then the number of character spaces available for processing on each fixation is also only 8. At normal reading distance for average type, 8 character spaces is just over 2° of visual angle—roughly the size of the fovea. If a reader can saccade 16 character spaces on the average, does this mean that he is processing twice as many characters or words during each fixation? Or, perhaps that his visual acuity is better for peripheral vision? I think not. Smith (1971) has noted most cogently that what a small saccade length permits the reader to do is to see each word several times, each time from a different perspective within the sentence as the eye progresses along the line. Thus, if the effective field of view is 40 character spaces, 20 on either side of the center of fixation, then 6 or 7 words would be available for some kind of processing during each fixation. If the average saccade size is 8 characters, then each word will in fact be visible in some form or other about 5 times. Near the forward (right) edge of this field of view, only the graphic features of the words may be picked up, but these will permit the reader to determine how many words there are, their length, and something about phrase structure. From these, plus what he has already processed from the left side of the visual field from the current and the last few fixations, he should have all he needs to infer the syntactic structure of the entire sequence of words in view. If his expectations about the meaning of what he is reading are sufficient, he can probably verify predictions about the presence of particular words from these graphic features plus the syntactic features he has already predicted.

The important point in this comment is that the effective field of view need not be limited to the average distance moved between fixations. Recognizing this makes more plausible the assertion that peripheral vision (information picked up from outside the $2°$ fovea, but within the effective field of view) is an important source of graphic features that can be used both as an aid to the processing of the meaning of the text, and as a guide to future fixation choices. It also makes plausible the finding that restricting peripheral vision reduces reading speed. McConkie and Rayner (1975), for example, found that this effect begins when peripheral vision is reduced below 30 to 50 character spaces in width. Thus, it seems obvious that rather wide reaches of peripheral vision are being used and that the effective field of view has to be larger than that given by simply the average distance moved during each saccade.

This also is quite consistent with Hochberg's (1970b) notion that the difference between good and bad readers is not something about their peripheral vision or their ability to perceive more features in each fixation, but rests in their ability to sample farther ahead in the text and to build more elaborate expectations that encompass more of the visual features available.

In summary, the critical differentiation of model 3 from models 2 and 1 is the prediction of a correlation between graphic features of the text and fixation choices. Specifically, words which are redundant or easily predicted can be verified by graphic features alone and will be less likely to draw fixations. Another version of this correlation is that a reader could correctly guess words not directly viewed if all the reader had were their graphic features. Thus, the eye—voice span should be larger if graphic features are present ahead of the eye than if nothing is there at all.

Empirical tests designed to differentiate the three models have not yet provided convincing evidence one way or the other. In this volume, one finds McConkie and Fisher providing more support for model 3 than for model 2;

Kolers arguing that 2 is sufficient and 3 unnecessary; and finally Hochberg seems to lean more strongly to 3 than 2. The four papers are united only in their rejection of model 1 as an alternative. The finally vote, of course, is not yet in. With the substantial effort currently being made, I expect that we will soon know much more about the interaction between the content of the text being read and the control of the eye movements made during the reading process.

DISCUSSION

NODINE: Would people be reading into the reading situations the notion that reading is visual search? I think the normal reading that Dr. Haber talked about, what we may not be achieving in the laboratory, is not visual search. By visual search I mean looking for or trying to detect a target.

Scanning behavior is really an attempt to input information. I think Dr. McConkie's data strongly support the view that there is little evidence that the eye is really attuned to information in the text beyond the limits of fixation.

So the hypothesis-testing model, or selective-attention model, seems to me to be nearly unsupportable, given Dr. McConkie's work and the realization that reading is not search, unless, of course, you structure the task that way, which many of us do, I am not denying that.

KOLERS: Reading is hypothesis testing, reading is search, reading is problem solving, reading is as many things as you want reading to be depending on what you are reading and why.

NODINE: And on how you structure the test.

HOCHBERG: There is a nonsequiter somewhere in the line. You have no forecasting, you have no peripheral vision at all in the original model that I tried to adapt, which is listening to somebody speaking. There you have got no periphery whatsoever, right? Yet that model will work as a hypothesis test or as an anticipation test or as a speech-string tester, with something as small as McConkie's nine-letter window.

So the fact that there is no peripheral processing would be totally irrelevant to whether you could use a speech-string tester. Anything you get from the periphery is gravy for that purpose.

Presumably what the periphery serves is to enable you to pursue a more selective listening—predicting task than you would have to if you were actually listening to speech. That is, you can select the rate at which the speaker is metaphorically speaking by skipping sections of it, the redundant sections.

But if you don't do that, if you have tunnel vision, then you are back to the same task that you face when you listen to somebody speak phoneme by phoneme, or whatever the short-term buffer may contain.

FISHER: I wanted to comment that many of the questions about contextual and physical effects on eye movements and fixation durations during reading were intensively studied by Tinker and his associates. McNamara, Paterson, and Tinker (1953) and Tinker and Paterson (1940; 1952) sought to determine optimal sizes using eye-movement records of adults and children. Tinker (1947; 1951) also compared pause durations for different forms of contextual material. He found that variability in duration of fixations depended upon the type of material, e.g., easy narrative versus algebra.

In his *Psychological Bulletin* review (Tinker, 1958), he hypothesized the operations of three mechanisms to account for fixation time: the reaction time of the eye to peripheral stimulation; the time taken when the eyes converge during saccades and diverge during fixation; and the nonvisual component of comprehension which is like what we call information processing. Of these, the first and second make up "perception time" and are fairly constant during reading, whereas the third varies with the material being read. I'm not sure how very much further along we've gotten today, and it seems to me that Tinker's efforts have provided the commonly accepted bases for the current research.

VI.6

References

Antes, J. R. The time course of picture viewing. *Journal of Experimental Psychology,* 1974, **103,** 62–70.

Brooks, V. An exploratory comparison of some measures of attention, Master's thesis, Cornell University, New York, 1961.

Buswell, G. T. An experimental study of the eye–voice span in reading. *Supplementary Educational Monographs,* **1920,** 17.

Buswell, G. T. Fundamental reading habits: A study of their development. *Education Monograph Supplement,* 1922, **21.**

Buswell, G. T. A laboratory study of the reading of modern foreign languages. New York: Macmillan, 1928.

Buswell, G. T. *How people look at pictures.* Chicago: University of Chicago Press, 1935.

Buswell, G. T. How adults read. *Supplementary Educational Monographs,* 1937, **45.**

Buswell, G. T. Perceptual research and methods of learning. *Scientific Monthly,* 1947, **64,** 521–526.

Fisher, D. F. Reading as search: A look at processes. Doctoral dissertation, University of Rochester, New York, 1973.

Fisher, D. F. Reading and Visual Search. *Memory and Cognition,* 1975, **3,** 188–196.

Fisher, D. F., & Lefton, L. A. Peripheral Information Extraction: A Developmental Examination. *Journal of Experimental Child Psychology,* 1976, **21.**

Geyer, J. Perceptual systems in reading: A temporal eye–voice span constant. Doctoral dissertation, University of California, Berkeley, 1966.

Gibson, E. J. Learning to read. *Science,* 1965, **148,** 1066–1072.

Glanzer, M., & Razel, M. The size of the unit in short-term storage. *Journal of Verbal Learning and Verbal Behavior,* 1974, **13,** 114–131.

Haber, R. N. Perceptual Components of Reading. Invited address at the Annual Convention of the American Psychological Association, Honolulu, August, 1972.

Hochberg, J. In the mind's eye. In R. N. Haber (Ed.), *Contemporary theory and research in visual perception.* New York: Holt, Rinehart & Winston, 1968.

Hochberg, J. Attention, organization and consciousness. In D. L. Mostofsky (Ed.), *Attention: Contemporary theory and analysis.* New York: Appleton–Century–Crofts, 1970. (a)

Hochberg, J. Components of literacy: Speculations and exploratory research. In H. Levin &

J. P. Williams (Eds.), *Basic studies on reading.* New York: Basic Books, 1970. Pp. 74–89. (b)

Hochberg, J. The representation of things and people. In E. H. Gombrich, J. Hochberg, M. Black, & M. Mandelbaum (Eds.), *Art, perception, and reality.* Baltimore: Johns Hopkins Press, 1972.

Hochberg, J., & Brooks, V. The prediction of visual attention to designs and paintings. *American Psychologist,* 1962, **17**, 7. (Paper at APA 1962–Abstracts.)

Hochberg, J., & Brooks, V. Reading as intentional behavior. In H. Singer & R. B. Ruddell (Eds.), *Theoretical models and processes of reading.* Newark, Delaware: International Reading Association, 1970.

Judd, C. H., & Buswell, G. T. Silent reading: A study of the various types. *Supplementary Educational Monographs,* 1922, **23**.

Keen, R. H. The effect on reading rate of the number of words used to express meaning. Doctoral dissertation, New York University, 1973.

Kolers, P. A., & Lewis, C. Bounding of letter sequences and the integration of visually presented words. *Acta Psychologica,* 1972, **36**, 112–124.

Latour, P. L. Visual threshold during eye movements. *Vision Research,* 1962, **2**, 261–262.

Mackworth, N., & Morandi, A. J. The gaze selects informative details within pictures. *Perception and Psychophysics,* 1967, **2**, 547–552.

Marshall, J. C. Some problems and paradoxes associated with recent accounts of hemispheric specialization. *Neuropsychologica,* 1973, **11**, 463–470.

McConkie, G. W., & Rayner, K. The span of the effective stimulus during fixations in reading. *Perception & Psychophysics,* 1975, **17**, 578–586.

McNamara, W. G., Paterson, D. G., & Tinker, M. A. The influence of size on speed of reading in primary grades. *Sight Saving Review,* 1953, **23**, 28–33.

Miller, G. A. The magical number seven, plus or minus two. *Psychological Review,* 1956, **63**, 81–97.

Neisser, U. *Cognitive psychology.* New York: Appleton, 1967.

Nelson, R. D. The combination of peripheral and foveal views. Doctoral dissertation, New York University, 1972.

Pollack, R., & Spence, D. Subjective pictorial information in visual search. *Perception and Psychophysics,* 1968, **3**, 41–44.

Rayner, K. The perceptual span and peripheral cues in reading. Unpublished doctoral dissertation, Cornell University, 1974.

Simon, H. A. How big is a chunk? *Science,* 1974, **183**, 482–488.

Smith, F. *Understanding reading.* New York: Holt, Rinehart & Winston, 1971.

Spragins, A. B. Eye movements in examining spatially transformed text: A developmental examination. Doctoral dissertation, University of South Carolina, Columbia, 1974.

Spragins, A. B., Lefton, L. A. and Fisher, D. F. Eye Movements While Reading and Searching Spatially Transformed Text: A Developmental Examination. *Memory and Cognition,* 1976, **4**, 36–42.

Stroop, J. R. Studies of interference in serial verbal reactions. *Journal of Experimental Psychology,* 1935, **18**, 643–662.

Taylor, S. Eye movements in reading: Facts and fallacies. *American Educational Research Journal,* 1965, **2**, 187–202.

Tinker, M. A. *Bases for effective reading.* Minneapolis, Minnesota: University of Minnesota Press, 1965.

Tinker, M. A. Fixation pause duration in reading. *Journal of Educational Research,* 1951, **44**, 471–479.

Tinker, M. A. Legibility of print for children in the upper grades. *American Journal of Optometry & Archives of American Acacdemy of Optometry,* 1963, **40**, 614–621.

Tinker, M. A. Recent studies of eye movements in reading. *Psychological Bulletin,* 1958, **55,** 215–231.

Tinker, M. A. Time relations for eye movement measures in reading. *Journal of Educational Psychology,* 1947, **38,** 1–10.

Tinker, M. A., & Paterson, D. G. Eye movements in reading a modern type face and Old English. *American Journal of Psychology,* 1940, **54,** 113–114.

Tinker, M. A., & Paterson, D. G. Reader preferences and typography. *Journal of Applied Psychology,* 1952, **26,** 38–40.

Warren, R. Stimulus encoding and memory. *Journal of Experimental Psychology,* 1972, **94,** 90–100.

Westheimer, G. H. Eye movement responses to horizontally moving visual stimulus. *Archives of Ophthalmology,* 1954, **52,** 932–943.

Wood, L. E. Visual and auditory coding in a memory matching task. *Journal of Experimental Psychology,* 1974, **102,** 106–113.

Woodworth, R. S. *Experimental psychology.* New York: Holt, 1938.

Part VII

EYE MOVEMENTS AND HIGHER MENTAL PROCESSES

Much of the foregoing material has been related to the way in which the eyes seek out and take in selected portions of the visual field, either to get information from a coherent world or to gain information from an ordered presentation of written material. This last session is concerned primarily with the way in which internal events within "the mind" are revealed by the ways in which people look at material presented to them or by the ways in which the eyes move even in the absence of visual stimuli. Thus, although some of the work is concerned with reading, emphasis is on the *internal representation* of the material that is read and the relationship of that material to the eye movements made during the reading as well as subsequent to it. *Visual form perception* and *visual imagery* are discussed, as is the relationship between that which is available to the eye and that which is done with the material observed. This work leads to a notion of an *active theory of visual form perception,* which is revealed by the nature of the distribution of fixation durations and locations. Another contribution relates eye movements to *interpersonal perceptions and needs* as well as to the basic structure and function of the central nervous system. *Memory* also is shown to depend upon eye fixations and movements per se rather than upon the total time spent in looking at material. This again favors an *active role* for the eye movement rather than a mere necessity dictated by the fixity of most objects in space. Finally, the question is raised as to whether eye movement data can improve our understanding of the way in which *material is encoded* for store in *memory*. In general, the thrust of all of these papers is that there is a strong, direct link between the way in which the eye moves and the fact of its moving at all, and the kind of perceptual and memory structure which is being used by the observer to store and organize information.

The chairman of the seventh session was Dr. Raymond C. Nickerson of Bolt, Beranek and Newman, Inc.

Part VII

EYE MOVEMENTS AND
HIGHER MENTAL PROCESSING

VII.1

Linguistic Influences on Picture Scanning [1]

Patricia A. Carpenter
Marcel Adam Just

Carnegie-Mellon University

Several speakers at this conference have discussed how people scan linguistic material while they are reading. The next research question that we might ask is: What do people do with that material once they have read it? Part of the answer is that they form an internal representation of the information that was just read, and that is the topic of central concern here. How is semantic information internally represented; what do the representations look like; and how are those representations manipulated? In particular, I will discuss some research that has focused on the semantic structure of negation, examining how negatives are internally represented and manipulated.

There are three main topics. First, I will explain the basic paradigm used to investigate how people read and process negative sentences. In these tasks, a subject reads a sentence and then decides if it is true or false with respect to an accompanying picture. Second, I will describe a model that accounts for the response latencies in these tasks (Carpenter & Just, 1975; Just & Carpenter, 1976). Third, I will present data that show that eye fixations are a valuable technique for discovering how people represent and process semantic structures.

In the experimental situation, the subject reads a linguistic stimulus, a phrase or a sentence, and then compares it to a picture to decide whether or not the sentence and picture agree. Or alternatively, the subject may be asked to read a question and then scan an accompanying picture for information to answer the

[1] This paper represents a collaborative effort and order of authors is arbitrary. The research was partially supported by the National Institute of Education, Department of Health, Education, and Welfare, Grant NIE-G-74-0016 and the National Institute of Mental Health, Grant MH-07722.

TABLE 1
Representations and Predictions for the Four
Information Conditions[a]

	True affirmative	False affirmative
Sentence:	The dots are red.	The dots are red.
Picture:	Red dots	Black dots
Sentence representation:	[AFF, (RED, DOTS)]	[AFF, (RED, DOTS)]
Picture representation:	(RED, DOTS)	(BLACK, DOTS)
	+ +	index = false −
	response = true	+ +
	k comparisons	response = false
		k + 1 comparisons

	False negative	True negative
Sentence:	The dots aren't red.	The dots aren't red.
Picture:	Red dots	Black dots
Sentence representation:	[NEG, (RED, DOTS)]	[NEG, (RED, DOTS)]
Picture representation:	(RED, DOTS)	(BLACK, DOTS)
index = false − +	index = false −
+ +	index = true − +
response = false	+ +
k + 2 comparisons	response = true
	k + 3 comparisons

[a]Plus and minus signs denote matches and mismatches of the corresponding constituents. Each horizontal line of plus and minus signs indicates a reinitialization of the comparison process.

question. We vary the semantic structure of the particular sentence or question to study the processing of different constructions.

In one study that was typical of many others, the subject was shown an affirmative sentence like *The dots are red*; or a negative sentence like *The dots aren't red*. Then he was shown a picture containing a group of red dots or a group of black dots, as shown in Table 1. We timed the subject while he read the sentence, looked at the picture, and decided whether the sentence was true or false. The main dependent variable was how long it took to respond "true" or "false."

The data from this experiment are shown in Fig. 1 (data from Just & Carpenter, 1971, Experiment II). There are two main results. First, there is an interaction between affirmation–negation and true–false. Affirmative sentences are easier to verify when they are true, but negative sentences are easier when they are false. Second, negative sentences take longer to verify than affirmative sentences. These results can be described in terms of two parameters: (1) falsification time, which is the absolute difference between true and false for the affirmatives averaged with the absolute difference for the negatives, and (2) negation time, the difference between affirmatives and negatives.

One of the first investigators to obtain these results, Gough (1965, 1966), suggested the basis of an explanation. He proposed that the information from the sentence and that from the picture are represented and then compared, and that the comparison process is easier when the color represented from the sentence matches the color represented from the picture. For example, affirmative sentences are easier when they are true because the color represented from the sentence matches the color that is encoded from the picture, e.g., *The dots are red* paired with a picture of red dots. Similarly, the color in a negative sentence like, *The dots aren't red* matches the picture in the false case (a picture of red dots), but not in the true case (a picture of black dots). In summary, a mismatch between the color predicates makes the processing take longer.

The difference in latencies between affirmative and negative sentences has been explained in very similar terms (Trabasso, Rollins & Shaughnessy, 1971; Chase & Clark, 1972; Clark & Chase, 1972). The explanation is that the negative sentence is represented as an affirmative core with an embedding negation marker. But pictures are represented affirmatively. So when the information from a negative sentence is compared to the information in the picture, there is a mismatch between the negative polarity marker in the sentence and the representation of the picture. Again, this kind of mismatch makes the processing take longer.

Here is a model that explains why mismatches are harder to process. First, the information in the sentence and that in the picture are represented in an abstract structure. The representation of a sentence like *The dots are red* must have several meaning components. The sentence concerns dots, it predicates that they are red, and furthermore, the predication is affirmative. The notation we will use to express these elements is a predicate-argument notation (AFF, (RED, DOTS)), or for a negative sentence (NEG, (RED, DOTS)), as shown in Table 1.

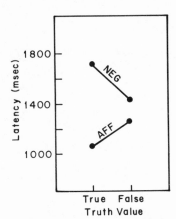

FIG. 1. Results from a typical verification experiment (data from Just & Carpenter, 1971, II.)

Similarly, when we then look at the picture we encode something about the dots, in one case that they are red, (RED, DOTS), or in the other case, that they are black (BLACK, DOTS). (Even though the affirmation marker isn't explicitly noted, the picture representations are assumed to be affirmative.) According to the model, the latency differences among the four conditions in Fig. 1 are due to the different amounts of time needed to compare the sentence and picture representations. The latencies are longer when corresponding constituents mismatch. The problem is to determine what extra mental operations underlie the longer latencies.

Figure 2 shows a model of what might be occurring when people are comparing sentences and pictures. First, there is a response index that records mismatches in the comparison stage. This index has two possible states, true and false. Its initial state is true, but each mismatch causes a change of its state. Next, there is a stage in which the sentence and picture are represented. Finally, the heart of the model is the comparison process in which each pair of constituents from the sentence and picture are retrieved and compared.

In the true affirmative case, the model says that pairs of constituents are compared, starting with the inner constituents. The inner constituents match and since both the sentence and picture are affirmative, the polarities also match. Thus, there are no mismatches and no extra operations. Therefore, the time for a true affirmative represents the base time it takes to represent the sentence and the picture and to compare corresponding constituents.

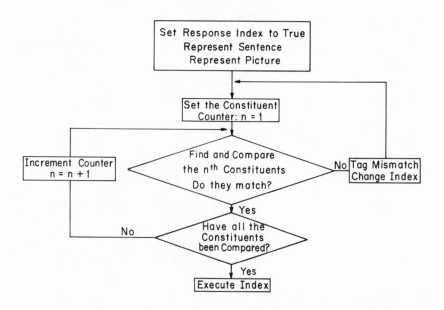

FIG. 2. A model of the processes in verification.

TABLE 2
A Trace of the Operations in Verifying a
False Affirmative

Operations	Stimulus sentence: The dots are red. Stimulus picture: A set of black dots
Initialize response index to *true*	
Represent sentence:	(AFF, (RED, DOTS))
Represent picture:	(BLACK, DOTS)
1. Compare first constituents	
Tag sentence constituent	(AFF, (M))
Tag picture constituent:	(M)
Change index to *false*	
Reinitialize comparison process	
2. Compare first constituents	+
3. Compare second constituents	+
Respond with content of index:	*False*
Number of comparisons:	$k + 1$, where $k = 2$

When there is a mismatch, there are extra operations that increase the latency. A mismatch causes the comparison process to begin again with the inner constituents. For example, in the false affirmative case, the sentence says *The dots are red,* but the picture shows black dots. The inner constituents mismatch and this has several consequences which are detailed in Table 2. (A plus under two constituents denotes a match; a minus denotes a mismatch.) The mismatch causes a change in the response index from true to false, and the two constituents are tagged so that they won't mismatch on future comparisons. The inner constituents are then recompared. Finally, the polarities are compared and found to match. This condition involves one more comparison operation than the true affirmative condition. A false negative has two more comparison operations than the true affirmative because of the mismatch between polarity markers. A true negative has three extra comparisons because of mismatches between both the inner constituents and the polarity markers.

Table 1 derives the predictions of this model for the four conditions. The model postulates a linear increase in the number of comparison operations, from true affirmatives to false affirmatives to false negatives to true negatives. If the response latency is a direct function of the number of comparison operations, there should be a corresponding linear increase in latencies in the four conditions.

Figure 3 shows the same results as Fig. 1, but now plotted a different way. The x axis represents the number of comparisons hypothesized for the four conditions. As predicted, the latencies show a linear increase. In fact, we have found this linearity in a large number of studies (summarized in Carpenter & Just,

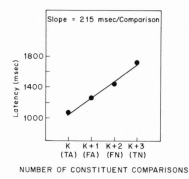

FIG. 3. Results from the verification experiment plotted according to the hypothesized number of operations (data from Just & Carpenter, 1971, II.)

1975). This supports the idea that there is an iterative "find and compare" operation and that mismatches cause reinitialization of the comparison process and, consequently, extra operations.

This model can explain the processing of explicit negatives—sentences with the *not* morpheme. In the next set of experiments, we used this paradigm and theory to investigate how implicit syntactic negatives are processed. A syntactically negative phrase can be identified by using what linguists call "cooccurrence rules." An example of such a rule is that negative clauses can *cooccur* with *either* (Klima, 1964). For example, one can say *Mary didn't go and John didn't go, either*; but one can't say *Mary went and John went, either.* Normally, you would say "too," rather than "either." Since "either" cooccurs only with negatives, it signals the presence of a negative; it acts as a sort of litmus test. This cooccurrence rule suggests that words like *few, hardly any,* and *seldom* are negative because phrases with these quantifiers can be "either-conjoined." For example, *Few boys went and few girls went, either* is an acceptable sentence. There are other quantifiers that can't be either-conjoined. For example, it's not acceptable to say *A minority of the boys went and a minority of the girls went, either.*

The linguist has presented some interesting cooccurrence rules pointing out a contrast between words like *few* and *hardly any* on the one hand and those like *a minority* on the other. Psychologists can now ask about the processing implications of this linguistic distinction. Are sentences with *few* or *hardly any* processed differently from those with *a minority*? The verification paradigm and the model allow us to determine how such sentences are internally represented and processed.

The experiment we ran to examine this question was a verification task where we presented our subjects with one of three kinds of quantified sentences. One kind of sentence had quantifiers like *few,* which the linguist would call syntactically negative. The psychological question is whether *few* is processed like a negative. A second kind of quantifier, like *many* and *most,* was affirmative and referred to a large subset. Notice that according to the cooccurrence rule they are affirmative, since one can't say *Many of the boys went and many of the girls went, either*. The third type of quantifier refers to a small subset, like *a minority* or *a small proportion*. These are also affirmative by the linguistic cooccurrence rule; you can't say *A minority of the boys went and a minority of the girls went, either*. In the experiment (Just & Carpenter, 1971), the subject read a sentence like *Many of the dots are red*. The display showed a large subset of dots of one color and two exceptions. For example, the large subset could be fourteen red dots and the small subset would be two black dots, or vice versa. The predictions can be derived by considering how the sentences are represented. The sentence *Many of the dots are red* presumably is internally represented as an affirmative. So just like the affirmatives discussed before, the true case should be easier than the false case. However, *Few of the dots are red* may be represented and processed like a negative. If it is, the false case should be easier than the true case.

The results in Fig. 4 show that our hypothesis was confirmed: *Many* is processed like an affirmative, while *few* is processed like a negative. The results for quantifiers like *few* can be contrasted with the results for quantifiers like *a minority*. Sentences with quantifiers like *a minority* were easier when they were true, supporting our hypothesis that such quantifiers are represented as affirmations about the smaller subset.

At this point, eye fixations provide a converging operation to further study the way these structures are represented and processed. In the first experiment, we investigated whether the locus of fixation would reflect on how these implicit negatives are represented. We set up a situation where we could monitor how the subject fixated the picture after reading the sentence (Carpenter & Just, 1972). If *few* is internally represented as a negation of *many,* a subject might fixate the larger subset after reading *few.* In contrast, if *a minority* is represented as an affirmative quantifier about the smaller subset, a subject should look at the smaller subset. Similarly, a sentence with *many* might cause the subject to look at the larger subset.

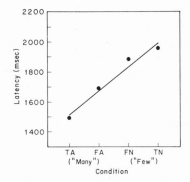

FIG. 4. Results from the verification experiment involving implicitly negative quantifiers (data from Carpenter & Just, 1972).

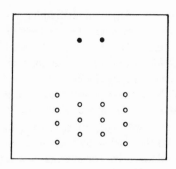

FIG. 5. Schematic represetnation of the relative positions of the sentence and the two sub-sets of dots in the picture.

In this experiment, the subject first read the sentence. Then the sentence disappeared and the picture was presented. We simply recorded the locus of the first fixation on the picture using a wide-angle reflection eye camera (Mack-worth, 1968). The picture was arranged as in Fig. 5. The larger set was always at the bottom; the smaller set was at the top. The subject knew the position of the two sets but didn't know which set would be red and which black. He would have to fixate a subset to determine its color. We hoped that the subject would fixate the subset that was in his internal representation of the sentence. If he did, then following a sentence like *Few of the dots are red*, he should fixate the larger subset. But following a sentence like *A minority of the dots are red*, he should look at the smaller subset.

The results, shown in Table 3, show the predicted interaction between quanti-fiers like *few* where subjects tended to look at the large subset, and quantifiers like *a minority* where subjects tended to look at the small subset. This interac-

TABLE 3
Locus of Fixation as a Function of Sentence Type[a]

Example of quantifier (proposed representation)	Subset fixated			
	Small subset (%)	Large subset (%)	Neither (%)	Errors (%)
"A minority" (Aff (small subset))	43%	23%	25%	9%
"Few" (Neg (large subset))	26%	36%	30%	8%
"Many" (Aff (large subset))	6%	59%	31%	4%

[a]Data from Carpenter and Just (1972).

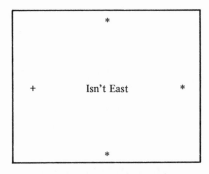

FIG. 6. Schematic drawing of a
typical stimulus display.

tion was consistent across our 18 subjects. And as expected, subjects looked at
the large subset following sentences with quantifiers like *many*.

The importance of this experiment is twofold. First, it confirms our hypothesis about the semantic structure of negatives. A sentence like *Few of the dots
are red* is represented as a negation of a proposition about the larger subset.
Second, the experiment makes an important methodological contribution. It
shows that the locus of an eye fixation can be used to investigate how people
represent linguistic information. In this case, superficially similar sentences like
Few of the dots are red and *A minority of the dots are red*, resulted in different
patterns of eye fixations. And in fact, the eye fixations reflected the hypothesized internal representations.

In a second experiment, we examined whether or not the durations of eye
fixations reflect the mental operations that underlie comprehension. To record
the duration of various fixations, we had subjects verify phrases like *Is East* or *Isn't
East* which referred to the location of a plus, as shown in Fig. 6. The plus could
be in one of four locations. The locations without the plus were filled by
asterisks. For example, if the plus were to the West of the sentence, there would
be asterisks in the North, South and East locations. The subject fixated a point
in the center of the screen and pressed a "ready" button to initiate the onset of
the display. Then he was timed and his eye fixations were recorded while he read
the sentence and responded.[2] The procedure assured that he initially fixated the
sentence. After that, he was free to scan anywhere on the display.

We can ask some simple questions about performance in this task. First, will
the total latencies resemble those for previous experiments? As shown in Fig. 7,
the total latency is beautifully linear; a straight line accounts for 99.9% of the
variance. So this experiment provides an independent confirmation of the
processing model.

The second question is whether the durations of eye fixations reflect the
mental operations we have proposed in the model of verification—operations
such as comparing predicates, comparing polarity markers, and doing extra

[2] We thank Chuck Faddis for designing the instrumentation.

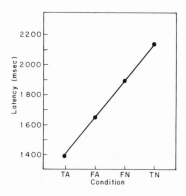

FIG. 7. Total latency in the verification experiment.

comparisons after encountering a mismatch between the sentence and picture representations. To answer this question, we computed the average duration that a particular part of the display was fixated in a trial. (For purposes of scoring, the screen was divided into a three-by-three matrix. All fixations within one of the nine squares were considered equivalent.) In this way, we broke down the total latency into four components. The first component is the duration of the initial fixation on the sentence. This was also the first fixation in a trial. The second component measured the duration of any subsequent fixations on the sentence if there were intervening fixations on other locations. The third component measured how long a person fixated the location mentioned in the sentence. For example, if the sentence said *Isn't East,* this component measured how long the East square in the display was fixated. Finally, the fourth component measured the time spent in any location other than the sentence or the location mentioned in the sentence.

As Fig. 8 shows, the amount of time a person fixated these various locations does reflect the proposed underlying operations. The duration of the first component, the initial fixation on the sentence, is influenced by whether or not there is a negation. The duration is significantly longer when the phrase is negative. The duration of subsequent fixations on the sentence is determined by whether or not there is a negative and whether or not there is a mismatch on the predicate. In other words, this duration is proportional to the hypothesized number of comparison operations. The third component, the time spent on the location mentioned in the sentence, is determined by whether the sentence is affirmative or negative. Again, the duration is significantly longer when the sentence is negative. Finally, the duration of the fourth component, fixations on other locations, is determined by whether or not there is a plus in the location mentioned in the sentence. This duration is significantly longer when there is no plus in the location mentioned in the sentence, namely in the false affirmative and true negative conditions. Thus, all four components reflect the very orderly effects of mismatches between corresponding constituents of the sentence and picture representations.

These results demonstrate two very important points: The total latency fits the model's predictions; moreover, each of the four component latencies reflect the kinds of processing stages postulated to underlie verification. It still remains to map the details of these results onto the model. However, the durations of the component latencies seem to reflect processes like comparing constituents. Thus, the duration of eye fixations, as well as the locus of fixations, as shown in the previous experiment, can be used to study comprehension.

What is exciting about this eye-movement research is that it is predicated on the hypothesis that eye fixations can be an externalization of the immediate processor. Eye fixations can be used to study what is being attended and encoded, and how it is being operated upon in immediate memory. We have shown that in these tasks, both the locus and duration of fixations reflect mental

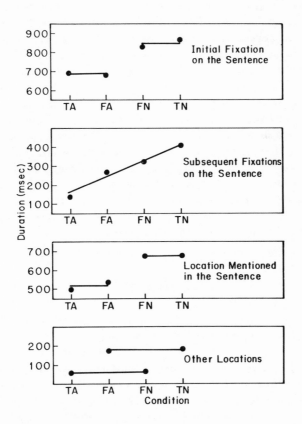

FIG. 8. Duration of fixations on various parts of the display.

operations like encoding and comparing representations. Thus, this represents a way of studying the extremely rapid mental operations in sentence comprehension.

The mental operations of encoding and comparing representations are not specific to tasks that involve visual scanning. In fact, the processing model presented above can explain sentence verification processes when the task requires that information be retrieved from semantic memory (cf. Carpenter & Just, 1975; Just, 1974). For example, the model can predict the latencies to verify sentences like *Seven isn't an even number,* or *Eight is an odd number,* which involve no visual scanning. The model is not concerned with whether the original source of information for a semantic structure is a visual display or previous knowledge of the world. While these sources will obviously entail somewhat different retrieval and encoding processes, it is the commonalities in processing that are of interest here. The model is concerned primarily with the general processes involved in representing and comparing abstract semantic structures. The results suggest that this research, including conclusions from the eye-fixation experiments, reflect many processes that are common to a variety of comprehension situations. Thus, this eye-movement research may provide a way of studying general comprehension processes—not only those that involve visual search.

In summary, there are two main points. The first one is that the locus and duration of eye fixations are systematically related to the underlying mental operations postulated for sentence verification. The second point is that we know how negatives are represented. A negative is represented as an affirmative core plus a negative tag. The difficulty of understanding negatives comes when that tag mismatches some other source of information. We now have the methodology and some of the answers. We can use this approach to investigate other interesting constructions, such as quantifiers and comparatives, to determine how such structures are represented and processed.

DISCUSSION

MONTY: I noticed you completely stayed away from any tendency to speak of the possibilities of subjects' translating from words to mental images. Was this deliberate?

CARPENTER: Mental images could be a possible format for certain kinds of processing. The difficulty is in understanding how someone would have a mental image that would correspond to a negative. That is probably why it is better to think of this task in terms of a comparison of abstract symbols. The other thing is that the abstract symbolic format suits cases where there may be no real images involved, for example, when you're retrieving certain kinds of information from long-term memory. For example, the model can predict the latency to verify sentences like *Seven isn't odd* or *Nixon isn't a Democrat* and I doubt that you generate images.

That doesn't preclude imaginal formats for other structures like comparatives, and there is a current controversy about that.

COOPER: Have you explored the possibility that whether a word like *few* is interpreted as a negative or a positive might depend upon surrounding verbal information? For example, if you consider the sentence *Although none of the dots in the group were red, few of the dots in group 2 were red.*

CARPENTER: Actually to make that sentence acceptable, you'd say . . . *a few of the dots in group 2 were red.* And *a few* is an affirmative whereas *few* is a negative. If you test it with the cooccurrence criteria, this distinction is clear. You can say: *Few of the boys went, and few of the girls went either,* but *A few of the boys went and a few of the girls went, either* isn't acceptable.

COOPER: Isn't it just possible that depending upon the surrounding words of the critical word, *few, few* might be interpreted either as a negative or as a positive?

CARPENTER: My tendency is to think that there are cases where people *convert* negatives like *few* into affirmatives like *a few* or *a minority*. Certainly we do that with explicit negatives. So we might take something like *John isn't home* and if we know there are only two alternatives we might internally convert it to *John must be at school.* That conversion process, the conditions under which people do it, how long it takes, and what mental operations are involved in transforming sentences, form an interesting question. Whether context encourages such transformations is an empirical question.

HABER: One of the morals suggested by an awful lot of data presented earlier was that, at least within the context of reading ability, you could not predict where the next eye movement was going to occur, and the durations of the movements were relatively independent of virtually anything that was tested or manipulated.

Yet you are presenting data which are showing an incredible effect of the kind of mental operations that are being performed on where and for how long the eye lands. Somehow reading ought to fit within the context of what you are discussing. Where is the contradiction?

KOLERS: I think you misrepresented the data from the previous session. Buswell's data showed clearly that when a person was stuck on a word he spent a large amount of time on it.

HABER: But he did it by making lots of fixations. You went to some length to suggest that the duration of these fixations was a relatively invariant phenomenon. Dr. Carpenter is showing that it isn't invariant.

CARPENTER: I want to be clear about one thing and then I will answer your question. These data are the average durations spent at a location during a trial, not the average duration of a single fixation.

More to the point is that the decoding component of reading is kind of a minor component in this task. People know what kind of semantic structures are possible. What I am really tapping and what I meant to tap are the kinds of operations that occur after initial decoding. I am using these operations to reflect on how people must represent information. For researchers who are interested in the original parsing process, this kind of approach has something to say about what kind of representation the parsing process must come up with.

You have to have parsing operations that derive the kind of structure that fits in with the results of these tasks. The representation of that parsing process is in that first box. However, we are mainly tapping another stage of the process: what you do with information once you have represented it.

VII.2

A Computer Implementation
of Constructive Visual Imagery
and Perception

Arthur M. Farley[1]

Carnegie-Mellon University

Classical or atomistic theory proposes that the visual perception of form is an "unconscious conclusion" realized by "unconscious inferences" which are based upon the values of the smallest discriminable or homogeneous patches of the stimulus field. This theory is the product of the traditional philosophy of perception and of the nineteenth century beliefs, now known to be invalid, as to the nature of the physiology of visual perception.

The Gestalt theory of visual form perception developed as a reaction to the failure of the Classical approach to adequately account for the effects of context upon the valuation (interpretation) of any part (atom) of the stimulus. Gestalt theory defines several organizational principles (figure–ground phenomena; laws of proximity, continuity, symmetry, simplicity) which are applied to the whole perceptual field (stimulation) during perception to yield the form perception (Koffka, 1935).

Gestalt theory, like atomistic theory, has proved to have its weaknesses. The organizational "laws" are not actually determinates of perceptual behavior, as they can be overriden by voluntary effort. These laws have also proved difficult to specify in quantitative or operational terms. The whole to which the laws are applied is apparently not specifiable either. Partial figure regions do have significant effects upon complete figural perceptions (Simon, 1967; Hochberg, 1968). Finally, Gestalt theory fails to consider that visual form perception

---

[1] Now at the University of Oregon.

normally involves multiple fixations of the eye and so provides no means for the integration of information from successive differing views.

The constructive theory of visual form perception has developed as an alternative to the Classical and Gestalt approaches. This theory proposes that an internal representation of the visual field is constructed by the integration of a succession of views of (fixations upon) the environment. This representation is both guide for and product of visual form perception. Hebb (1949) began the modern psychological formulation of this theory, describing "cell assemblies" joined together by (into) "phase sequences" as its basic functional elements. Hochberg (1968, 1970a) has recently continued the investigation. He proposes "schematic maps" as the underlying structural organizations which make possible the selective attention to and the successive integration of the visual environment.

The research which is reported here is a further investigation and specification of the constructive theory of visual form perception. More specifically, the goals have been: (1) to investigate the nature of the processes and memories which are involved in the fixation and integration of successive views of the environment; (2) to investigate the nature of the internal representation (symbolic visual image) which is capable of embodying the necessary partial and complete perceptions; (3) to specify the results of the investigations in the form of an operational, computer-implemented visual imagery and perception system (VIPS). VIPS is the name of such a program which has been implemented in LISP 1.6 on a Digital Equipment Co. PDP-10 at Carnegie Mellon University.

Motivation for the two investigative goals is abundant. The need is best expressed by the following two statements: (1) by Haber and Hershenson (1973), "There is little evidence to guide our thinking on how these integrations and constructions take place. In fact, . . . little attention has been paid to how such processes occur at all [p. 174]"; and (2) by Hochberg (1968), "What we need is a set of operations for defining and studying the kind of visual storage that will build up the structures of perceived forms out of momentary glimpses [p. 322]."

As for the goal of specifying the results in the form of a computer-implemented model, I believe that one major factor which has contributed to the fluid state of affairs at the theoretical level is the failure to attempt complete specifications and implementations of the imagery and perceptual processes implied by a stated theory. Descriptive theories of perception often employ easily expressible, intuitively understood, but difficult-to-realize operations. Accepting the view that perception and imagery are basically symbolic information-processing activities, the computer and several existing programming language systems (i.e., LISP) now provide a valuable means for the further investigation of theoretical proposals. Not only can some light be shed on the sufficiency questions for any proposal, but through implementation design and subsequent actual system behavior, other theory implications possibly not realized earlier appear for consideration. What control information is necessary and can it be feasibly included? Is the information representation concise enough to fit into a limited active memory, yet rich enough to afford the inferences which subjects display? These are only two of the many questions which cannot really be answered for a perceptual (cognitive) theory until a completely operational specification and implementation has been realized, or at least attempted, for a reasonable subset of activity. Experimental research in psychology has provided the necessary critical mass of design-relevant information to attempt an initial implementation of the theory such as VIPS.

The implementation goal here has been more extensive (inclusive) than that of achieving simple input–output equivalence or correspondence. VIPS employs a number of memory components and perceptual processes which explicitly contain all of the symbolic information involved in the perceptual system's operation. The memory components (icon, short-term and long-term memory) and their associated characteristics have been inferred from experimental results of cognitive psychology. Thus, the model attempts to realize correspondence at a less superficial, internal level. The programmed system's output is a trace of active memory contents at selected points of processing. A common criticism of computer-implemented models (simulations) of human cognitive behavior has been that they necessarily employ many hidden computer-oriented nonpsychological operations to achieve input–output equivalence. VIPS and other recently implemented systems (Newell, 1972; Moran, 1973) attempt to make theoretical implications explicit in the implementation to a greater extent than before and to explore (confront) the consequences. This report is based upon research done as a Ph. D. thesis in computer science at Carnegie-Mellon University. A more complete discussion of the work appears in the thesis which is available as a published report from that department (Farley, 1974).

Two experiments were conducted to provide data from which to infer characteristics of the visual image representation and the rules of the perceptual processes. The first experiment presents subjects with a task situation which forces them to perform what is primarily perceptual activity over an extended (cognitive) time frame. The VIPS has been implemented to explain this behavior. The second experiment presents a task situation which is nearer to that of "normal" visual form perception. These results are considered in light of the theory embodied by VIPS and as the basis for its necessary extension and modification.

The first part of Experiment I had subjects simply view a line drawing (of approx 25° visual angle extent) until they were capable of verbally describing and drawing it from memory. At the subject's signal, the drawing was removed and the subject proceeded first to describe, then to draw the picture. Four students (one senior and three graduate) of Carnegie-Mellon University participated as subjects in Experiment I. Figure 1 shows the line drawings used. This part familiarized the subjects with the classes of drawings to be used in the main

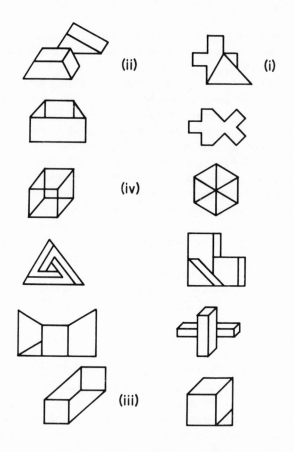

FIG. 1. Stimuli of Experiment I, part 1. Four classes of line drawings: (i) two dimensional with overlay; (ii) three dimensional projections; (iii) three dimensional, impossible; (iv) three dimensional, reversing.

experiment part. The transcribed verbal descriptions and the drawing behavior were used as bases for image representation specification.

The main task of Experiment I presented the subject with a line drawing taped to a table which was covered by a large paper mask with a hole in it. The hole (of approx. $3°$ visual angle extent) allowed the subject to view at most one vertex at a time. The subject's task was to move the hole over the drawing until he was capable of verbally describing and drawing the complete picture. The subject was also instructed to "think aloud" during the hole-movement sequence. This task is an extension and modification of the partial, sequential viewing task described by Hochberg (1968).

The protocols were videotaped. Table 1 indicates the line drawings used and the degree of consideration given each protocol during analysis. The protocols

TABLE 1
Stimuli of Experiment I and the Degree of
Consideration Given each Protocol as System Design Basis

Stimulus / Subject	[1][a]	[2][a]	[3][a]	[4][a]	[5]	[6]	[7]	[8]	[9]	[10]
B	T	–	T	T	N	N	N	N	N	N
G	I	N	T	T	N	N	N	N	N	N
P	–	I	T	T	N	N	N	N	N	N
S	I	I	–	T	N	N	N	N	N	N

[a]I, implemented, thoroughly analyzed; T, transcribed, thoroughly analyzed; N, not transcribed, considered generally; –, behavior protocol not taken.

served as a basis for perceptual-process-rule specification, for the structure of recognition long-term memory, and, together with the verbal descriptions and the drawings, for image-representation specification. Table 2 is the initial segment of a transcribed protocol.

Something must be said concerning the relevance of the verbal data to the specification of the visual image and perception system. The protocol verbalizations indicate internal states (goals, confirmations) and as such do form a reasonable basis for process-rule specification. These verbalizations are not introspective assertions as to the nature and course of activity. The visual image which is constructed by the perceptual activity serves as the semantic basis for the subsequent verbal description. As such, the verbal description indicates information that must be contained in or be readily derivable from that visual image.

Experiment II was conducted upon a corneal reflecting eye-movement tracking and recording (video-taping) system. Two subjects participated; both had been subjects for Experiment I which had been conducted one month earlier. In the first part, a line drawing (of approx. 25° visual angle extent) was presented for 250 to 350 msec. while the subject fixated a preset point of the visual field. The eye-movement recording provided the means of assuring that only a single fixation occurred. Immediately upon removal of the picture, the subject simulta-

TABLE 2
A Segment of Transcribed Protocol

View seen through hole	Direction if any	Associated verbalization
(1)		looks like the corner [SI] this part right here looks like the corner of a uh [S2] of a square [S3] now, lets see if I can... [S4]
	→ RT	if it is to be a square [S5] this would be the bottom of the square [S6]
(3)		aha! [S7] looks like we might have a triangular object [S8] this would be
	↖ UL	the second side of the triangle [SI0] (slowly)
(8)	↖ UL	(through vertex 8)
	↖ UL	
(2)		
	↓ DO	and this is the third side [SII]
		okay [SI2]

neously proceeded to describe and to draw what he now knew of the line drawing.

In the second part, the subject was again given a preset initial fixation point. A line drawing (approx. 25°) was presented, and the subject was allowed to view (scan) the line drawing until he was capable of verbally describing and drawing it from memory. The picture was removed at the subject's signal and the subject proceeded first to describe and then to draw the line drawing. Several of the line drawings used had been previously used in the hole-movement task (those starred in Table 1). The eye movements were videotaped and the verbal descriptions were audiotaped.

Imagery recently has returned as a concept under investigation in cognitive psychology. One result of this renewed interest is the need for an adequate scientific definition of imagery. An image is defined here to be an internal, semantic, symbolic representation of information which is capable of determining (guiding) behavior and which has an internal modality characteristic. The internal modality characteristic distinguishes images from other forms of internal representations by requiring that the image be structured so that it can be (is) accessed by processes isomorphic to those which access the external environment for the given sensory modality (Simon, 1972). With regard to a perceptual image, semantic means that meaning, but not necessarily the order of the information acquisition, is represented. By further specification, a visual image is an internal semantic representation of visual feature and spatial relation information consisting of symbols and relations which are structured so as to be straightforwardly retrievable by internal processes isomorphic to those which access the visual environment during visual perception. A visual image is capable of guiding motor and cognitive behavior with regard to the visual environment that it represents. A primary example of such behavior is visual form perception. On the other hand, visual form perception is a primary source of visual images. A visual image is classified as a "perception" when it bears sufficient correspondence to external events and environment.

The basic unit of meaningful visual image information within VIPS is the image chunk. An image chunk is a semantic structure of interrelated symbol elements. An image chunk represents a visual concept. VIPS uses five types of image chunks (concepts) in its representations of the line-drawing environment, these being the VERTEX, OBJECT, LINE, SIDE, and FACE types.

An image chunk consists of one Chunk Header element, one or more Position elements, and several Image Body elements. The Chunk Header serves to indicate the chunk's type and to afford a means of access to the chunk's structure of Image Body elements. A Position element serves to indicate the perceived location of the Image Body elements which reference it. This position is in terms of a seven-by-seven locational area grid which is bound to the current area of interest within the visual environment. All Image Body elements reference a Position element. This binds the Image Body structure, and thus the visual image, to locations in perceptual (imaginal) space. Perceptual space is not retinally based, but rather is bound to an area of current interest within the visual field. This plays a significant role in the maintenance of a stable visual world in spite of the varying retinal states which occur with changing fixations during visual form perception.

The Image Body elements form a nonhierarchical symbol structure which embodies the spatial configuration of visual features of the visual concept represented by the chunk. This structure is a doubly directed circular list of elements. The relational links between Image Body elements have directional or space-traversal (direction and distance) meaning. Thus, the allowed means of accessing the image, which is by traversal of existing structural links, is isomorphic in meaning to a visual search or scan of the external visual environment. This feature of visual imagery is the internal modality characteristic for vision.

Five types of Image Body elements (XIT, ANGLE, INTERNAL, END, and QUICKSEE) are used to represent the concepts embodied by image chunks. Each element type is defined by the role it plays in the Image Body structure (the features and relations it embodies). These five element types also form a straightforward basis for generalization of the image representation. Figure 2

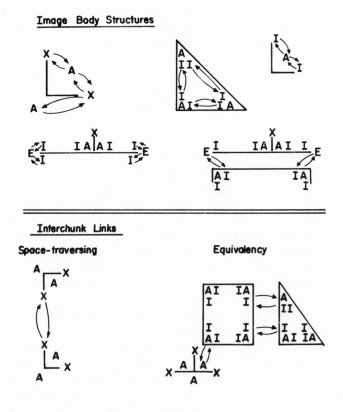

FIG. 2. Pictorial representations of exemplar image chunk structures.

pictorially illustrates the use of these elements in representative examples of the different chunk-type Image Body structures. A VERTEX chunk consists of alternating XIT and ANGLE elements. An OBJECT chunk consists of "corner configurations" made up of INTERNAL and ANGLE elements. An INTERNAL differs from an XIT element in that it has only one internal vertex direction and link to an ANGLE element. This is the image representation's embodiment of the figure—ground phenomenon of visual perception. To traverse around the "outside" of an object corner, another chunk must be accessed (attended). The LINE and SIDE chunks introduce the use of the END element. A SIDE chunk is always associated with an OBJECT chunk.

A visual image is a semantic structure of interrelated image chunks. An Image Body element of one image chunk may be linked to one of another chunk by one of two basic relation types. One type has space-traversal meaning, relating the two elements in terms of a direction and distance defined within the imaginal space. The other type is an equivalency relation. This type of link relates two elements of differing chunks which represent the same actual component of the external visual field. Thus, that component is embodied within two visual-image concepts (chunks). For example, a line segment shared by two adjacent objects is represented within (by) both of the OBJECT chunks. The INTERNAL elements which embody the line segment are linked by equivalency relations. Equivalency links introduce a certain degree of redundancy and reflect the semantic character of the image representation.

The perceptual system of VIPS consists of six memories and four processes, as shown by Fig. 3. In the figure, an arrow from a process to a memory indicates

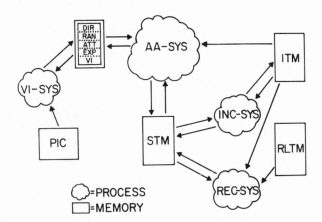

FIG. 3. VIPS system architecture. An arrow from a process to a memory indicates that the process can alter the memory contents. An arrow from a memory to a process indicates that the process can access the memory contents.

that the process can alter the memory's contents, while an arrow from a memory to a process indicates that the process can access the memory's contents. The characteristics of the system at the overview (general) level result primarily from a consideration of relevant research results and theoretical proposals of cognitive psychology.

Since perceptual activity involves the interaction of organism and environment, VIPS must represent both. As such, PIC (PICture) is the environment, defined in terms of the visual modality, and it consists of a list of vertex-feature lists. Each vertex-feature list represents the detectable visual features at one of the line-drawing vertices (the observed points of "hole fixation"). The Current Picture Pointer (CPP) is associated with PIC and references one vertex-feature list, being equivalent to the current hole position.

The five cells of the Visual Register (VR) serve as communication registers between the VI-SYS and AA-SYS processes. The cells of VR are set prior to VI-SYS activation by AA-SYS. VI-SYS accesses PIC according to the VR cell specifications and appropriately alters the cells of VR prior to the return of control to AA-SYS upon deactivation.

The VI (Visual Information) cell is the iconic visual image (Neisser, 1967). It is constructed automatically as a result of the new hole positioning, being always set to null prior to VI-SYS activation. The representation of visual information in VI is that of an image chunk. It is as yet unrelated to any existing image contents produced by prior perceptual activity. Its form is not affected by any active perceptual goal.

When specified, EXP (EXPectation) and ATT (ATTention) make possible the application of preattentive functions by VI-SYS to the newly accessed PIC information. EXP can be specified either as an angle code or as a vertex type and specification. Upon VI-SYS deactivation, EXP will be YES, NO, or CON (CONtained), indicating the relationship of expectation to realization. ATT can be specified as a direction code symbol. VI-SYS will then move through an encountered vertex which is straight (has 180° angle) on the ATT side of the line being traversed.

The value of DIR (DIRection) specifies the direction of the hole movement to be effected by VI-SYS. The value of RAN (RANge) specifies the range of that move. RAN is a returned value of VI-SYS in VIPS (hole movement), whereas during saccadic (ballistic) eye-movement behavior, it would be prespecified by AA-SYS. The values of these cells may be incorporated into the image by AA-SYS. This reflects the intrinsic role of motor (efferent) activity in visual perception and imagery.

Short Term Memory (STM) consists of an ordered list of nine chunks, being the limited amount of active memory available to the perceptual (cognitive) system for image construction (Miller, 1956). An STM chunk is an image chunk or an image chunk with a Special type element (GOL, LAST, COM, or OGOL) appended. STM chunks are accessed according to Image Body element containment or Special element appendment. STM is the memory in which the visual image (perception) is constructed. STM and VR are the active memory components or "mind's eye" during visual form perception. During recall and drawing involving imagery, only STM is active as the mind's eye.

There are three components of long-term memory in VIPS. LTM is the universe of symbols used in VIPS. The symbols are interrelated, forming a semantic network of symbols and relations. The use of any symbol in an active memory or by a process rule is an activation of that LTM element. (In the implementation in LISP 1.6, it is a pointer to that element.) A symbol of LTM is said to be in a memory when it plays the appropriate processing role. As such, any active memory entity (VR cell or STM chunk) is only pseudoself-contained. Every symbol instance implies the possible use of all of its LTM relations and related symbols by the active process. The symbol remains effectively imbedded in the LTM structure when activated.

Recognition Long-Term Memory (RLTM) is an n-ary discrimination net. The discrimination structure is determined by angle symbols and the objects which angle configurations determine. It is used to recognize complete object images and to hypothesize known objects from incomplete images. Image-generating functions are associated with the memory and are used by REC-SYS to complete hypothesized object images.

Intermediate-Term Memory (ITM) is the memory into which selected STM chunks are incorporated. Meaningful results of the perceptual activity are transferred to this memory as the current meaningful processing context. The contents of ITM are recallable into STM for use by the perceptual process. As chunks are incorporated, new links are added between image-chunk Chunk Header elements. These new links indicate a chunk's immediate imaginal context (related image chunks) and the temporal order of OBJECT chunk incorporations. Thus, the final perceptual image, which is found in ITM is a heterarchical symbol structure. Hunt (1973) and Wickelgren (1972) discuss different reasons for the likely existence of ITM as part of the human cognitive system.

All four processes are implemented in the form of a production system (Newell & Simon, 1972). A production system consists of an ordered list of condition–action pairs. The system is cyclic in operation. With each cycle, the first rule found which has its *condition* satisfied is said to "fire," resulting in the *action's* being executed. Rule firings depend upon and alter only active memory contents, reflecting the contextual nature of human cognition.

The Assimilation–Accommodation process (AA-SYS) is named for the two basic types of behavior associated with it (Piaget, 1968). This process either can assimilate the contents of VR into the image as found in STM or must accommodate that current image in light of the conflicting contents of VR. AA-SYS is the "main" process: it is the source of most goals; it sets VR and activates VI-SYS so as to access new PIC contents; it activates REC-SYS to aid in its image construction activity; it activates INC-SYS to incorporate satisfactory and meaningful segments (chunks) of the image into ITM.

As the primary source of current goals and their transitions, AA-SYS embodies the perceptual strategy in the VIPS implementation. Two over-all strategies have been inferred from the protocol data, resulting in two corresponding AA-SYS implementations. One strategy is that of successively recognizing objects until having represented the whole line drawing. The other is that of first attempting to scan and represent the entire line drawing outline and then linking up unknown inward-directed exits. The second strategy diverts to the first in a number of circumstances.

The other three processes are supplementary perceptual processes. The basic activity and function of VI-SYS has already been described in the VR discussion. REC-SYS traverses appropriate image chunks of STM, and recognizes or hypothesizes known objects. INC-SYS incorporates chunks into ITM and can improve the image in certain ways. It also adds links between Chunk Header elements which indicate interacting chunks during chunk incorporation.

Each rule of AA-SYS, REC-SYS, and INC-SYS has the name of the current goal as the primary consideration of its condition. Visual form perception is a goal-determined activity which consists of a sequence of goal-related episodes. The current goal is the primary determinant of what current visual (VR) and image (STM) information is of interest, what external information is to be accessed (fixated) next, and into what class of image structures the new information is to be integrated and then represented. Figure 4 is a goal episode chart

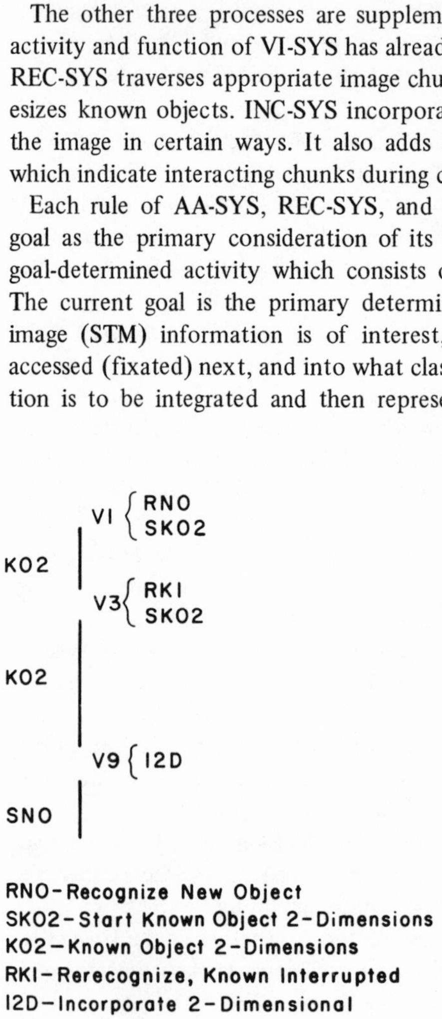

```
              ⎧ RNO
         VI  ⎨
              ⎩ SKO2
  KO2   │
              ⎧ RKI
         V3 ⎨
              ⎩ SKO2

        │
  KO2   │

        │
         V9 ⎰ I2D

  SNO   │
```

RNO – Recognize New Object
SKO2 – Start Known Object 2 – Dimensions
KO2 – Known Object 2 – Dimensions
RKI – Rerecognize, Known Interrupted
I2D – Incorporate 2 – Dimensional

FIG. 4. A goal episode chart for the behavior transcribed as Fig. 2.

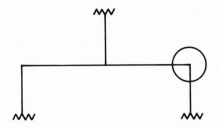

FIG. 5. A partial line drawing with the hole positioned over the right-angle vertex to the right.

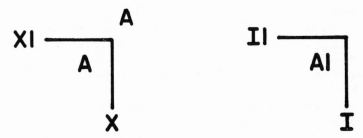

FIG. 6. The image contents of VI (icon) given fixation upon the vertex visible through the hole in Fig. 5.

FIG. 7. The initial phase of OB-JECT image construction given the icon of Fig. 6.

which illustrates the inferred goal sequence for the protocol segment of Table 2. Goals to the right (in brackets) of a protocol frame number are active at (during) that "hole fixation." A goal to the left of a vertical line is active during the hole-movement sequence occurring between the protocol frames indicated.

Examples of the activity of VIPS in several hypothetical situations indicate the nature of assimilation–accommodation and the effects of active goals upon the perceptual process and the resultant perception.

Figure 5 presents a partial line drawing. Suppose that the hole is initially positioned at the circled vertex and that the strategy is that of successively recognizing objects. Figure 6 pictorially illustrates the initial contents of VI (icon), indicating that it is a VERTEX chunk. AA-SYS assimilates VI by simply making it a chunk of STM, and then activates REC-SYS with a current goal of RNO (Recognize New Object). REC-SYS traverses the new VERTEX chunk in STM, moves CRMP in RLTM according to the right angle encountered, and begins construction of a new object chunk, as illustrated by Fig. 7. Since there is no more relevant information in STM, then REC-SYS applies an image-generating function which is indicated by the RLTM node referenced by CRMP, completing a square or rectangle image chunk as illustrated by Fig. 8. Subject behavior indicates that this is the usual hypothesis, given a right angle as the only relevant information. REC-SYS deactivates, and control returns to AA-SYS.

AA-SYS uses this new OBJECT chunk to determine new Visual Register settings prior to VI-SYS activation requesting new visual information. The current goal (NAME of GOL) is now KO2 (Known Object 2 dimensions). Another property of the Special element GOL (which is now appended to the OBJECT chunk) is CR (Current Reference). The CR of GOL is now set to I1 (see Fig. 8). DIR is now set to LE (LEft), according to the direction of I1's link to I2. Then ATT is set to DO (DOwn), according to I1's link to A1, and EXP is set to RTA (RighT Angle), according to the ANG (ANGle) property of A2. RAN and VI are set to null and VI-SYS is activated. VI-SYS moves the hole (CPP) to the left, going past the vertex where the vertical hits the horizontal from above, due to ATT being DO. The hole comes to rest at the other right-angle vertex, as shown in Fig. 9. EXP is set to YES as the right angle is found on the down side of the newly fixated vertex as expected. RAN is set to a distance symbol and VI contains new image contents, as illustrated by Fig. 10. This illustrates the use of a QUICKSEE element in VIPS when a vertex is moved through during hole movement. A QUICKSEE element partially represents that vertex by indicating only the number of vertex exits leaving the line at that point (in this case, 1).

With the return of control, AA-SYS notes that EXP is YES and that the image in VI is a LINE type chunk. This causes a rule to fire which accommodates that LINE chunk to a new SIDE chunk and places it in STM, binding it to the OBJECT chunk as shown in Fig. 11. As a hypothesized object is confirmed visually, the appropriate image elements are "marked" by a special property. Elements I2, A2, and I3 are now so marked and CR of GOL is updated to I3. The goal remains KO2 and the image is used to determine new VR settings as discussed above, the next movement direction being down. If EXP had been NO (say an acute angle was found on the bottom vertex side), then REC-SYS would

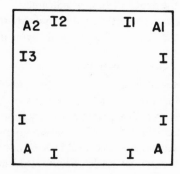

FIG. 8. The completed square image as hypothesized from the icon of Fig. 6.

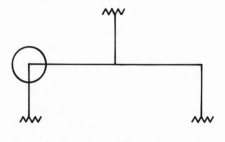

FIG. 9. The resultant new hole fixation realized by using the image of Fig. 8 to guide the hole movement.

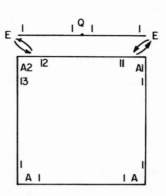

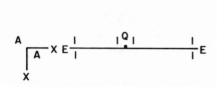

FIG. 10. The image contents of the icon (VI) as a result of the hole movement to the location indicated in Fig. 9.

FIG. 11. The resultant image in STM after assimilation of the new Visual Register contents.

have been reactivated with goal RKI (Rerecognize, Known Interrupted) to accommodate the proposed object image in light of the new visual information. This can be seen in the goal–episode chart of Fig. 4 accounting for the protocol behavior of Table 2.

We reconsider this from the initial situation (Fig. 5) given that the strategy is now first to scan the exterior outline of the line drawing. Again VI is initially as in Fig. 6, the icon affected only by Visual Register and Picture contents. AA-SYS again assimilates this information simply by making this VERTEX chunk into a chunk of STM. The GoI element is appended to this chunk, CR of GOL is set to X1, and PDIR (Prime DIRection) of GOL is set to UP, PDIR being the perceived outside direction relative to CR of GOL. The current goal (NAME of GOL) is SEO (SEarch Outside). AA-SYS sets DIR to LE (LEft) according to the vertex exit-direction property of X1. The other VR cells are set to null and VI-SYS is activated.

VI-SYS moves the hole (CPP) left, stopping at the vertex where the vertical hits the horizontal from above, as shown in Fig. 12. When only DIR is specified, the first vertex encountered in that direction is fixated. RAN is set to a distance symbol and the vertex chunk illustrated in Fig. 13 is realized in VI. VI-SYS deactivates, returning control to AA-SYS.

AA-SYS assimilates this new information by entering it as a new chunk in STM and linking it to the first chunk as shown in Fig. 14. This new link incorporates the value of RAN as a range-specification property. The fired rule of AA-SYS then appends the Special element LAST to this chunk, indicating to the next system cycle that that chunk represents the visual information seen last. CR of the Chunk Header element of that chunk is initially set to X2, that being the exit that the hole movement entered. The chunk is now traversed in the UP (PDIR of GOL) direction, reaching X3. CR of LAST is set to X3, and PDIR of GOL is updated to RT (RighT), now being the perceived outside direction

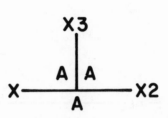

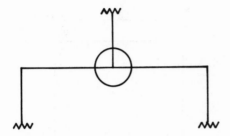

FIG. 12.   The resultant hole fixation point when moving from that
of Fig. 5 with the goal to scan the
figure boundaries.

FIG. 13.   The resultant new VI
contents at the fixation point of
Fig. 12.

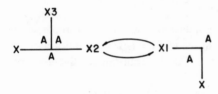

FIG. 14.   The image in STM as a
result of the assimilation of Visual
Register contents produced by
the hole movement.

relative to CR of LAST. The next hole movement would be up, being the vertex
exit direction of CR of LAST (X3).

These examples illustrate the current goal's effect upon the hole-movement
sequence undertaken and the representation (perception) of the visual information which is encountered. The basic nature of image construction based upon a
succession of input views is also illustrated. How the image serves both as guide
for and product of perceptual behavior is shown. This assimilation—
accommodation activity typifies man's interaction with the environment during
perceptual behavior. VIPS is implemented to explain four selected protocols,
although consideration was given to all protocols. In terms of hole-movement
correspondence, VIPS is above 80% for three of the protocols (65% on the
other), which is significantly better than uniformly random or uniformly random with no backtracking hole-movement generators. Consideration of the
behavior in terms of goal-related sequences allows VIPS to regain hole-movement
correspondence after brief periods of activity which do not exactly match the
protocol. VIPS consistently has sufficient active memory to serve as a basis for
the observed perceptual inference and verbal behavior.

The behavior which was observed and recorded as data from Experiment II has
been considered only on a general descriptive level (up to the time of this
report). No perceptual system has been implemented which produces corre-

sponding behavior and which could then serve as an operative theoretical explanation of the behavior. This general consideration of the data has been favorable to the proposition that VIPS can be straightforwardly transformed into a sufficient explanation of that behavior.

The verbal descriptions and partial drawings obtained as data in part I of Experiment II provide the basis for inferring the state of the mind's eye following processing of the initial fixation by the perceptual system. The data indicates that the initial fixation serves the perceptual system as a source (basis) of inferences and hypotheses. General characteristics of the total extent of the line drawing are consistently inferred, thus determining (delimiting) the current area of perceptual interest. Object hypotheses are generated for regions (areas bounded by spatially disjoint features) within that extent of the visual field. Such processing of the initial fixation is consistent with an active assimilation–accommodation theory of visual form perception as is embodied by VIPS.

Much of the initial processing is based upon visual information's lying in the periphery of the visual field. This input must be sensed by the means and processes of peripheral vision. The data indicate that peripheral information at positions of up to $25°$ of visual angle from the fixation point contributes to the initial inferences and hypotheses. Some observed-object hypotheses relate visual information which must have been entirely peripheral. Although a sufficient basis for object hypothesis, peripheral vision consistently failed to allow subjects correctly to infer the particulars of object interactions (interrelationships).

The hole-movement task's situation masked peripheral vision information. Therefore, the representation and utilization of peripheral vision's input are not part of VIPS and are most basic and necessary extensions to the system. A class of elements which embody the position of irregularities or discontinuities in the periphery shows promise as a possible symbolic representation. The position information would necessarily be retinally based and, as such, would be relative (direction and distance) to the current fixation point. Uhr (1973) discusses a means of detecting and locating discontinuities by use of simple psychologically and physiologically feasible and readily implementable differencing operators. Such elements appear to be an adequate supplement to foveal (feature) elements as a basis for the observed inferences, hypotheses, and eye-movement behavior.

The recorded eye-movement sequences obtained in Experiment II have been considered in terms of fixation durations and locations. Fixation durations varied from approximately $\frac{1}{8}$ sec to over 1 sec. The distribution was neither uniform nor normal but was skewed, most fixations being less than $\frac{1}{3}$ in length. The variation in fixation length favors an active theory of visual form perception which requires differing amounts of information processing at fixations. The initial fixation was significantly longer in duration than those immediately following it (see Table 3), thus upholding its role as a highly processed source of inferences and hypotheses. The exception is a sequence during the perception of a line drawing with several overlaid objects (as perceived) and initially could have

TABLE 3
Fixation Durations[a] (1/60 sec)

Eye-movement sequence	Fixation number			
	1	2	3	4
SI	24	10	15	24
PI	40	10	12	34
S2	35	13	11	17
P2	34	15	11	15
S3	33	10	32	11
P3	24	26	21	15
S4	42	10	21	26
P4	43	11	20	12
MEAN	34.4	13.1		
A.D.	5.6	3.8		

[a]For the initial four fixations upon the line drawings starred in Table 1.

involved continuous image accommodation. In general, the eye-movement sequences consisted of an initial over-all scan of the line drawing, perception relying heavily upon peripheral input, followed by a rescan which concentrated primarily upon object-interaction areas.

In conclusion, VIPS has been implemented to account directly for four hole-movement protocols. An evaluation of protocol program-trace correspondence is favorable to the perceptual theory embodied by the system. Extensions are discussed which transform the system into a more inclusive perceptual theory. A comparison of studies yields the proposal that human information representation in active memory is flexible, being as suited to the task as possible in light of the existing symbols, relations, and structure of an evolving long-term memory upon which all cognition is based (Farley, 1974).

The research which has been reported here has resulted in a speculative theoretical specification of the constructive theory of visual form perception. It is not meant to be a conclusion and this report does not really have one. As an initial implementation, VIPS can now have modifications and extensions applied (some are discussed above) to represent better the perceptual activity it is meant to explain. Being a theoretical statement, it can serve as a source of experimental questions, the resulting experimental findings being the basis for subsequent specification improvement.

VII.3

Eye Movement Fixations and Gating Processes[1]

Robert J. Hall

University of Nevada, Las Vegas

The concept of gating processes or intermittency in perception is not new and the idea that the brain operates by taking successive samples of sensory information at different points and times is supported by the discrete nature of perception. This gating process (i.e., the tendency for incoming information to be perceptually grouped in time) is supported by the very nature of eye movements (fixation sequences) and evoked potentials (Harter, 1967).

In a discussion of eye movements, evoked responses, and visual perception, White (1969) pointed out that in a number of studies dealing with the activity of the visual system, 250–300 msec appears to be a critical duration. This critical period was derived from studies measuring fixation duration during visual search, evoked cortical potential patterns, and the temporal limitations in perceiving sequential events. All of this suggests that this critical period is related to certain aspects of the processing and the assimilation of visual information.

My interests here are: (1) what eye movements may indicate about interpersonal perceptions and needs, and (2) what eye movements may indicate about the processing of sensory data by the CNS.

A review of the eye movement literature (Hall & Cusack, 1972) has led me to the conclusion that the difficulty of relating eye movements to interpersonal needs and cognitive processes has been due largely to the lack of adequate apparatus and techniques for processing the large volumes of data generated by eye movement trackers. The apparatus used in the following studies incorporated data processing techniques for partitioning and analyzing eye movement data.

[1] The work reported here was supported in part by the U.S. Army Human Engineering Laboratory and by the Advanced Research Projects Agency.

491

I will summarize a series of experiments conducted while the apparatus, described earlier by Lambert (Also see Lambert, Monty, & Hall, 1974; Monty, 1975) was under development. Among the primary dependent variables to be discussed here are: fixation duration and variability, number of fixations, and mean distance between fixations.

The purpose of a series of experiments conducted by Hall, Rosenberger, and Monty (1974a) and by Monty, Hall and Rosenberger (1975) was to determine if the eye movements of heroin addicts differed from nonaddicted matched controls. I will discuss only a part of the data here. Briefly, eye movements were tracked and recorded at the rate of 60 frames per second, without the subject's knowledge and without interfering with his visual behavior, yielding a total of 129,600 frames of eye movement data for each of 46 subjects.

The first experiment was designed specifically to examine visual search behavior during visual learning and later recognition. To accomplish this, both groups of subjects were required to examine word sets, some of which would be presented in a subsequent recognition session. Eye movements were monitored continuously throughout the learning process. Three categories of words were employed: *neutral words, drug jargon,* and *dirty words,* in the expectation that the words would reveal differences between addicts and control subjects. Various combinations of these word types were projected four at a time in the approximate center of each of the quadrants of a 1 m X .76 m viewing surface. The words themselves subtended an angle of approximately 1° X 3° at the eye. During the learning session the mean number of fixations of 100 msec or longer falling within each quadrant was recorded. The data are shown in the upper portion of Fig. 1. It can be seen that the number of fixations was somewhat higher for the upper right and upper left than for the lower left and lower right positions for both groups, and that controls had consistently more fixations than addicts. These differences may reflect position preferences of the subjects or possible differences in system accuracy at various portions of the field.

The average durations of these fixations are shown in the lower half of Fig. 1. The mean fixation durations are longer than we might expect, for example, greater than 500 msec. This occurs because the size of the area or the boundary criterion used to define a simple fixation in each quadrant tended to combine successive fixations that were close to one another. A comparison of the upper and lower halves of the figure indicates that the number of fixations per position was greater for the controls than for the addicts, and, of course, the average duration of fixation was greater for the addicts than the controls. In other words, both groups were attending to the words but the control subjects tended to scan more frequently between words.

To determine if there were any difference between addicts and controls in terms of their reaction to emotionally loaded words (i.e., *drug* or *dirty words*) each subject's fixation duration for each *drug* or *dirty word* was subtracted from his or her own mean fixation duration for neutral words occurring in the same

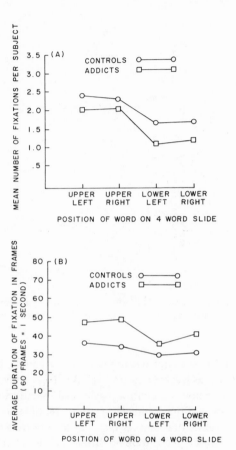

FIG. 1.   Mean number of fixations (A) and average duration of fixation (B) during the learning process on the word recognition task. (after Monty, Hall & Rosenberger, 1975.)

position. This was done to avoid confounding with possible subject preferences or apparatus artifacts associated with position. These results are shown in Fig. 2. It can be seen that addicts spent substantially more time looking at drug and dirty words relative to neutral words than did controls. However, differences between addicts and controls exist even for the neutral word category. This suggests that there may be two types of differences between addicts and controls: differences produced by the motivational aspect of the drug and dirty words, and differences caused by some more basic phenomenon stemming from the rate at which information is processed.

A second session was run in the same manner as the first, except that each slide contained four objects, one in each quadrant of the slide. The objects were

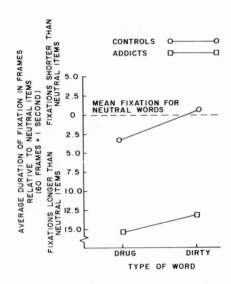

FIG. 2. Average duration of fixation in frames on drug words and dirty words relative to neutral items during the learning process on the word recognition task. (After Monty, Hall, & Rosenberger, 1975.)

either drug related (such as apparatus for injecting heroin, tie offs, or tourne-quets) or neutral (such as wallets or ash trays). A typical array is shown in Fig. 3. During the learning session the controls again made significantly more fixations than the addicts. In addition, addicts spent more time looking at the drug objects relative to the neutral objects than did the controls. In contrast to the first experiment, however, there were no differences between groups in the time spent looking at neutral objects.

Taken together, these results suggest that two factors are operating: motivational or interest factors associated with the nature of the stimulus material, for example, drug versus neutral items, and possible differences in reading skill and the ability to manipulate printed material as indicated by the differences noted between words and objects. However, the observation that fixation durations are generally substantially longer for addicts than for controls suggests that there are also basic differences in the physiological and central nervous system processes that regulate eye movement or an underlying information processor.

In a parallel investigation of cutaneous sensitivity Hall, Rosenberger, and Monty (1974b) found that the time taken to detect the direction of movement of a stylus drawn across the volar surface of the forearm is greater for heroin addicts than for nonaddicts. Perception of nontemporal dimensions such as stylus pressures were not affected, suggesting that the effects of heroin addiction are highly specific and alter the rate of central nervous sytem processes.

In summary, when the visual data and the cutaneous data are considered together, there is support for the speculation that addicts have a slower rate of CNS functioning, which manifests itself as a slower visual scanning rate in our studies. They also appear to have an altered interest pattern which reflects their concern with acultural ideas.

The next series of experiments dealt with eye movements during a simple detection and threat evaluation task. A 75-min simulated tactical display was devised which involved surveillance, tracking, and threat evaluation of targets. During this task the amount of eye movement data generated and analyzed for one subject equals 270,000 frames of eye-movement data or 2,970,000 frames for the 11 subjects used.

The simulated tactical display consisted of two concentric circles in which the outer circle indicated the effective missile range and the inner circle represented the defended area as shown in Fig. 4. The subject's task was to watch the targets which appeared at the periphery of the display and moved in the general direction of the defended area. The subject had to decide if the target was a hostile missile which would enter the defended area or a decoy which would bypass it. The subject was given two buttons: (1) a detection button that he or she pressed as soon as he saw a target appear on the screen; and (2) a "fire" button that he pressed to launch his missile if he decided that the target was a hostile one. The subject was instructed to let decoys pass by.

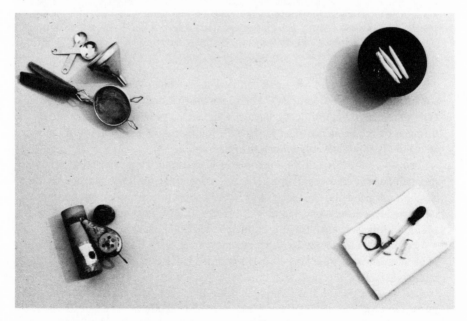

FIG. 3. Typical array of objects used in the learning session of drug recognition task.

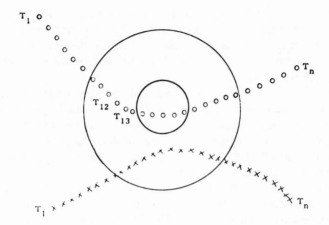

FIG. 4. This figure represents the simulated tactical display which was presented to the subject. The outer circle represents the effective missile range; the inner circle represents the defended area. The series of (o) ($T_1 - T_{35}$) represents the various positions of a hostile target at 2-sec intervals and the (X) sequence illustrates the course of a decoy target. The first (o) in the upper left T_1 (o) is the beginning of a hostile target sequence on the display screen. T_{12} (o) represents the approximate point at which the subject may decide that the target is hostile and fire a missile at it. T_{13} (o) represents the approximate point at which the target disappeared, the target sequence was terminated and followed by a blank period during which there were no targets. T_n (o) represents the end of the program for the hostile track's course or the starting point when the hostile track is run in the reverse direction. T_1 (X) through T_n(X) indicates the sequence of a decoy target's course.

The targets consisted of small colored dots which were either white (high contrast) or red (low contrast). There was no relationship between color and type of target (i.e., hostile or decoy). The targets moved at a constant speed throughout the sequence. The initial position of the target course was random-ized and distributed evenly among the quadrants.

Figure 4 illustrates the time courses of hostile and decoy targets which were programmed by the computer. The sequence (o's) outlines the course of a hostile target and the sequence of (X's) the course of a decoy target. During any target sequence only one target was present at any time and appeared at each position in the sequence for approximately 2 sec.

As expected, the detection and eye-movement data on target and nontarget sequences showed that the red (low-contrast) targets were not detected as rapidly as the white ones. As time on watch increased, the detection of red targets became poorer and false detections increased. The analysis of eye-move-ment data (mean distance between successive fixations and mean fixation durations) did not provide any indication of fatigue or impaired performance. However, the variance of fixation durations was much smaller during search periods when no targets were present than when the individual was observing and evaluating targets.

To summarize briefly, one finds longer fixation durations for drug materials than for neutral material in addicts but not in controls. In threat evaluation experiments fixations were less variable during search when no targets were present on the display than when threatening targets appeared on the scope. These data demonstrate the influence of motivational factors on eye movement behavior.

Further, the fact that the fixation durations of addicts were substantially longer than those of controls may be interpreted as suggesting that for the addict there is a slowing of CNS processes. The assumption that locus of the slowing is in the central nervous system is justified by the fact that the effects are specific and longlasting, but not easily observable on complex tasks.

Teichner (1973) in discussing his attempt to develop quantitative models for predicting human visual perceptual–motor performance states: "We have been frustrated for three years in our attempt to establish a data base of studies which might allow us to develop relationships between parameters of ocular behavior and measures of performance [p. 1]."

I feel that Teichner's frustration stems from two principle causes: (1) inadequate apparatus and procedures to measure eye movements and process the data, and (2) the mistaken belief that a simple response measure (e.g., pushing a button when a target is detected) will reveal information about the complex information seeking and organizing processes of the visual system.

The effect of subtle changes in visual processing time is not readily observable in many complex tasks because of the small amount of visual data for critical items. For example, if the task requires the subjects to observe and locate 10 critical pieces of information during a 1-hr watch, a 10–50 msec difference in mean fixation duration may not affect the outcome if the performance measure is mean number of targets detected. Hence, in a 60-min task that requires the subjects to recognize a series of objects, a subject using 300 msec per average fixation may be able to process the information just as accurately as a subject who only requires 250 msec per fixation. The point is that many subtle differences in visual behavior are not revealed by measures of dependent variables like button pushing to indicate target detection. Therefore, if an experimenter wishes to measure differences in human visual perceptual processes and study the relationship between eye-movement behavior and performance, he must employ a high speed oculometer system and processing techniques which can handle the large volumes of data that are generated. In other words, the complexity and capacity of the recording device *must* approximate that of the performance to be recorded.

Results from these studies involving high data acquisition rates and the analysis of substantial volumes of data suggest that the eye movements associated with fixation sequencing reflect changes in CNS temporal processes. For example, the major differences between the eye movements of addicts and controls were reflected in fixation frequency and duration, not in their task performance as measured by the subject's recognition memory for previously seen words and objects. Such results suggest that eye movements (fixation number and duration) may be a sensitive measure of gating and timing processes that group incoming sensory data, and that these data are not easily detected by conventional performance measures, such as, the percentage of targets seen and identified.

VII.4

A Framework for a Theory of Picture Recognition[1]

Geoffrey R. Loftus

University of Washington

As suggested by the title, I do not intend to present a full-blown theory of picture recognition. Rather, I want to suggest a framework within which such a theory might be couched, concentrating primarily on how information from a visual scene is encoded. Within this framework, eye fixations play a dual role. First, the pattern of eye fixations over a picture provides a powerful, ecologically valid, overt measure of the parts of a picture to which the observer is attending. Second, it is suggested that the processes involving acquisition of information within a single eye fixation should be viewed as a central component in any theory of picture memory.

Picture Recognition versus Recognition of Verbal Material

Since we currently have some fairly sophisticated theories of recognition memory for verbal material (Bernbach, 1967; Kintsch, 1970; Anderson & Bower, 1972), I'd like to start with some preliminary remarks on the question of why a theory dealing specifically with picture recognition is needed in the first place. To answer this question, I'll discuss what I consider to be two fundamental differences between verbal stimuli (e.g., words, digits, letters, etc.) and pictorial stimuli. I will then argue that these *stimulus* differences have some logical implications vis-à-vis *processing* differences.

What stimulus is processed? Consider a verbal stimulus, such as a word which a subject knows he will eventually be asked to remember. Common to most

[1] This research was supported, in part, by National Science Foundation Grant GB39615 to the author.

theoretical frameworks is the notion that after a fairly early processing stage, the continued physical presence of the to-be-remembered stimulus becomes unnecessary. This is because a pattern-recognition process is assumed to operate on the physical stimulus which results in the activation of some preformed representation of the stimulus from long-term store. Subsequent processing may then be done on this representation rather than on the physical stimulus itself. A picture, on the other hand, is a genuinely "new" stimulus in the sense that the observer has presumably never seen it before. Lacking a preformed representation of the picture, all processing must be done on the physical stimulus itself. This fact has at least two implications. First, if the physical stimulus is removed, processing must halt. This notion has been confirmed in several experiments (Potter & Levy, 1969; Shaffer & Shiffrin, 1972; Loftus, 1974). The second implication is that, when presented with a new picture, the observer is faced not only with the task of encoding information about the picture into long-term memory, but also with the task of "exploring" the picture in order to decide which aspects of it deserve attention (foveal processing) and which do not. (This is not to say that a period of exploration is followed by a period of encoding. Probably both processes are carried out simultaneously.)

Time-tag information versus isomorphic-stimulus information. In theories and experiments dealing with memory for verbal stimuli, the physical form of the stimulus generally assumes little, if any, importance. That is to say, the to-be-remembered information can be presented to a subject in an infinite variety of physical forms. It can be presented visually in any number of writing styles or type faces; it can be presented auditorially by a man or a woman or a computer or a parrot. It is then typically the case that the memory test does not require information about the physical form of the stimulus, but rather only the information that the stimulus, in some physical form or another, occurred in the study phase of the experiment. Therefore, at the time the information is originally presented, it is the task of the subject simply to tag it as having occurred at that particular time (cf. Anderson & Bower, 1972). Again, the situation is quite different when pictures rather than verbal material are used as stimuli—here, the physical form of the stimulus is of paramount importance. Suppose, for example, that during a picture-recognition test, an observer is looking at a picture of a mountain, trying to decide whether to classify the picture as "old" or "new." The observer's decision is one of whether or not he has previously seen the *identical physical* stimulus which he is now looking at. This means that encoding of a picture should consist, at least in part, of formulating a memorial representation of the picture which is, in some sense, isomorphic to the original stimulus—as opposed to simply *tagging* some already-stored information as having occurred in the experimental situation.

Bearing all this in mind, let me now proceed to my vision of what a theory of picture recognition might look like. Figure 1 sketches this framework, which is

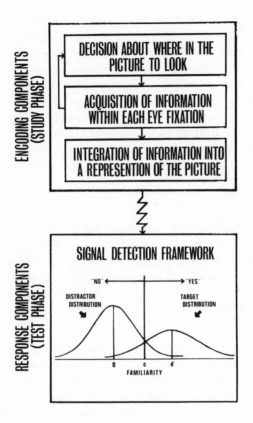

FIG. 1. A general framework for a theory of picture memory.

initially broken down into components involving encoding processes (top box) and components involving response processes (bottom box).

Response Processes

At the time a subject is deciding whether to respond "old" or "new" to a test picture, a great deal of processing is undoubtedly going on. However, due to time and knowledge limitations, I'm going to give short shrift to response processes and say only that I believe that at a rather general theoretical level, the theory of signal detection provides a good working framework. The application of signal detection theory to recognition memory is well documented (e.g., Egan, 1958; Kintsch, 1968; 1970; Freund, Loftus, & Atkinson, 1969) and I won't dwell on it here except to make a few brief comments on the construct of "familiarity." In terms of ultimately generating a more specific theory of picture recognition, it seems reasonable to postulate visual "features" which may be extracted from a picture at the time it is originally viewed. Then, instead of talking about distributions of "amount of familiarity" possessed by target and distractor pictures, we can talk about distributions of "numbers of features." I prefer to think of things this way because a feature seems to be a somewhat more tangible entity than a "unit of familiarity" as a candidate for something that can be extracted from a picture. If we talk about features from pictures, then we can also talk about (1) distributions of number of features that may be extracted during an eye fixation and (2) sets of features that are shared by targets and distractors. This second notion could serve to clarify the effects on recognition performance of target—distractor similarity.

Encoding Processes

Three encoding processes have been included in the top box of Fig. 1. First, as noted earlier, a decision must be made as to which parts of the picture should be processed (attended to). At any given time, this corresponds to a decision about where the next eye fixation should be. Second, once a particular area of the picture is being fixated, information must be extracted from that area and processed during the fixation. Finally, the information extracted during a series of fixations must be integrated into some over-all representation of the picture.

Where to look. Since the pioneering work of Buswell (1935) it has been clear that eye fixations are not distributed randomly over the picture. Rather, a large majority of the fixations are made on a rather small number of "areas of general interest" in the picture. This makes intuitive sense. If I show you a picture of the New York skyline under a clear blue sky, you are more likely to fixate on, say, the Empire State Building than somewhere in the middle of the clear blue sky.

Following Buswell's work, there have been attempts to specify the notion of an "area of general interest" somewhat more precisely. Berlyne (1958) presented subjects with pairs of pictures of the sort shown in Fig. 2. In each case, one member of the pair was defined as "informative" (in an information–theoretic sense) whereas the other member of the pair was defined as relatively less informative. Subjects tended to spend more time looking at the informative as opposed to the noninformative member of the pair. More recently, the work of Mackworth (Mackworth & Morandi, 1967; Mackworth & Bruner, 1970; cf. also Pollack & Spence, 1968) has dealt with the notion of informative areas within a complex, naturalistic scene. The procedure used in these experiments was to divide a picture into an 8 X 8-in grid. A group of subjects then rated how informative was each individual square, following which an independent group of subjects was permitted to view the entire picture. Eye-fixation patterns were recorded from the second group, and the results indicated a strong positive correlation between the informativeness rating of a particular square and the number of fixations made on that square.

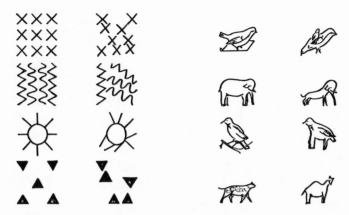

FIG. 2. Stimuli used in the Berlyne (1958) experiments. For each pair, one member is defined as "informative" (in an information–theoretic sense) whereas the other member is noninformative.

Mackworth's work has been valuable in confirming the existence of informative areas in pictures, but his definition of *informativeness* is highly empirical—an area is informative to the extent that other people say it is informative. Combining Mackworth's results with those of Berlyne, however, it seems reasonable to expect that subjects tend to look at areas of pictures which may be specified a priori as being informative in an information–theoretic sense. More precisely, I would like to offer the following definition of an informative area (or object) in a picture: An object in a picture is informative to the extent that it has a low conditional probability of being there given the rest of the picture and the subject's past history. As an example of what I mean by this, consider Figs. 3 and 4. Figure 3 shows a picture of a farm and contains a number of objects—the farmhouse, wagon, tractor, etc.—which most of us would agree belong on a farm. Figure 4 depicts exactly the same scene with one exception: an octopus has been substituted for the tractor. According to my proposed definition of informativeness, this octopus would constitute an informative object to any person whose experience with farms has not included the presence of an octopus.

If subjects do, in fact tend to fixate on areas of pictures which are informative by this definition, then they are carrying out the most efficient strategy possible in terms of subsequently being able to recognize the picture. Recognition of a picture involves being able to *discriminate* the picture from other similar pictures.[2] Therefore, the most valuable aspects of a picture to encode are those

[2] This notion naturally assumes that the picture being viewed is a member of some known, reasonably well-defined class of pictures. In a typical picture-recognition experiment, the class quickly becomes apparent to a subject via experimental instructions, warm-up pictures, or the first few pictures of the study sequence. Thus, the class of pictures might be naturalistic scenes, faces, common objects, etc.

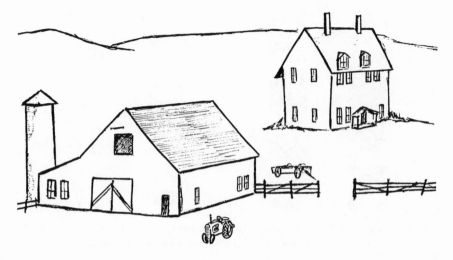

FIG. 3.   A picture containing several noninformative objects.

aspects that are least likely to be common to other pictures being viewed. If a subject were looking at Fig. 4 trying to encode it for subsequent recognition, he would be in good shape by encoding the presence of an octopus, since any potential distractor pictures of farms would be unlikely to contain an octopus— i.e., the octopus provides the best discriminative cue.

These speculations suggest an obvious experiment that we are currently carrying out. We have created a large number of pairs of picture similar to the pair of Figs. 3 and 4. Each subject views a series of pictures, half of which contain an

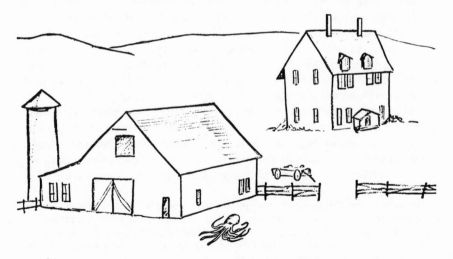

FIG. 4.   A picture which contains one informative object—the octopus.

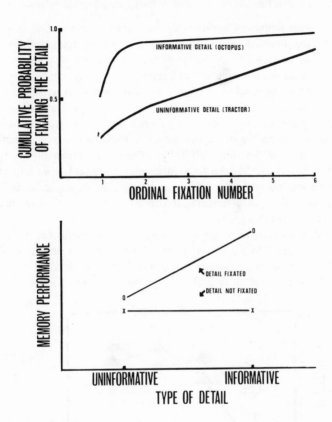

FIG. 5. Hypothetical results. The top panel depicts expected results for eye movements and the bottom panel depicts expected results for recognition performance.

informative object (like Fig. 4) and the other half of which do not contain an informative object (like Fig. 3). Eye fixations are recorded during initial viewing and the pictures are later tested in a yes–no recognition procedure. The data have not yet been collected, so I have created them instead. Figure 5 shows the pattern of results we expect (i.e., hope) to get. The top panel shows the cumulative probability of having fixated an object as a function of the ordinal fixation number on the picture. If my definition of an informative object corresponds to what Mackworth's subjects called an informative object, then a given object in the picture should be fixated sooner when it is informative than when it is not informative.

The predicted relationship between informativeness and subsequent recognition performance is depicted in the bottom panel of Fig. 5. When an informative detail is fixated, it should aid recognition performance relative to cases where an informative detail is not fixated or where the fixated detail is not informative.

Processes occurring within a fixation. We now arrive at the second encoding component. Having decided where to fixate and having fixated there, the observer must now extract information from the fixated area. A good place to go for clues as to what is happening within a fixation is the voluminous literature on the information available within a single brief visual presentation. Research in this area has proceeded under the rationale that an understanding of the processes taking place during a controlled tachistoscopic presentation will in turn provide an understanding of the processes occurring within an eye fixation. Indeed, a classic paper by Sperling (1960) begins with the statement, "... [the question of how much can be seen in a single brief exposure] is an important problem because our normal mode of seeing greatly resembles a series of brief exposures ... [and] the eye assimilates information only in the brief pauses between saccadic movements [p. 1]."

A paradigm that simulates a single eye fixation using a tachistoscope is one introduced by Sperling (1963). This paradigm involves the presentation of an array of verbal stimuli (e.g., letters) for a brief, variable amount of time, followed by a visual noise mask. Figure 6 shows Sperling's results. The amount

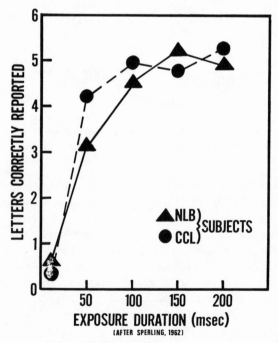

FIG. 6. Memory performance (number of items correctly reported) as a function of exposure time of the letter array. (After Sperling, 1963.)

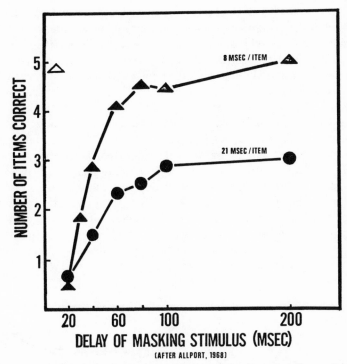

FIG. 7. Memory performance (number of items correctly reported) as a function of the exposure time of the stimulus array. The top curve represents data when letters are used as stimuli and the bottom curve represents data when Landolt C's are used as stimuli. (After Allport, 1968.)

of information acquired from the array (as measured by the number of letters reported) increases with the exposure time of the array up to about 100 msec and then asymptotes. A question of some potential importance is: Why does there appear to be no further acquisition of information after 100 msec? One possibility is that the onset of a new visual stimulus activates a pattern recognizer—or more generally, a visual information-acquisition process—that operates for only about 100 msec following the onset of a visual stimulus and then stops and is idle until the eye is presented with a new stimulus. Carrying this notion over to an eye fixation, this would mean that within a given eye fixation, information from the stimulus being fixated would be acquired for only the first 100 msec or so following the onset of the fixation.

A second somewhat less interesting explanation for the asymptote in Fig. 6 is that the five items acquired in the first 100 msec fill up short-term store. However, other data do not support this possibility. Figure 7 shows data collected by Allport (1968). Allport used the same paradigm as did Sperling but used two types of stimuli. The top curve in Fig. 7 shows the results when letters were used as stimuli whereas the bottom curve shows the results when Landolt C's were used. If the asymptote were due to a filling up of short-term store, then it is difficult to imagine why different stimuli would produce different asymptotic levels, in view of the fact that the number of items which can be held in short-term store is relatively independent of what the items are (Miller, 1956). Even more compelling data have been gathered by Sperling, Budiansky, Spivak, and Johnson (1971). In their experiment (which simulates a series of eye fixations) subjects were shown a series of letter arrays which appeared in rapid succession on a cathode-ray tube. The size of the arrays varied from 2 to 25 letters, and the time each array remained on the screen varied from 10 to 320 msec. Embedded somewhere in one of the arrays was a digit, and it was the subject's task to report the digit's location. Using this procedure, it is possible to estimate the number of locations scanned in each array. Figure 8 shows this measure of visual information processing as a function of how long each array was presented (labeled ISI). Again, these functions all asymptote at around 100 msec. Since this paradigm almost completely eliminates short-term memory limitations, these results support the notion that the asymptote is due to a limit

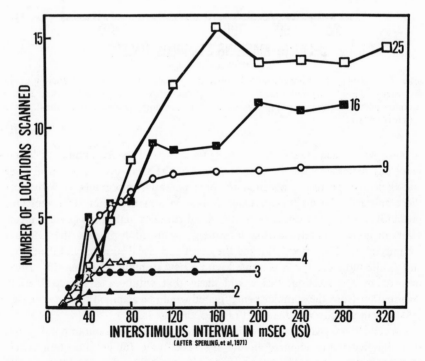

FIG. 8. Estimated number of locations scanned as a function of exposure time of the stimulus array (ISI). The curve parameter is the number of letters in each array. (After Sperling et al., 1971.)

LOFTUS (1972) EXPERIMENT I

STUDY PHASE ·· 90 PAIRS OF PICTURES
Each Trial ·· Each member of the upcoming pair is assigned
1, 5, or 9 points

For example:
1. Experimenter reads, "ONE, NINE"
2. A pair of slides is shown for 3 seconds

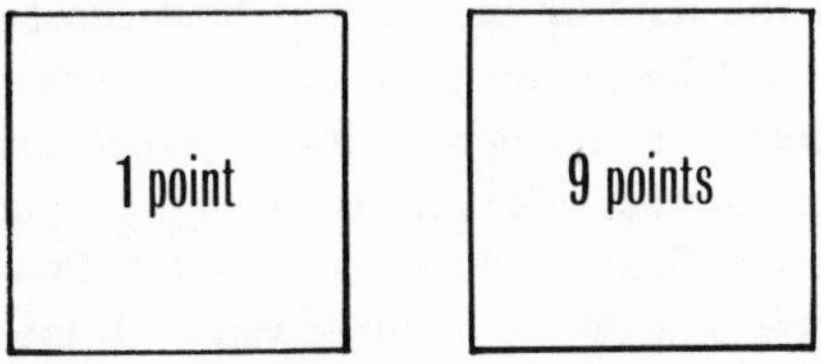

| 1 point | 9 points |

TEST PHASE ·· 360 PICTURES SHOWN INDIVIDUALLY
180 Targets from the study phase
180 Distractors
Points earned:

		value assigned at study			distractor
		1	5	9	distractor
S's response	'yes'	GAIN 1 PT	GAIN 5 PTS	GAIN 9 PTS	LOSE 5 PTS
	'no'	LOSE 1 PT	LOSE 5 PTS	LOSE 9 PTS	GAIN 5 PTS

FIG. 9.   Design of Experiment 1 of the Loftus (1972) study.

in how long the "visual information acquisition" program will operate following the onset of a new visual stimulus.

A series of picture-recognition experiments that I have reported (Loftus, 1972) provides evidence that the information acquisition process within an eye fixation follows the same time course as that depicted in Figs. 6–8. Figure 9 shows the design of Experiment 1 of this study which was originally motivated by the question: What is the relationship between the number of fixations made on a picture and subsequent recognition-memory performance for that picture? In an initial study phase of the experiment, subjects were shown 90 pairs of pictures for 3 sec per pair. Eye fixations were recorded during this study phase. To gain some control over the number of fixations per picture, each member of the pair was assigned a value of 1, 5, or 9 points prior to the onset of the picture. This value was directly related to the amount of money the subject would gain if, during the subsequent recognition test, the subject correctly recognized the picture. It was thus expected that more fixations would be made on high-valued pictures than on low-valued pictures.

The results of this experiment showed that both number of fixations and subsequent recognition-memory performance were increasing functions of value. Figure 10 shows memory performance (hit rate) as a function of the number of fixations made on the picture at the time of study. The curve parameter is the value of the picture. Two aspects of these results are of interest. First, the more fixations accorded the picture, the higher is subsequent recognition performance. Second, with the number of fixations held constant, memory performance is independent of the picture's value. The implications of this result is that the higher memory performance on higher-valued pictures is completely mediated by the greater number of eye fixations on these pictures.

Table 1 shows average fixation duration as a function of the number of fixations on the picture and of the picture's value. Of interest is the fact that (for unknown reasons) the greater the value of the picture, the longer was the average duration of fixations made on the picture. However, as Fig. 10 shows, the extra time per fixation on the high-valued pictures did not add anything in terms of memory performance. Making the reasonable assumption that memory performance reflects the amount of information extracted from the picture, we are left with the conclusion that no extra information was acquired in the

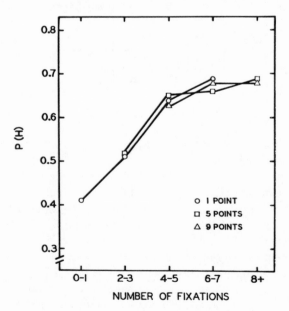

FIG. 10. Memory performance (hit rate) as a function of number of fixations accorded the picture at time of study. The curve parameter is the value of the picture.

TABLE 1
Average Fixation Duration as a Function of
Value for Pictures over *i* Fixations

| Value (points) | Average fixation duration (sec) | | | | |
	$i = 3$	$i = 4$	$i = 5$	$i = 6$	$i = 7$
1	.292	.292	.290	.279	.300
	(117)[a]	(111)	(69)	(49)	(26)
5	.325	.311	.312	.304	.300
	(85)	(92)	(93)	(88)	(69)
9	.350	.369	.336	.308	.311
	(35)	(59)	(92)	(111)	(25)

[a]Numbers in parentheses are the sample sizes for each cell.

additional time per fixation on the higher-valued pictures. This result suggests that a hypothetical function relating the amount of information acquired to fixation duration would resemble the curve shown in Fig. 11. The correspondence between Fig. 11 and Figs. 6–8 should be fairly obvious—it appears to be the case that the same information-processing mechanisms operate following the

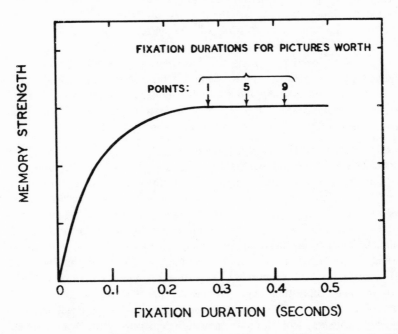

FIG. 11. A hypothetical function representing acquisition of information as a function of fixation duration for a single eye fixation.

onset of a new visual stimulus either when the visual stimulus is initiated by the observer (with an eye movement) or when it is initiated by the experimenter (with a tachistoscope).

Experiment 2 in the Loftus (1972) study provides some confirmation of this notion. In Experiment 2, single pictures were displayed in the study phase at exposure times varying from 300 to 5000 msec. Again, eye movements were recorded during the study phase, and the pictures were subsequently tested in a yes–no recognition test. Two results of interest emerged from this study. First, with exposure time held constant, memory performance was a strongly increasing function of number of fixations made on the picture at study—for example, after a 3-sec exposure, fifteen 200 msec fixations produced considerably better performance than ten 300-msec fixations. The second result was that with the number of fixations held constant, performance was independent of exposure time; for example, if 12 fixations were made during a 3-sec exposure, performance did not differ from the case when 12 fixations were made during a 5-sec exposure. Taken together, these results suggest that each fixation results in the acquisition of one "chunk" of information about the picture—and within a fixation, all the information germane to subsequent recognition memory is acquired rather quickly following the onset of the fixation.

The most intriguing question to come out of all this is: Why does it seem that the last part of each fixation is wasted time? One possibility which has been suggested by Gould (1969) is that the last part of a given eye fixation is spent computing where the next fixation will be made. I believe that this is an appealing possibility. Under this view, an eye fixation would be divided into two major (possibly overlapping) stages. The first stage would involve wide, peripheral processing to determine where the next fixation should occur. The second stage would probably be somewhat task specific (cf. Yarbus, 1967). Thus, for example, in scanning a picture, informative areas would be identified; in a visual search task, a potential target would be sought out, etc.

Integration of Information over Successive Fixations.   Information integration seems to be a two-stage process. The first stage is *getting the big picture*. At least three lines of research have suggested that within a very short time after a picture has appeared, an observer has some notion of what the "gist" of the picture is. First, Mackworth's work, already discussed, shows that observers look at "informative areas" very quickly—within the first one or two fixations on the picture. In order to do this, some processing must have taken place to provide information about which areas of the picture are informative to begin with. Second, Potter (1972) has reported an experiment in which a series of pictures is shown in rapid succession (e.g., one picture per 100 msec). Subjects were instructed to press a button when they saw a picture whose gist was defined in some very vague way (for example, "a picture depicting a game") and were able to do this with no difficulty. Finally, an experiment by Biederman (1972) utilized a procedure in which subjects were shown a picture for a brief period of time. Following the exposure, they were asked to name an object from the picture whose location was specified by a visual marker. There were two conditions: in a "jumbled" condition, the picture was cut into six sections which were spatially scrambled, thereby making identification of the gist very difficult. The second condition was a control condition in which the normal, complete, unscrambled picture was shown. Object detection in the jumbled condition was poorer than in the normal condition, suggesting that rapidly acquired information about gist was being used to aid detection.

The second stage of information integration is *getting informative details*. It seems likely that, following the early acquisition of this "gist information," successive eye fixations are utilized to acquire information from informative areas in the picture, as discussed above. To make a stab at exploring this process, Susan Bell and I have conducted a picture-recognition experiment in which subjects were asked, at the time of recognition, to identify the bases of their responses. Specifically, they were asked to make one of two choices: (1) they were responding because they remembered some specific detail in the picture or (2) they were responding merely on the basis of the "general familiarity" of the picture. Exposure time was varied from 60 to 500 msec at the time the pictures were originally viewed. Several results of interest emerged from this experiment. First, consider the function relating the probability of naming a specific detail from a picture to the original exposure time of the picture. Ninety-six percent of the variance in this function was accounted for by a model which assumed that, during each eye fixation, the probability of an informative detail is encoded with some constant probability α. Second, when a detail was named, performance (measured in terms of d') was increased by about 1.5 relative to when a detail was not named.

To recapitulate, it appears that some general information about a picture is acquired very quickly after the picture is first exposed. Following the acquisition of this initial information, the task of each eye fixation is to encode more precise information about what is in the picture. In terms of picture *recognition*, a simplistic view—but one that seems to work—is that with each eye fixation, there is some constant probability that a detail will be encoded which will serve to distinguish the picture from other pictures and upon which a recognition response may be based.

VII.5

Visual Memory for Letters and Random Dot Patterns: Could Eye-Movement Data Help Us Understand It Better?[1]

Raymond S. Nickerson

Bolt, Beranek, and Newman, Inc.

This paper may be unique among the papers comprising this conference in that it does not present any data on eye movements or eye fixations at all. What I would like to do is raise a question as to whether such data might be used to advantage in some specific experimental situations designed to study certain aspects of human memory. Eye-movement and eye-fixation recording techniques have not been used in the situations that I will discuss, and the question is whether they should be.

The hypothesis that visually presented information is often recoded into an auditory or articulatory form for storage in short-term memory is a familiar one (Conrad, 1964; Sperling & Speelman, 1970; Wickelgren, 1966). Presumably, auditory or articulatory representations are more amenable to rehearsal than are visual representations. The evidence that such recoding occurs is quite compelling. What seems less certain, however, is whether, when such recoding does occur, a visual representation of the stimulus is also retained. Or, to ask a slightly different question, is the recoding done because the information cannot be retained in visual form, or are auditory representations simply easier to remember and recall? Or might it be that one often can remember *either* visual or auditory representations, and which he chooses to retain depends somewhat on the nature of the task?

[1] The experiments described in this report were supported by the United States Air Force Office of Scientific Research under Contract F44620-69-C-0115. The assistance of Barbara Noel Freeman in collecting data is gratefully acknowledged.

I will describe three experimental paradigms that I have used recently in an effort to collect some data that would help to answer questions such as these. The results of several experiments in which these paradigms have been used have been published elsewhere, so they will be only briefly summarized here. The question that I wish to raise concerning the possible utility of eye-movement data in this research stems not so much from the objective results that have been obtained as from some subjective impressions that one gets from performing these tasks.

In the first paradigm (Nickerson, 1972), the subject saw two visual patterns on each trial. Each pattern was composed of a subset of the dots of a seven-by-five-dot matrix of the type that is sometimes used to construct letters for presentation on a point-plotting cathode-ray tube. Figure 1 illustrates the types of patterns that were used. Under one condition, both of the patterns presented on each trial formed letters, as is illustrated by the patterns in the top row of the figure. On a random half of the trials, the second pattern was the same as the first; and on the other half, it was different. Under a second and a third condition, the patterns were randomly selected 12-dot subsets of the 35-dot matrix, as is illustrated in the bottom two rows of Fig. 1. The difference between the second and third conditions was in the degree to which nonidentical patterns differed: in the second condition (easy discrimination), the two patterns either were the same or they differed with respect to the positions of eleven dots ($\Delta = 11$ dots); in the third condition (difficult discrimination), the two patterns either were the same or they differed with respect to the position of a single dot ($\Delta = 1$ dot). In each case, the two patterns were the same on half of the trials and they differed on the other half.

The random-dot patterns that were used in this experiment were generated by a computer on each trial, and the probability of seeing exactly the same pattern

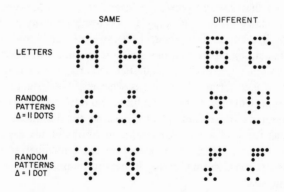

FIG. 1. Types of patterns used in the first experimental paradigm discussed. Each condition is described in its respective row.

on more than one trial was exceedingly small. This is an important point because the intent was to preclude the possibility that initially novel patterns would become familiar—and possibly labeled—as a result of frequent exposure during the experiment.

The experimental procedure was as follows. On each trial, the subject was shown the first of the two patterns that was to be presented on that trial. The exposure duration of this pattern was varied from .25 sec to 4.0 sec. At some period of time, which varied from 0 to 8.0 sec, following the termination (by superimposition of the 35-dot matrix) of the first pattern, the second pattern was presented. The subjects' task was to indicate as quickly as possible whether the second pattern was the same as the first.

The question of interest was whether the relationship between performance (measured in terms of response time and error rate) and the duration of the retention interval would be different for the letters that were assumed to be easily encoded auditorily, than for the random patterns, for which auditory encoding was assumed to be much less likely. The results did not support the idea that the memory representations of these two types of stimuli decayed at different rates. More specifically, subjects performed much more poorly with "difficult" random patterns than with either "easy" random patterns or letters, but evidence of an interaction between stimulus type and retention interval was not obtained.

In the second paradigm that was used (Nickerson & Pew, 1973), the subject saw two *pairs* of visual patterns on each trial. Again, the patterns were composed from subsets of seven-by-five-dot matrices and, again, under some conditions the patterns formed letters and under other conditions they did not. As in the experiment described above, the intent was to have some stimuli that would be easy to encode auditorily, and some that would not.

A trial began with the simultaneous presentation of one pair of patterns (the target stimuli). After these patterns had been exposed for 2 sec, each was masked by superimposition of the entire 35-dot matrix. One-half sec following the onset of the masks, the second pair of patterns (the probe stimuli) was displayed directly below the location of the first pair. Figure 2 shows the sequence of events, and illustrates the two types of patterns that were used.

The subject's task was to make a decision as quickly as possible concerning whether or not the two pairs of patterns that were presented on a given trial corresponded in a specified way. Three different decisions were required: (1) whether the two pairs had *any* (at least one) items in common, (2) whether they had *both* items in common, and (3) whether they were identical (same items in same positions). Any given subject made only one type of decision and worked exclusively with letters or with random patterns.

One of the things of interest in this experiment was the extent to which spatial-position effects would be found with the two types of patterns. There are various ways in which the two pairs might relate to each other with respect to

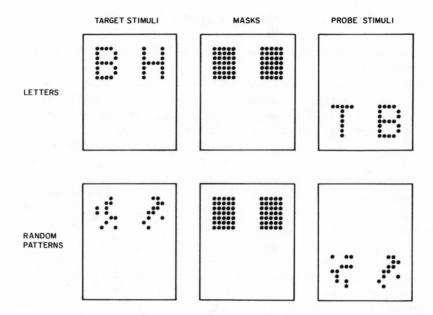

FIG. 2. This figure illustrates the stimuli that were used in the second experimental paradigm, and the sequence of events constituting a trial. Target patterns were displayed for 2 sec, after which they were masked by the full dot matrices as shown in the middle column. One-half sec following this onset, the marks were erased and the probe stimuli were presented.

the positions of matching items. They might, for example, have both items in common and occupying the same positions, both items in common but in opposite positions, one item in common and in the same or opposite position, or no items in common. One would expect that such spatial relationships would be more likely to play a significant role in determining decision times if the decisions were based on visually encoded representations than if the memory representations on which these decisions were based were auditory. Strong position effects were in fact obtained both with the letters and with the random-dot patterns. For example, given the first decision task (whether the pairs had at least one item in common), performance with stimulus pairs which had a single item in common was better (response time was shorter and error rate smaller) when the matching items occurred in the same positions in both pairs than when they occupied different positions. The results were taken to be consistent with the assumption that the matching process made use of visually encoded information, both in the case of the random-dot patterns and in that of the letters, although it was concluded that the letters may have been encoded in auditory as well as in visual form.

In the third paradigm that I want to mention (Nickerson, in press), the stimuli again were patterns formed from subsets of the dots of a seven-by-five-dot matrix. In this case, however, each pattern was a composite of a letter and a noise pattern, composed of several randomly positioned dots. On each trial, the subject saw two such patterns, and his task was to indicate whether both patterns contained the same letter. In some cases the two patterns were presented simultaneously, and in other cases the onset of one of the patterns followed the offset of the other by an interval of from 0 to 8 sec. When the patterns were presented sequentially, the exposure duration of the first pattern was 2 sec.

The independent variable of primary interest had to do with the way in which the noise patterns that were used on a given trial related to each other. Under one condition the noise patterns were identical, and under the other they were different. The noise patterns were said to be correlated in the first case and uncorrelated in the second. Figure 3 illustrates the effects of both correlated and uncorrelated noise patterns when superimposed on letters that are the same and when superimposed on letters that are different. The important thing to notice about the stimuli in these figures is that when the noise is correlated, the judgment concerning whether the two letters of a pair are the same or different can be made on the basis of a test for visual congruence. It is not necessary to identify the letters; one can be sure that they are the same if the patterns—noise and all—look the same. When the noise is uncorrelated, however, a test for congruence does not suffice inasmuch as, even when the letters of a pair are the

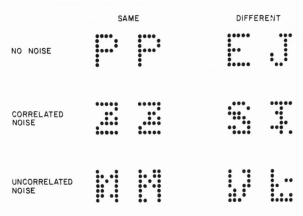

FIG. 3. This figure illustrates the types of stimuli that were used in the third experimental paradigm discussed. Under the "correlated-noise" condition, the same noise pattern was superimposed on the two letters that occurred on a given trial, whether or not the letters were the same. Under the "uncorrelated-noise" condition, different noise patterns were superimposed on the two letters than occurred on a given trial.

same, the different noise patterns assure that the composite patterns look different.

The rationale for using this paradigm was as follows. If, in performing the same–different task, a subject does not retain visual information, but remembers only the name of the first letter, and decides whether it is the same as or different from the name of the second, performance should be independent of whether the noise patterns used on the two letters of a pair are correlated. As it turned out, performance was much better (response times were shorter and error rates smaller) when the noise was correlated than when it was not, and this difference was relatively independent of the duration of the retention interval over the range of intervals studied. It was concluded that visual information about the composite letter-plus-noise patterns was indeed preserved in short-term memory and used in the performance of this task.

On balance, the results of these experiments suggest that visual patterns can be retained, at least for several seconds, in a form that preserves visual properties. This does not rule out the possibility that some of these patterns, especially those that are easily encoded in another way, are *also* retained in another form. In particular, the names of letters, especially when the letters are readily identified, are undoubtedly retained, and perhaps often used in the decision-making process.

What does this all have to do with eye fixations or eye movements? Perhaps nothing. On the other hand, it is perhaps worth raising the question of whether eye-fixation data would shed any light on the way in which these patterns are encoded for retention in memory. Recall that the reason for using nonrecurring random-dot patterns in the first place was to preclude the possibility that subjects would learn to give the patterns names, and thereby be able to recode them auditorily. It is not clear after the fact, however, that recoding of the patterns into a nonvisual form is impossible. Unfortunately, the only evidence we have on this point so far is subjective. One gets the impression, from performing this task, that there is more than one strategy that can be brought to bear on it. One can, if one chooses, be a relatively passive observer, simply "looking at" the target patterns as they are presented. On the other hand, if one wishes, one can "do something" with a pattern in addition to simply looking at it. What is done is difficult to describe. It appears to involve implicit motor activity of a sort. For example, if a pattern happens to have isolatable segments—perhaps several sets of dots, each of which can be thought of as a "part" of the pattern having some integrity—one may find oneself making subvocal "sounds" or implicit gestures that correspond in some vague way to the components into which one has decomposed the pattern. I would like to know more about these "things that one can do with a pattern" in order to increase one's chances of remembering it, and the question is whether eye-fixation or eye-movement data would be informative in this regard.

Would scan records provide useful clues concerning how a pattern is decomposed (if it is) into memorable parts? Would they provide any insights concerning what constitute "informative areas" in such patterns (Mackworth & Morandi, 1967)? Does a representation of the scan path itself, or of the neural commands for the scan movements, or of the proprioceptive feedback from the movements constitute part of the memory code for a pattern?

One of the things that becomes apparent as a result of working with random patterns such as those used in some of these experiments is that some of them are considerably easier to remember than others. Why that is the case is not so apparent. My guess is that what makes a pattern memorable is closely related to what makes it perceptually "good" in the sense in which Garner (1966) has used that word. That is to say, I would expect that patterns that would be given a low rating on Garner's goodness scale (the lower the rating, the better the pattern) would tend to be remembered better than those given a high rating. It might be of interest to determine whether patterns that are easy to remember, or are judged to be good patterns, are scanned in a different way than are those that are difficult to remember, or are judged to be poor patterns. A particularly intriguing question is whether a study of scanning behavior would provide any clues concerning why some patterns are more readily encoded and retained than others.

VII.6

Language behind the Eye:
Some Findings, Speculations,
and Research Strategies

Stanley F. Wanat

State University of New York at Stony Brook

One of the most fascinating areas of research into the higher mental processes deals with linguistic communication and, more specifically, with the question of how the reader extracts meaning from written language. I will discuss research on the role that language plays in guiding the reader's eyes. The two major issues to be considered here are (1) whether the reader selectively allocates his visual attention in extracting meaning from written language; and (2) if so, whether areas of relatively greater or lesser visual attention are predictable from the linguistic structure of the material being read. The research to be presented here was designed to examine the eye-fixation patterning of proficient readers while they read materials that contained specific kinds of linguistic features considered central to comprehension.

I studied the reader's allocation of visual attention by monitoring where he looked when he was reading. There were five component measures of visual attention: (1) number of forward fixations, (2) time spent on forward fixations, (3) number of regressions from areas in the sentence, (4) number of regressive fixations to areas in the sentence, and (5) time spent on regressive fixations. These measures were obtained for each sentence as a whole and for each area within the sentence. The eye movements of 12 mature readers were recorded while each read 80 test sentences. A Mackworth wide-angle reflection eye camera was used to record the reader's eye movements. For every comparison made of contrasting linguistic features, each subject read eight examples of the first linguistic type and eight examples of the contrasting linguistic type. (Also, additional numbers of simple active and simple passive sentences were read.)

Each subject read one member of each test pair at each of two test sessions, so that if he read the left-embedded (subject-modifying) form, "On the picnic the girls that Bill teased saw the child," at the first test session, he would get the corresponding right-embedded (object-modifying) form, "The girls saw the child that Bill teased on the picnic," at the second test session one week later. For every comparison made between two contrasting linguistic features, 192 sentence readings were analyzed—2 linguistic features $\times$ 8 sentences per linguistic feature per subject $\times$ 12 subjects. The subjects were instructed to read the sentences naturally and to attend to their meaning. To insure that the subject attended to the meaning of the sentences, he was told that after he read a sentence, he might be asked to paraphrase it. There were 18 such requests for paraphrase on randomly selected sentences for each subject.

In this investigation, semantic and syntactic features at three levels of linguistic structure were studied: sentence level, phrase level, and word level.

At the sentence level, one structural feature is the sentence's immediate constituent analysis—the way the sentence is divided into component parts. It is possible to take a set of phrases and combine them one way to get one sentence, and then combine the same phrases another way to get another sentence:

Comparison A. Type RE: The gang/beat the guard that Mike called at the airport. Type LE: At the airport the gang that Mike called/beat the guard. The RE stands for right embedding—a relative clause follows and modifies the sentence object. The LE stands for left embedding—a relative clause follows and modifies the sentence subject. The slanted lines indicate the dividing point in each sentence between subject and predicate. Sentences of this type were written and used as test materials to see if differences in a sentence's immediate constituent analysis would affect the way the reader allocated his attention.

At the sentence level, it is possible for one sentence structure to be more predictable than another. Levin, Grossman, Kaplan, and Yang (1972) presented subjects with a set of sentences with certain parts deleted: "The soldier _____ during the morning service." They asked the subjects to fill in the missing parts. They found that when they gave the subjects a sentence frame in which either a left embedding or a right embedding is possible, there were over three times as many right embeddings as left embeddings. In other sentence-completion tasks, when just the left embedding was deleted, 33% of the items written in by subjects were left embeddings. But when just the right embedding was deleted, 78% of the items written in by subjects were right embeddings. Thus, a sentence containing a right embedding is more predictable than a sentence containing a left embedding.

In another comparison of contrasting linguistic features, this time at the phrase level, the immediate constituent analysis was kept constant while the structural predictability of phrases inserted into that frame was varied. The sentence frame was of the form: noun phrase + verb phrase + prepositional phrase. . . Following the procedure of holding the immediate constituent analysis constant while varying the structural predictability of phrases that are inserted into that framework, one comparison dealt with the visual-attention scores for active-sentence constituents inserted into this immediate-constituent-analysis frame, versus passive-sentence constituents inserted into the same frame:

Comparison B. Active sentence: noun phrase (*The poet*) + verb phrase (*was writing*) + prepositional phrase . . . (*in the studio . . .*). Passive sentence: noun phrase (*The ship*) + verb phrase (*was beached*) + prepositional phrase . . . (*by the helper . . .*).

Another comparison involved test materials in which the immediate constituent analysis of sentences was held constant while the structural predictability of phrases inserted into that framework was varied. In this case, two kinds of prepositional phrases differing in their structural predictability were inserted into the same passive sentence frame:

Comparison C. Agent-included passive: noun phrase (*The ship*) + verb phrase (*was beached*) + prepositional phrase . . . (*by the helper . . .*). Agent-deleted passive: noun phrase (*The Ship*) + verb phrase (*was beached*) + prepositional phrase . . . (*by the harbor . . .*). The first passive form in Comparison C is referred to as an agent-included passive, since it gives information about who performed the action. The second passive form is referred to as an agent-deleted passive, since the linguistic cue indicating who performed the action is deleted (in its place is a prepositional phrase that gives information on location). The agent-versus-nonagent difference is signaled by a content word (*helper* versus *harbor*).

Still another comparison in the present study dealt with structural predictability at the word level. In this test, the agent-included-passive versus agent-deleted-passive comparison (Comparison C immediately above) was redone using a function word to signal the agent-versus-nonagent difference:

Comparison D. Agent-included passive: noun phrase (*The note*) + verb phrase (*was brought*) + prepositional phrase . . . (*by the leader . . .*). Agent-deleted passive: noun phrase (*The note*) + verb phrase (*was brought*) + prepositional phrase . . . (*to the leader . . .*).

When the visual-attention scores from D are compared to the visual-attention scores from C, it is possible to gain some insight about the relative effect of content-word cues versus function-word cues to the same within-sentence semantic relations.

In Comparisons B, C, and D, every one of the sentences being compared line up word for word, and they also line up letter for letter. This was done to gain as precise control as possible of the test materials. The test materials presented in Comparisons C and D were designed so that the two linguistic structures being compared differed from one another only by the word that served to signal differences in the sentence structures. (Since the sentences in Comparison A differ in their immediate constituent analysis, by definition, then their constituents cannot line up.)

Also considered in the present study is the mode of reading; that is, whether the material was read silently or orally. Half of the test materials of each type were read orally and half silently. This was done to see if the reader's allocation of visual attention was different for oral reading than for silent reading.

Findings. Oral reading requires significantly more visual attention than silent reading. It was initially thought that this would be the case because of the belief that oral reading requires the reader to process more information in the text, hence it requires more visual attention. Also, it was felt that the reader's eye–voice span (the distance between where the eye is and where the voice is in oral reading) would act as a brake on his visual scanning. This view was confirmed. Significant differences were found between the oral and silent reading scores for the same linguistic materials. For example, the oral reading time for left-embedded and right-embedded sentences averaged 920 msec per sentence while the silent reading time averaged 720 msec per sentence. This difference was significant at the .001 level. (It should be noted that, with respect to the linguistic features discussed below, the effects of differences in linguistic features on visual attention was generally more pronounced in oral reading than in silent reading.)

A second finding in the present study was that readers selectively allocate their attention to different areas of the sentence. This was expected to be the case, given the Mackworth and Morandi (1967) finding demonstrating selectivity of attention in the visual scanning of pictures, and given linguistic research indicating that some structures within sentences play a relatively more central role in sentence comprehension. This was confirmed by the findings on all five component measures of visual attention. There were significant differences in the scores for individual sentence areas in all these cases at the .01 level or better.

A third finding dealt with whether a sentence type which is structurally less predictable requires more visual attention. This hypothesis was based upon the Levin et al. (1972) finding that the structurally less predictable left-embedded sentence type significantly limited the amount of information the reader could process, as measured by the eye–voice span. The visual-attention measures here reported employed the same two sentence types that Levin et al. compared in their study. The total time spent on forward fixations in reading the less predictable LE form was significantly greater than the total time spent on forward fixations in reading the more predictable RE form ($p < .005$). (The average *number* of forward fixational pauses for LE and RE sentences was the same, and none of the three measures of regressive eye fixations showed any significant differences between LE and RE forms.)

A fourth finding dealt with whether or not a sentence's immediate constituent analysis affects the way that the reader's visual attention is distributed across the sentence. This inquiry was based upon Kennedy's (1967) reexamination of some of Buswell's (1920) data, suggesting that regressions are more likely to take place within, rather than across, phrase boundaries. Both the Kennedy and the Mehler, Bever, and Carey (1967) studies provided provocative (but inconclusive) data about the sensitivity of the reader's visual scanning to a sentence's immediate constituent analysis.

In the present study, the following reasoning was used. From the discussion in an earlier paragraph, it is known that both LE and RE sentences each have, on the average, the same number of forward fixations per sentence. It is also known that LE and RE sentences have different immediate constituent analyses. Therefore, if the analyses of variance of the eye-fixation scores indicated a significant *sentence-area* X *sentence-type* interaction, this would indicate that there is significant variability in the way that the same amount of visual attention is distributed across these sentence types that differ in their immediate constituent analysis. This was confirmed to be the case, since there was a significant sentence-area X sentence-type interaction $(p < .01)$, indicating that the distribution of forward fixations across the sentence areas was not the same for the two sentence types.

A fifth question was whether or not differences in the structural predictability of phrases that are inserted into the same immediate-constituent framework significantly affect the amount of visual attention required, with structurally less predictable phrases requiring more visual attention. This question stemmed from Levin & Kaplan's (1968) and Wanat & Levin's (1968, in preparation) findings that varying the structural predictability of phrases while maintaining the same immediate constituent framework significantly affected the amount of information the reader could process, as measured by his eye–voice span. This viewpoint was confirmed by the present research, since there were significant differences in the visual-attention scores for sentences with such linguistic characteristics (active sentences, agent-included passive sentences, and two different kinds of agent-deleted passive sentences). For the sentence structures with these characteristics there were significant differences in the visual-attention scores for time spent on regressive fixations $(p < .025)$, for the number of regressions from sentence areas $(p < .05)$; and for the number of regressive fixations to sentence areas $(p < .05)$. Interestingly, the scores among which there were significant differences all involved regressive-eye-fixation patterning. Neither of the two measures of forward fixations showed significant differences among the scores for these active and passive sentence types.

A sixth problem is whether or not different word classes require different amounts of visual attention. Put another way, do different surface structure cues to the same kinds of underlying sentence relations require different amounts of visual attention? This question stemmed from research findings indicating that some linguistic features within sentences play a relatively more central role in sentence comprehension. Also considered here was research suggesting different reader-error rates for different word categories, including Kolers' (1970, 1972) research dealing with adult readers, and a reanalysis of some of Weber's (1970) research dealing with beginner readers. In the present study, this question was explored by comparing the visual-attention scores for the agent-deleted passive in which the agent deletion is signaled by a content word, versus the visual-attention scores for the agent-deleted passive in which the agent deletion is signaled by a function word. When the visual-attention scores are broken down for individual areas of the sentence, the pattern of scores suggests that different surface-structure cues to the same underlying relations are processed differently by the reader's eye. This suggests that, although the reader's goal is understanding—getting to the meaning—of what he is reading, we ought not to forget that the reader gets at the writer's meanings by plowing through surface structure. While some linguists take the view that "deep structure" and "surface structure" are one and the same, there may be a number of alternative surface-structure realizations of a particular underlying structure. Line-of-sight studies of how the reader allocates his visual attention to different linguistic structures can provide important insight into the readability of different kinds of structures, and can truly pinpoint specific features affecting readability.

The seventh question explored in this study dealt with possible differences in the control mechanisms for the reader's forward-visual-scanning behavior, and for his regressive-visual-scanning behavior. This question was posed because of Hochberg's (1970b) constructs of peripheral search guidance and cognitive search guidance and his discussion of how they might operate to guide the reader's information extraction; and because of Goldman-Eisler's (1969) finding that there are two kinds of pauses in spontaneous speech, one reflecting conventional parsing, and the other reflecting cognitive planning, searching, and testing. If there are these two functionally distinct types of pauses in productive processes for communicating by language, perhaps there would be two parallel types of pauses in receptive processes for communicating by language. Also, Weber's (1970) analyses of the kinds of oral-reading errors made by young children learning how to read indicates that the skill of going back and correcting linguistically inappropriate guesses is an important step in becoming a mature reader. Thus, a number of strands of research dealing with linguistic communication suggested that somewhat different kinds of attentional guidance factors, performing somewhat different kinds of meaning-extraction tasks, might be at work in reading. Examination of the results in the present research indicated that forward-eye-fixation patterning tends to be related to the sentence's immediate constituent analysis; whereas regressive-eye-fixation patterning tends to be related to the structural predictability of constituents within the sentence frame. This position is supported by the findings that the LE/RE structural differences—which were differences in immediate constituent analysis—affected forward-eye-fixation patterning, but not regressive-eye-fixation patterning; whereas the active/passive structural differences—which were differences in the structural predictability of constituents within the sentence frame—affected regressive fixations but not forward fixations.

In summary, analysis of motion picture records of 12 mature readers, each reading 80 test sentences, indicates that

1. oral reading requires more visual attention than silent reading;

2. the reader selectively allocates his attention to different areas of the sentence;

3. a sentence type which is structurally less predictable requires more visual attention;

4. a sentence's immediate constituent analysis affects the way the reader's visual attention is distributed across the sentence;

5. differences in the structural predictability of phrases inserted into the same immediate constituent framework affect the amount of visual attention required;

6. different kinds of linguistic cues to the same underlying semantic structure appear to require different amounts of visual attention;

7. differences in the immediate constituent analysis of sentences affect forward scanning; differences in the structural predictability of items within a given immediate constituent framework affect regressive scanning.

In conclusion, the line-of-sight approach promises to be a very sensitive measure for studying the kinds of perceptual strategies that good readers—and poor readers—use to extract meaning from written language. I view this research as a promising beginning. We need to do these same tests with sentences presented within a paragraph context, and we need to examine the visual-scanning behavior of readers at different stages in the development of reading skill. The research that I have discussed here provides no final answers, but it does, I believe, raise some interesting questions about the role of language behind the eye.

VII.7

References

Allport, D. A. The rate of assimilation of visual information. *Psychonomic Science,* 1968, **12,** 221–232.

Anderson, J. M., & Bower, G. H. Recognition and retrieval processes in free recall. *Psychological Review,* 1972, **79,** 97–123.

Berlyne, D. E. The influence of complexity and novelty in visual figures on orienting responses. *Journal of Experimental Psychology,* 1958, **55,** 289–296.

Bernbach, H. A. Decision processes in memory. *Psychological Review,* 1967, **74,** 462–480.

Biederman, I. Perceiving real-world scenes. *Science,* 1972, **177,** 77–80.

Buswell, G. T. An experimental study of the eye–voice span in reading. *Supplementary Educational Monographs,* 1920, **17.**

Buswell, G. T. *How people look at pictures.* Chicago: University of Chicago Press, 1935.

Carpenter, P. A., & Just, M. A. Semantic control of eye movements during picture scanning in a sentence–picture verification task. *Perception and Psychophysics,* 1972, **12,** 61–64.

Carpenter, P. A., & Just, M. A. Sentence comprehension: A psycholinguistic processing model of verification. *Psychological Review,* 1975, **82,** 45–73.

Chase, W. G., & Clark, H. H. Mental operations in the comparison of sentences and pictures. In L. W. Gregg (Ed.), *Cognition in learning and memory.* New York: Wiley, 1972, 205–232.

Clark, H. H., & Chase, W. G. On the process of comparing sentences against pictures. *Cognitive Psychology,* 1972, **3,** 472–517.

Conrad, R. Acoustic confusions in immediate memory. *British Journal of Psychology,* 1964, **55,** 75–84.

Egan, J. P. Recognition memory and the operating characteristic. Indiana University, Hearing and Communication Laboratory, Tech. note *AFCRC-TN-58-51,* 1958.

Farley, A. M. VIPS: A visual imagery and perception system; The result of a protocol analysis. Doctoral thesis, Carnegie-Mellon University, Computer Science Department, Pittsburgh, 1974.

Freund, R. D., Loftus, G. R., & Atkinson, R. C. Applications of multiprocess models for memory to continuous recognition tasks. *Journal of Mathematical Psychology,* 1969, **6,** 576–594.

Garner, W. R. To perceive is to know. *American Psychologist,* 1966, **21,** 11–19.

Goldman-Eisler, F. *Psycholinguistics: Experiments in spontaneous speech.* New York: Academic Press, 1969.

532 REFERENCES

Gough, P. B. Grammatical transformations and speed of understanding. *Journal of Verbal Learning and Verbal Behavior,* 1965, 5, 107–111.

Gough, P. B. The verification of sentences: The effects of delay of evidence and sentence length. *Journal of Verbal Learning and Verbal Behavior,* 1966, 5, 492–496.

Gould, J. D. Eye movements during visual search. Research report #RC2680. Yorktown Heights: IBM Thomas J. Watson Research Center, 1969.

Haber, R. N., & Hershenson, M. *The psychology of visual perception.* New York: Holt, Rinehart & Winston, 1973.

Hall, R. J. and Cusack, B. L. The measurement of eye behavior: Critical and selected reviews of voluntary eye movement and blinking. *Technical Memorandum 18-72,* U.S. Army Human Engineering Laboratory, Aberdeen Proving Ground, Maryland, 1972.

Hall, R. J., Rosenberger, M. A., & Monty, R. A. An experimental investigation of the visual behavior of young heroin addicts and matched controls. *Journal Supplement Abstract Service,* 1974, 4, 7. (a)

Hall, R. J., Rosenberger, M. A., & Monty, R. A. Cutaneous perception of heroin addicts: Evidence of an altered temporal process. *Bulletin of the Psychonomic Society,* 1974, 3, 352–354. (b)

Harter, M. R. Excitability cycles and cortical scanning: A review of two hypotheses of central intermittency in perception. *Psychological Bulletin,* 1967, 68, 47–58.

Hebb, D. O. *The organization of behavior.* New York: Wiley, 1949.

Hochberg, J. E. In the mind's eye. In R. N. Haber (Ed.), *Contemporary theory and research in visual perception.* New York: Holt, Rinehart & Winston, 1968. Pp. 309–331.

Hochberg, J. E. Attention, organization, and consciousness. In D. L. Mostofsky (Ed.), *Attention: Contemporary theory and analysis.* New York: Appleton, 1970. (a)

Hochberg, J. Components of literacy. In H. Levin and J. P. Williams (Eds.), *Basic studies on reading.* New York: Basic Books, 1970. (b)

Hunt, E. B. The memory we must have. In R. C. Schank and K. M. Colby (Eds.), *Computer models of thought and language.* San Francisco: W. H. Freeman and Co., 1973.

Just, M. A. Comprehending quantified sentences: The relation between sentence–picture and semantic memory verification. *Cognitive Psychology,* 1974, 6, 216–236.

Just, M. A., & Carpenter, P. A. Comprehension of negation with quantification. *Journal of Verbal Learning and Verbal Behavior,* 1971, 10, 244–253.

Just, M. A., & Carpenter, P. A. Verbal comprehension in instructional situations. In D. Klahr (Ed.), *Cognition and instruction.* Hillsdale, New Jersey: Lawrence Erlbaum Associates, 1976.

Kennedy, J. M. Regressive eye movements may depend on syntax. Manuscript, Cornell University, Department of Psychology, Ithaca, New York, 1967.

Kintsch, W. An experimental analysis if single-stimulus tests and multiple-choice tests of recognition memory. *Journal of Experimental Psychology,* 1968, 76, 1–6.

Kintsch, W. Models for free recall and recognition. In D. A. Norman (Ed.), *Models of human memory.* New York: Academic Press, 1970.

Klima, E. S. Negation in English. In J. A. Fodor & J. J. Katz (Eds.), *The structure of language.* Englewood Cliffs, New Jersey: Prentice-Hall, 1964. Pp. 246–323.

Koffka, K. *Principles of Gestalt psychology.* New York: Harcourt-Brace, 1935.

Kolers, P. A. Three stages of reading. In H. Levin and J. P. Williams (Eds.), *Basic studies on reading.* New York: Basic Books, 1970. Pp. 90–118.

Kolers, P. A. Experiments in reading. *Scientific American,* 1972, 227, 84–91.

Lambert, R. H., Monty, R. A., & Hall, R. J. High-speed data processing and unobtrusive monitoring of eye movements. *Behavior Research Methods and Instrumentation,* 1974, 6, 525–530.

Levin, H., Grossman, J., Kaplan, E., & Yang, R. Constraints and the eye–voice span in right and left embedded sentences. *Language and Speech,* 1972, **15**, 30–39.

Levin, H., & Kaplan, E. Eye–voice span within active and passive sentences. *Language and Speech,* 1968, **11**, 251–258.

Loftus, G. R. Eye fixations and recognition memory for pictures. *Cognitive Psychology,* 1972, **3**, 525–551.

Loftus, G. R. Acquisition of information from rapidly presented verbal and nonverbal stimuli. *Memory and Cognition,* 1974, **2**, 545–548.

Mackworth, N. H. The wide-angle reflection eye camera for visual choice and pupil size. *Perception and Psychophysics,* 1968, **3**, 32–34.

Mackworth, N. H., & Bruner, J. S. How adults and children search and recognize pictures. *Human Development,* 1970, **13**, 149–177.

Mackworth, N. H., & Morandi, A. J. The gaze selects informative details within pictures. *Perception and Psychophysics,* 1967, **2**, 547–552.

Mehler, J., Bever, T. G., & Carey, P. What we look at when we read. *Perception and Psychophysics,* 1967, **2**, 213–218.

Miller, G. A. The magical number seven, plus or minus two. *Psychological Review,* 1956, **63**, 81–97.

Monty, R. A. An advanced eye-movement measuring and recording system featuring unobtrusive monitoring and automatic data processing. *American Psychologist,* 1975, **30**, 331–335.

Monty, R. A., Hall, R. J., & Rosenberger, M. A. Eye movement responses of heroin addicts and controls during word and object recognition. *Neuropharmacology* 1975, **14**, 693–702.

Moran, T. P. The symbolic nature of visual imagery. *Proceedings of the Third International Joint Conference on Artificial Intelligence,* Stanford, California, 1973.

Neisser, U. *Cognitive psychology.* New York: Appleton–Century–Crofts, 1967.

Newell, A. A theoretical exploration of mechanisms for coding the stimulus. Carnegie-Mellon University, Department of Computer Science, Pittsburg, 1972.

Newell, A. and Simon, H. A. *Human Problem solving.* Englewood Cliffs, New Jersey: Prentice-Hall, 1972.

Nickerson, R. S. Auditory codability and the short-term retention of visual information. *Journal of Experimental Psychology,* 1972, **95**, 429–436.

Nickerson, R. S. Short-term retention of visually presented stimuli: Some evidence of visual encoding. *Acta Psychologica,* in press.

Nickerson, R. S., & Pew, R. W. Visual pattern matching: An investigation of some effects of decision task, auditory codability and spatial correspondence. *Journal of Experimental Psychology,* 1973, **98**, 36–43.

Piaget, J. *Structuralism.* Paris: Presses Universitaires de France, 1968 New York: Basic Books, 1970.

Pollack, I., & Spence, D. Subjective pictorial information and visual search. *Perception and Psychophysics,* 1968, **3**, 41–44.

Potter, M. C. What memory and detection of picture sequences tell us about visual processing during eye fixations. Paper presented at *Meetings of the Eastern Psychological Association,* Boston, 1972.

Potter, M. C., & Levy, E. I. Recognition memory for a rapid sequence of pictures. *Journal of Experimental Psychology,* 1969, **81**, 10–15.

Shaffer, W. O. and Shiffrin, R. M. Rehearsal and storage of visual information. *Journal of Experimental Psychology,* 1972, **92**, 292–295.

Simon, H. A. An information-processing explanation of some perceptual phenomena. *British Journal of Psychology,* 1967, **58**, 1–12.

Simon, H. A. What is visual imagery? An information-processing interpretation. In L. W. Gregg (Ed.), *Cognition in learning and memory.* New York: McGraw-Hill, 1972, Pp. 183–204.

Sperling, G. The information available in brief visual presentations. *Psychological Monographs,* 1960, **74,** 1–29.

Sperling, G. A model for visual memory tasks. *Human Factors,* 1963, **5,** 19–31.

Sperling, G., Budiansky, J., Spivak, J., & Johnson, M. C. Extremely rapid visual search. *Science,* 1971, **174,** 307–311.

Sperling, G., & Speelman, R. G. Acoustic similarity and auditory short-term memory: Experiments and a model. In D. A. Norman (Ed.), *Models of human memory.* New York: Academic Press, 1970.

Teichner, W. A. Final status report: Quantitative models for predicting human visual perceptual/motor performance. New Mexico State University, Department of Psychology, September 1973.

Trabasso, T., Rollins, H., & Shaughnessy, E. Storage and verification stages in processing concepts. *Cognitive Psychology,* 1971, **2,** 239–289.

Uhr, L. *Pattern recognition, learning, and thought.* Englewood Cliffs, New Jersey: Prentice-Hall, 1973.

Wanat, S. F., & Levin, H. The eye–voice span: Reading efficiency and syntactic predictability. In H. Levin, E. J. Gibson, & J. J. Gibson (Eds.), *The analysis of reading skill: A program of basic and applied research.* U. S. Office of Education Final Report, *Project #5-1213.* Ithaca: Cornell, 1968. Pp. 237–253.

Wanat, S. F., & Levin, H. The eye–voice span in sentences containing different amounts of information. (in preparation).

Weber, R. M. First graders' use of grammatical context in reading. In H. Levin & J. P. Williams (Eds.), *Basic studies on reading.* New York: Basic Books, 1970, Pp. 147–163.

White, C. T. Eye movements, evoked responses and visual perception: some speculations. *Acta Psychologica,* 1967, **27,** 337–340.

Wickelgren, W. A. Short-term recognition memory for single letters and phonemic similarity of retroactive interference. *Quarterly Journal of Experimental Psychology,* 1966, **18,** 55–62.

Wickelgren, W. A. Coding, retrieval, and dynamics of multitrace associative memory. In L. W. Gregg (Ed.), *Cognition in learning and memory.* New York: McGraw-Hill, 1972.

Yarbus, A. L. *Eye movements and vision* [translated by Basil Haigh]. New York: Plenum Press, 1967.

Author Index

W

Wanat, S. F., *201, 368,* 527, *534*
Warren, R., 413, *455*
Webb, I. B., 308, *369*
Weber, R. M., 528, *534*
Weiss, A. D., 35, *65*
Weisstein, N., 81, *154*
Wempe, J., 197, *202*
Westheimer, G. H., 26, 27, 57, 58, 59, 62, 63, *69, 70,* 446, *455*
Wheeless, L., 40, *70*
White, C. T., 330, *367, 369,* 491, *534*
Whiteside, J. A., 109, *151*
Wickelgren, B. G., 25, *69*
Wickelgren, W. A., 483, 515, *534*
Wiersma, H., 289, *300*
Wiesel, T. N., 112, *152,* 231, *300*
Williams, J. P., *454, 532, 534*
Williams, L. G., 324, *369*
Wilson, M. E., 231, 242, *302*
Wilson, P. D., *299*
Winterson, B. J., 129, 143, *152, 154*
Wood, L. E., 393, *455*
Woodworth, R. S., 73, 115, *154,* 405, *455*
Wright, J. C., 178, *201*

Wurtz, R. H., 48, *66, 70,* 231, 232, 233, 234, 235, 236, 237, 238, 239, 240, 241, 242, 243, *300, 301, 302, 303*
Wyman, D., 40, *69,* 129, 132, 133, 134, 146, 147, 148, *154*

Y

Yagi, N., 14, *67*
Yakimoff, N., 74, 80, 83, 98, *153*
Yamamoto, M., 10, 14, *67*
Yang, R., 524, 526, *533*
Yarbus, A. L., 111, *154,* 188, 191, *202,* 328, 329, 344, 358, *369,* 512, *534*
Yasui, S., 33, *70*
Yeates, H., 74, *154*
Young, L. R., 6, 14, 33, 35, 36, 40, *66, 68, 70,* 147, *154,* 157, 188, 191, *202*
Young, R. A., 40, *67*

Z

Zeidner, J., 364, *369*
Zinchenco, V. P., 331, 334, 343, 355, *369*
Zuber, B. L., 41, *70,* 74, 77, 83, 94, *154*

Subject Index